Care of Older People with Diabetes

Care of Older People with Diabetes: A Manual for Healthcare Practice

Edited by

Alan J. Sinclair
Ahmed H. Abdelhafiz

WILEY Blackwell

This edition first published 2025

Registered Offices
John Wiley & Sons, Inc., 111 River Street, Hoboken, NJ 07030, USA
John Wiley & Sons Ltd, New Era House, 8 Oldlands Way, Bognor Regis, West Sussex, PO22 9NQ, UK

For details of our global editorial offices, customer services, and more information about Wiley products visit us at www.wiley.com.

The manufacturer' s authorized representative according to the EU General Product Safety Regulation is Wiley-VCH GmbH, Boschstr. 12, 69469 Weinheim, Germany, e-mail: Product_Safety@wiley.com.

Wiley also publishes its books in a variety of electronic formats and by print-on-demand. Some content that appears in standard print versions of this book may not be available in other formats.

Library of Congress Cataloging-in-Publication Data Applied for:

Paperback ISBN: 9781394205035

Cover Design: Wiley
Cover Images: © Tama2u/Shutterstock, © PamelaJoeMcFarlane/Getty Images, © adamkaz/Getty Images, © andreswd/Getty Images, © Ground Picture/Shutterstock

Set in 11.5/13.5 STIXTwoText by Straive, Pondicherry, India

Contents

Contributors xxvii

Foreword xxxiii

Preface xxxv

About the Companion Website xxxvii

Characteristics and Care Needs xxxix

Ahmed H. Abdelhafiz, Ann Middleton and Alan J. Sinclair

Introduction xxxix

Characteristics xli

Care Needs xliii

Physical Function xliii

Mental Function xliii

Care Delivery xlvi

Family Support xlvi

Care Organisation xlvii

Continuity of Care xlvii

Care Homes xlviii

Conclusion xlix

Clinical Practice Question xlix

References xlix

1 Epidemiology and Pathophysiology 1

Sarah L. Sy

Introduction 1

Epidemiology 2

Pathophysiology of Diabetes in Older Adults 3

Age-related Alterations in Glucose Metabolism 3

Genetics 5
Lifestyle and Environmental Factors 5
Other Factors 6
What Are the Key Issues? 6
Prevention of Diabetes in Older Adults 6
Hypoglycaemia 7
Management 7
Summary 7
Clinical Practice Question 9
References 9

2 Screening and Diagnosis 11
Isabelle Bourdel-Marchasson
Introduction 11
Background 12
Key Issues 14
Screening 14
Diagnosis 16
Clinical Practice Questions 17
References 18

3 Lifestyle Interventions 21
Abdiazizi Yusuf and Ahmed H. Abdelhafiz
Introduction 21
Impact of Lifestyle Changes 22
Lifestyle Intervention 23
Nutrition 24
Exercise 25
Synergy Between Nutrition and Exercise 27
Care Homes 27
Summary 28

Clinical Practice Question. 28
References 29

4 Oral Hypoglycaemic Therapy 31
Nahian Kazi and Ahmed H. Abdelhafiz
Introduction 31
Hypoglycaemic Agents 32
Low Hypoglycaemia-Risk Agents 32
Metformin 32
Dipeptidyl Peptidase-4 Inhibitors 34
Sodium Glucose Transporter-2 Inhibitors 34
Glucagon-like Peptide-1 Receptor Agonists. 35
Thiazolidinediones 35
Alpha-glucosidase Inhibitors 36
High Hypoglycaemia Risk Agents 36
Sulfonylureas 36
Meglitinides. 37
Therapeutic Approach 37
Summary 38
Future Perspectives. 39
Clinical Practice Question. 39
References 40

5 Insulin Therapy. 41
Giuseppe Maltese
Introduction 41
Basal Insulin Analogues 42
Rapid-acting Analogues 44
Treatment Regimens 45
Summary 47
Clinical Practice Question. 47
References 47

6 Use of Continuous Glucose Monitoring in Older People with Diabetes 49
Giuseppe Maltese
Introduction 50
Continuous Glucose Monitoring 50
Patient Assessment 52
Challenges 54
Clinical Practice Question 54
References 55

7 Education: Key Features for Achieving Success 57
Kirsty Winkley and Angus Forbes
Introduction 57
Key Issues 58
Diabetes Complications 59
Other Comorbidities Not Specific to Diabetes 60
Polypharmacy 60
Anti-diabetes Oral and Injectable Agents 60
Hypoglycaemia 62
Risk of Falls and Fractures 63
Cognitive Impairment 63
Nutrition 64
Management 64
Determine Frailty Risk 64
Deprescribing and Optimisation 65
Glucose Monitoring and Insulin Delivery Technologies 66
Physical Exercise 66
Healthy Diet 67
Diabetes Self-management Education for Older People 67
Clinical Practice Question 68
References 68

8 Carers and Care Needs 71
Puja Merwaha and Ahmed H. Abdelhafiz
Introduction 71
Care Needs 72
Carer Groups 73
Role of Carers 73
Benefit of Care on Outcomes 74
Caring for Carers 74
Carers' Burden 75
Supporting Carers 75
Summary 76
Clinical Practice Question 78
References 78

9a Macrovascular Complications: Peripheral Arterial Disease 81
Leocadio Rodríguez-Mañas, Rubí E. Sandoval-Santoyo and Marta Castro-Rodríguez
Epidemiology 81
Risk Factors 81
Prevalence 82
Pathogenesis 82
Consequences of Peripheral Arterial Disease 83
Investigations 83
Anamnesis 83
Physical Examination 84
Non-invasive Tests 84
Invasive Tests 85
Management 85
Risk Factor Modification 85
Exercise Rehabilitation 85
Foot Care 86

Pharmacological Therapy 86
Antiplatelet Therapy 86
Cilostazol 86
Revascularisation 86
Clinical Practice Question. 86
References 87

9b Macrovascular Complications: Coronary Arterial Disease. 89

Leocadio Rodríguez-Mañas, Rubí E., Sandoval-Santoyo and Marta Castro Rodríguez

Epidemiology 89
Pathogenesis 90
Medical Treatment 90
Indications for Revascularisation 91
Management of Cardiovascular Risk Factors According to Baseline Functional and Cognitive Status. 92
Effect of Glycaemic Control on Cardiovascular Events. 92
Effect of Blood Pressure Control 92
Lipid Monitoring. 93
Physical Exercise and Diet 93
Frailty Management 93
Management 93
Summary 95
Clinical Practice Question. 95
References 96

9c Macrovascular Complications: Cerebrovascular Disease. 97

Abubakhr Subkhan, Arshad Majid and Ali Ali

Introduction 97
Epidemiology 98
Risk Factors 98

Aetiology and Pathophysiology 99
Presentation 99
Stroke and Transient Ischaemic Attack.... 101
Cerebral Small Vessel Disease and Dementia 101
Management of Cerebrovascular Disease 102
Acute Stroke 102
Management of Risk Factors 104
Prognosis 105
Summary 106
Clinical Practice Question.... 106
References 107

10a Microvascular Complications: Diabetic Eye Disease 109
Archith Kamath and Nachiketa Acharya
Introduction.... 110
Epidemiology.... 110
Presentation.... 110
Pathophysiology 111
Management 113
Primary Care.... 113
Secondary Care.... 115
Summary 117
Clinical Practice Questions.... 117
References 118

10b Microvascular Complications: Diabetic Kidney Disease.... 119
Mohsen El Kossi
Introduction.... 119
Diabetic Kidney Disease.... 120
Definitions and Diagnoses.... 120
Management 121

Lifestyle ... 121
Glycaemic Control ... 122
Blood Pressure Control ... 122
Lipid Control ... 123
Diabetic Kidney Disease-related Complications ... 124
Anaemia ... 124
Mineral Bone Disorder ... 124
Metabolic Acidosis and Fluid Retention ... 125
Nephrology Referral ... 125
Summary ... 126
Clinical Practice Question ... 127
References ... 127

10c Microvascular Complications: Peripheral Neuropathy ... 129
Mitra Tavakoli
Introduction ... 130
Prevalence and Risk Factors ... 130
Clinical Manifestations and Complications ... 131
Diagnosis and Assessment ... 132
Management of Diabetic Neuropathy ... 135
Diabetes Foot Care in Care Homes ... 136
Summary ... 138
Clinical Practice Question ... 138
References ... 139

11a Vascular Risk Factors: Hypertension ... 141
Pann Ei Hnynn Si and Ahmed H. Abdelhafiz
Introduction ... 141
Age-related Blood Pressure Changes ... 142
Definition ... 142
Diagnosis ... 144

Types 144
Management 145
Recommended Targets 145
Medications 146
Considerations in Older People 147
Orthostatic Hypotension 147
Falls 148
Systolic Hypertension 148
Frailty 148
Dementia 149
Comorbidity 149
Polypharmacy 149
Summary 149
Clinical Practice Question 151
References 151

11b Vascular Risk Factors: Dyslipidaemia 153

Pann Ei Hnynn, Si and Ahmed H. Abdelhafiz

Introduction 153
Ageing and Lipid Profile 154
Diabetes and Lipid Profile 154
Diabetes and Risk of Atherosclerotic Cardiovascular Disease 155
Atherosclerotic Cardiovascular Disease Risk Reduction 156
Lipid-lowering Agents 157
Goals of Therapy in Old Age 160
Recommendations from Guidelines 160
Goals in Frailty 162
Summary 162
Clinical Practice Question 162
References 164

12a Metabolic Decompensation: Hyperglycaemic Crisis.....165
Puja Merwaha and Ahmed H. Abdelhafiz
Introduction 165
Epidemiology 166
Precipitating Factors 166
Pathogenesis 168
Clinical Presentation 168
Diagnosis 169
Management 171
Correction of Hypovolaemia 172
Correction of Hyperglycaemia 173
Correction of Acidosis 174
Correction of Electrolytes 175
Complications 175
Prevention 176
Clinical Practice Question 176
References 177

12b Metabolic Decompensation: Hypoglycaemia...........178
Srikanth Bellary, Ahmed H. Abdelhafiz and Alan J. Sinclair
Introduction 179
Definition 179
Recognition 179
Epidemiology 180
Pathophysiology 180
Clinical Consequences 181
Impact on Cognition 182
Impact on Frailty 182
Management 183
Summary 185
Clinical Practice Question 185
References 186

13a Management of Diabetes in Hospital 189
Julie Lewis and Chris Cottrell
Introduction 189
Fundamentals of Care 190
Key Considerations for Effective Inpatient Care for Older People with Diabetes 192
The Inpatient Setting 192
Pressure Damage and Footcare Assessment 193
Planning Care 193
Key Considerations to Reduce Unscheduled Admission to Hospital 193
Monitoring Requirements 196
Education and Training 196
Summary 197
Clinical Practice Questions 198
References 199

13b Management of Diabetes in Care Homes 201
Lynne Reedman and Alan J. Sinclair
Introduction 201
Important Considerations for Diabetes Care 203
Importance of Monitoring Glucose Levels 207
Other Management Issues 207
Hypoglycaemia 208
Diabetes Foot Disease 209
Nutritional Deficiency and Weight Loss 209
Frailty 210
Education 210
Communication and Collaboration 211
Use of Audit 211
Measuring Outcomes 212
Summary 212

Clinical Practice Question. 213
References 214

14 Nutrition 215
Rihan Said and Grace Zaman
Introduction 215
Nutritional Deficiencies 216
Causes of Malnutrition in the Elderly 216
Recommendations 217
Specific Recommendations for Older People with Diabetes 218
Practical Steps for Nutritional Care in the Elderly 218
Screening 218
Assessment 219
Intervention 219
Enteral Nutrition 221
Types of Enteral Tubes 221
Types of Feeds 221
Enteral Feed Delivery Options 221
Management of Blood Glucose 221
Parenteral Nutrition 222
Management of Blood Glucose 223
General Considerations for Patients on Nutritional Support 224
Summary 224
Clinical Practice Questions 225
References 226

15 Sexual Health 229
Pann Ei Hnynn Si and Ahmed H. Abdelhafiz
Introduction 229
Ageing and Sexual Function 230
Diabetes and Sexual Dysfunction 230

Sexual Dysfunction in Men 231
Aetiology and Pathogenesis 231
Diagnosis 232
Treatment 233
Sexual Dysfunction in Women 236
Aetiology and Pathogenesis 236
Diagnosis 237
Treatment 237
Summary 238
Clinical Practice Questions 238
References 239

16a Special Issues in Old Age: Frailty 241
Alan J. Sinclair and Ahmed H. Abdelhafiz
Introduction 241
Frailty–diabetes Inter-relationship 242
Effect of Diabetes on Frailty 244
Effects of Frailty on Diabetes 245
Outcome Effects 249
Metabolic Effects 249
Sarcopenic Obese Phenotype 254
Anorexic Malnourished Phenotype 254
Prevention and Management 255
Screening 255
Non-pharmacological Therapy 256
Pharmacological Therapy 257
Special Considerations 259
Glycaemic Control 259
Choice of Hypoglycaemic Agent 260
Sarcopenic Obese Phenotype 260
Anorexic Malnourished Phenotype 260
Goals of Therapy 261
Summary 262

Future Perspectives. 262
Clinical Practice Question. 263
References 264

16b Special Issues in Old Age: Multimorbidity 266
Alan J. Sinclair and Ahmed H. Abdelhafiz
Introduction 266
Multimorbidity 267
Multimorbidity–Frailty Interaction 268
Multimorbidity Effects on Diabetes 268
Clusters of Multimorbidity 269
Clinical Implications 270
Summary 272
Future Perspectives. 272
Clinical Practice Question. 273
References 273

16c Special Issues in Old Age: Type 1 Diabetes Mellitus 275
Alex M. Summerbell and Ahmed H. Abdelhafiz
Introduction 275
Epidemiology and Diagnosis 276
Management 276
Insulin Therapy. 278
Monitoring 279
Reducing Hypoglycaemia 280
Goals of Therapy 282
Summary 282
Clinical Practice Question. 282
References 283

16d Special Issues in Old Age: Cognitive Health Agility, Cognitive Dysfunction, Dementia and Diabetes 285

Tali Cukierman-Yaffe

Introduction 286

Population Studies Demonstrating the Relationship Between Cognitive Dysfunction, Dementia and Diabetes 286

Implications of the Relationship Between Diabetes and Cognitive Dysfunction 287

The Effect of Cognitive Dysfunction on Self-care Capacity in Older People with Diabetes 288

Assessment of Cognitive Health Agility in Older People with Diabetes 290

Prevention and Treatment of Cognitive Dysfunction in Older People with Diabetes 291

The Effect of Current Diabetes Pharmacological Agents on Cognitive Dysfunction 291

Glucose Control 292

Insulin 293

Dipeptidyl Peptidase-4 Inhibitors 294

Glucagon-like Peptide-1 Receptor Analysts 294

The Multidomain Approach 295

Summary, Knowledge Gaps and Future Research 296

Clinical Practice Question 296

References 298

16e Special Issues in Old Age: Depression 299

Sara-Louise Wylie

Introduction 299

Depression and Diabetes 300

Presentation 300

Evaluation . . . 302
Screening . . . 302
Diagnosis . . . 303
Assessment . . . 304
Management . . . 307
Lifestyle . . . 307
Pharmacological Therapy . . . 308
Psychotherapy . . . 309
Collaborative Care . . . 310
Summary . . . 310
Clinical Practice Question . . . 310
References . . . 311

16f Special Issues in Old Age: Foot Care . . . 313
Solomon Muzulu
Introduction . . . 313
Epidemiology . . . 314
Pathogenesis . . . 314
Ageing and Diabetic Foot Ulcer Disease . . . 315
Assessment of a Diabetic Foot . . . 316
Testing for Peripheral Sensory Neuropathy . . . 316
10-g Monofilament Test . . . 317
128-Hz Tuning Fork . . . 318
Ipswich Touch Test . . . 318
Checking for Peripheral Vascular Disease . . . 318
Management . . . 318
Offloading . . . 320
Debridement . . . 320
Dressings . . . 320
Infection Control . . . 320
Ischaemia Relief . . . 321
Glycaemic Control . . . 322

Prevention 322
Summary 323
Clinical Practice Question. 323
References 324

16g Special Issues in Old Age: Skin Care 326

Grace Keegan and Sarah Mahmoud

Introduction 326
Age-related Skin Changes 327
Diabetes Mellitus-related Skin Conditions 327
Primary Skin Conditions 328
Acanthosis Nigricans 328
Necrobiosis Lipoidica 328
Diabetic Dermopathy 329
Bullous Eruption of Diabetes Mellitus 329
Diabetes-related Skin Infections 330
Bacterial Infections 330
Fungal Infections 331
Diabetes Medications-related Skin Adverse Effects 334
Insulin 334
Sodium Glucose Transporter-2 Inhibitors 334
Summary 334
Clinical Practice Question. 335
References 335

16h Special Issues in Old Age: Falls and Bone Health 336

Nandkishor V. Athavale

Introduction 336
Epidemiology 337
Pathophysiology of Fracture Risk in Diabetes 337
Pathophysiology and Risk Factors for Falls in Diabetes 338
Assessment of the Risk of Falls in the Community 339

Assessment of Bone Health in Community . . . 340
Management and Prevention . . . 344
Falls . . . 344
Fractures . . . 345
Summary . . . 345
Clinical Practice Question . . . 345
References . . . 346

16i Special Issues in Old Age: Avoiding Hospitalisation . . . 347
Demelza Emmerton and Ahmed H. Abdelhafiz
Introduction . . . 347
Risk Factors for Hospitalisation . . . 348
Avoiding Hospitalisation . . . 349
Patient-Related Interventions . . . 349
Physical Function . . . 349
Mental Function . . . 351
Polypharmacy . . . 351
Healthcare System-related Interventions . . . 352
Community Setting . . . 352
Care-home Setting . . . 353
Emergency Setting . . . 353
Summary . . . 355
Clinical Practice Question . . . 355
References . . . 356

16j Special Issues in Old Age: Use of Technology . . . 357
Anna Kahkoska, Aastha Dubal, Josh Weinstein and Ruth S. Weinstock
Introduction . . . 358
What Is Diabetes Technology? . . . 358
What Is Remote Patient Monitoring? . . . 359
Diabetes Technology and Remote Patient Monitoring in Older Adults . . . 360
Management . . . 362

Continuous Glucose Monitoring 362
What Is Continuous Glucose Monitoring? 362
What Is the Evidence for Continuous Glucose Monitoring as Part of Management for Older Adults with Diabetes? 362
What Are Challenges for Continuous Glucose Monitoring Use in Older Adults? 363
Automated Insulin Delivery Systems 363
What Is Automated Insulin Delivery? 363
Evidence on Automated Insulin Delivery for Older Adults 364
Clinical Guidelines for Automated Insulin Delivery Usage among Older Adults with Type 1 Diabetes 364
What Are Challenges for Automated Insulin Delivery Use in Older Adults? 364
Integration of Diabetes Technologies with Remote Patient Monitoring 365
What Are the Key Issues? 366
Clinical Practice Questions 368
References 369

16k Special Issues in Old Age: Annual Reviews 371
Puja Merwaha and Ahmed H. Abdelhafiz
Introduction 371
Diabetes Phenotype in Older People 372
Multimorbidity 372
Geriatric Syndromes 373
Frailty 373
Functional Implications 373
Annual Review Contents 374
Demographics 374
History 374
Physical Examination 374
Vascular Complications 376
Sexual Function 376

Cognition and Mood 376
Physical Function and Frailty 377
Foot Care 377
Diet and Nutrition 377
Medication Review 377
Infection Prevention 378
Summary 378
Clinical Practice Question 378
References 380

16l Special Issues in Old Age: Mouth Care 381
Nali Ahmed and Ahmed H. Abdelhafiz
Introduction 381
Age-related Oral Changes 382
Diabetes-related Oral Changes 382
Common Oral Conditions in Older People with Diabetes 384
Periodontal Disease 384
Dental Caries 384
Dry Mouth 385
Candida 386
Oral Cancer 386
Taste Impairment 387
Mouth Care 387
Education 387
Glycaemic Control 388
Preventative Measures 388
Summary 389
Clinical Practice Question 390
References 390

16m Special Issues in Old Age: Pain Management 392
Pann Ei Hnynn Si and Ahmed H. Abdelhafiz
Introduction 392
Aetiology 393

Assessment 393
Pain in Care-home Residents 396
Management 397
Non-pharmacological Therapy. 397
Pharmacological Therapy 398
Prevention 401
Clinical Practice Question. 401
References 402

17 Deintensification of Therapy. 405
Antoine Christiaens
Introduction 405
Key Issues. 407
Management 407
Identifying Patients Who Might Benefit 407
Deintensifying Glucose-lowering Treatment in Older Patients 409
Implementing Deintensification in Daily Clinical Practice 410
Clinical Practice Questions. 411
References 412

18 Diabetes in End-of-Life Care 413
June James
Introduction 413
Background 414
What is End of Life and How is the Need for End-of-life Care Identified? 414
Management of Diabetes in End-of-Life Care. 419
Medicines Management and De-escalation of Therapies. 419
Steroids and Cancer. 422
Nutrition and Enteral Feeding 424
Advanced Care Planning 424
Treatment Withdrawal 424

Workforce Training and Competencies 424
Summary 425
Clinical Practice Questions 425
References 426

Answers to Clinical Practice Questions 429

Index 445

Contributors

Ahmed H. Abdelhafiz
Department of Geriatric Medicine, Rotherham General Hospital
Rotherham, UK

Abdiazizi Yusuf
Department of Geriatric Medicine, Rotherham General Hospital
Rotherham, UK

Nachiketa Acharya
Directorate of Ophthalmology, Royal Hallamshire Hospital, Sheffield
Teaching Hospitals NHS Trust, Sheffield, UK

Nali Ahmed
Department of Geriatric Medicine, Rotherham General
Hospital, Rotherham, UK

Ali Ali
Department of Geriatrics and Neurosciences, Royal Hallamshire
Hospital, Sheffield Teaching Hospitals NHS Foundation Trust, and
the University of Sheffield, Sheffield, UK

Nandkishor V. Athavale
Department of Geriatric Medicine, Rotherham General
Hospital, Rotherham, UK

Srikanth Bellary
Diabetes and Endocrinology, University Hospitals NHS Trust
Birmingham, Birmingham, UK
Metabolic Medicine, School of Biological Sciences, Aston University,
Birmingham, UK

Isabelle Bourdel-Marchasson
Center for Magnetic Resonance of Biological Systems, University
of Bordeaux, Bordeaux, France
Gerontological Department, University Hospital of
Bordeaux, Bordeaux, France

Marta Castro-Rodríguez
Geriatric Medicine Department, University Hospital of Getafe
Madrid, Spain

Antoine Christiaens
Clinical Pharmacy and Pharmacoepidemiology research group
Louvain Drug Research Institute, Université catholique
de Louvain, Brussels, Belgium
Fund for Scientific Research, Brussels, Belgium

Tali Cukierman-Yaffe
Center For Successful Aging With Diabetes, Division of Endocrinology and Metabolism, Sheba Medical Center, Ramat Gan, Israel
Epidemiology Department, School of Public Health, Faculty of Medicine, Herczeg Institute on Ageing, Tel-Aviv University, Tel Aviv, Israel

Aastha Dubal
Division of Endocrinology and Metabolism, University of North Carolina at Chapel Hill, Chapel Hill, NC, USA

Mohsen El Kossi
Nephrology Department, Doncaster Royal Infirmary
Doncaster, UK

Demelza Emmerton
Department of Geriatric Medicine, Rotherham General Hospital
Rotherham, UK

Angus Forbes
Florence Nightingale Faculty of Nursing and Midwifery
King's College London, London, UK

June James
Leicester Diabetes Centre, University Hospitals of Leicester NHS Trust, Leicester, UK

Anna Kahkoska
Division of Endocrinology and Metabolism, University of North Carolina at Chapel Hill, Chapel Hill, NC, USA
Department of Nutrition, Gillings School of Global Public Health
University of North Carolina at Chapel Hill, Chapel Hill NC, USA
UNC Center for Aging and Health, University of North Carolina at Chapel Hill, Chapel Hill, NC, USA

Archith Kamath
Princess Alexandra Eye Pavilion, NHS Lothian, Edinburgh, UK

Nahian Kazi
Department of Geriatric Medicine, Rotherham General Hospital
Rotherham, UK

Grace Keegan
Dermatology Department, Rotherham General Hospital
Rotherham, UK

Julie Lewis
Primary and Community Care, Betsi Cadwaladr University
Health Board, Bangor, UK

Sarah Mahmoud
Dermatology Department, Rotherham General Hospital Rotherham, UK

Arshad Majid
Department of Geriatrics and Neurosciences, Royal Hallamshire
Hospital, Sheffield Teaching Hospitals NHS Foundation Trust, and
the University of Sheffield, Sheffield, UK

Giuseppe Maltese
School of Cardiovascular Medicine and Sciences, King's College
London, London, UK
Department of Diabetes and Endocrinology, Epsom and St Helier
University Hospitals, Surrey, UK

Puja Merwaha
Department of Geriatric Medicine, Rotherham General Hospital
Rotherham, UK

Ann Middleton
Person living with diabetes
Diabetes UK Research Steering Group, Droitwich Spa, UK

Solomon Muzulu
Department of Diabetes and Endocrinology, Rotherham General
Hospital, Rotherham, UK

Lynne Reedman
DUET Diabetes Ltd, Cambridge, UK

Leocadio Rodríguez-Mañas
Geriatric Medicine Department, University Hospital of Getafe
Madrid, Spain

Rihan Said
Department of Diabetes and Endocrinology, Rotherham General Hospital, Rotherham, UK

Rubí E. Sandoval-Santoyo
Geriatric Medicine Department, University Hospital of Getafe
Madrid, Spain

Pann Ei Hnynn Si
Sheffield Kidney Institute, Sheffield Teaching Hospitals
Sheffield, UK

Alan J. Sinclair
King's College London, London, UK
Foundation for Diabetes Research in Older People
Droitwich Spa, UK

Abubakhr Subkhan
Department of Geriatrics and Neurosciences, Royal Hallamshire Hospital, Sheffield Teaching Hospitals NHS Foundation Trust, and the University of Sheffield, Sheffield, UK

Alex M. Summerbell
Leeds Teaching Hospitals NHS Trust, Leeds, UK

Sarah L. Sy
Division of Geriatric Medicine, Department of Medicine, University of British Columbia, Vancouver, BC, Canada

Mitra Tavakoli
Exeter Centre of Excellence for Diabetes Research
National Institute for Health and Care Research
University of Exeter Medical School, Exeter, UK

Josh Weinstein
Department of Health Policy and Management, Gillings School of Global Public Health, University of North Carolina at Chapel Hill, Chapel Hill, NC, USA

Ruth S. Weinstock
Division of Endocrinology, Diabetes and Metabolism
Department of Medicine, SUNY Upstate Medical University, Syracuse, NY, USA

Kirsty Winkley
Florence Nightingale Faculty of Nursing and Midwifery
King's College London, London, UK

Sara-Louise Wylie
General Practice, Clinical Commissioning Group, Sheffield, UK

Grace Zaman
Department of Nutrition and Dietetics, Rotherham General Hospital
Rotherham, UK

Foreword

Although we all agree that longevity is one of the most important achievements of modern societies, an ageing population remains one of the main challenges facing medicine in the twenty-first century, because of its associated increased risk of chronic diseases and disability. Diabetes, a common illness in older adults, can cause severe complications, leading to loss of physical and cognitive function and premature death. A prompt diagnosis and appropriate management, through both pharmacological and lifestyle interventions, are essential in the control of the disease and its impact. In this perspective, this *Manual* provides the reader with an accessible, updated, practical source of consultation, written by outstanding authors of international repute, who bring a wealth of clinical experience and scientific expertise in their chapters. It is intended for diabetologists, geriatricians and general practitioners, but it is also a resource not easily obtained elsewhere for all members of the healthcare team who care for older people with diabetes, including nurses, dietitians and other paramedical staff, as well as students in these various disciplines.

A specific chapter is devoted to comprehensive geriatric assessment, the multidimensional diagnostic process focused on determining the medical, psychological and functional capacity of the older patient, which allows a targeted, coordinated and integrated plan for interventions. The treatment goal for patients with diabetes at advanced age is not just survival but maintaining function, reducing complications and improving quality of life, and all these aspects are discussed extensively in dedicated sessions.

I sincerely congratulate the editors and the authors of the individual chapters for the outstanding contributions they have made, as I am confident that this *Manual* will prove to be an invaluable reference guide on the care of older people with diabetes.

Stefania Maggi, MD, MPH, PhD
Research Director CNR Aging Branch-IN Italy
Member, Diabetes Special Interest Group for Older People, International Diabetes Federation 11th Edition Atlas Group
Past President, European Geriatric Medicine Society

Preface

We are delighted to present this *Manual* as a natural development after four editions of the textbook, *Diabetes in Old Age*. We felt it was important, if not essential, to produce a clinician-friendly book (manual) that has more practical examples of management and less detailed literature of each subject area.

This *Manual* provides a general introduction to the domains of geriatric diabetes and establishes the key aims of diabetes care and its related priorities. The *Manual* comprises over 30 chapters and covers a wide range of topics from epidemiology, screening for diabetes, treatment strategies, complications (both microvascular, macrovascular), metabolic emergencies, inpatient care and management of diabetes in care homes. There are also other important topics, including frailty, foot care and avoiding hospitalisation. In this first edition, we have included areas dealing with technology, deintensification of treatment and the end of life.

In this first edition of the *Manual*, we have assembled a list of distinguished international, local and regional authors working full-time in clinical practice. This combination provides the right amount of insight and expertise that is warranted in the pursuit of unravelling the complexities of geriatric diabetes. The generalist and the specialist should both benefit from this guidance, which should aid rational and effective decision making in everyday clinical scenarios involved in the diabetes care of the older person.

Management of geriatric diabetes can be challenging, particularly if we consider those with significant renal impairment or cardiovascular disease, with or without frailty, as well those with other medical comorbidities that have contributed to functional loss, disability and reduced life expectancy. Metabolic target or goal setting is limited by lack of randomised controlled trials of interventions in diabetes care of older people, but the guidance put forward in this *Manual* has synthesised the data, extrapolated from younger counterparts where necessary, and provided an additional expert viewpoint.

In the book, you will find key messages listed at the start of each chapter and clinical practice questions at the end of the chapter; these elements provide examples of clinical issues in management and how they should be addressed. Ten key references are included in the printed book; a full reference list is available online.

We hope you enjoy reading this *Manual of Diabetes Care for Older People* and that it will stimulate you to seek a more in-depth review of the subject in due course.

A. J. Sinclair
A. H. Abdelhafiz
April 2024

Acknowledgements

We would like to thank Caroline Sinclair for her devoted clerical and administrative contributions to this *Manual*.

We would like to thank Wiley-Blackwell publishers and the managing editors, Moyuri Handique and Harini Arumugam, for supporting this work, particularly in the transition from a textbook format to a *Manual*.

About the Companion Website

This book is accompanied by a companion website:

www.wiley.com/go/sinclair/1e

The website includes:

- Full list of References for each chapters
- Multiple Choice Questions
- Case Studies

Characteristics and Care Needs

Ahmed H. Abdelhafiz[1], *Ann Middleton*[2] *and Alan J. Sinclair*[3,4]

[1] *Department of Geriatric Medicine, Rotherham General Hospital, Rotherham, UK*
[2] *Person living with diabetes; Diabetes UK Research Steering Group, Droitwich Spa, UK*
[3] *King's College London, London, UK*
[4] *Foundation for Diabetes Research in Older People, Droitwich Spa, UK*

Key Points

- Diabetes prevalence is increasing in older people.
- Diabetes in old age is associated with related complications and morbidities.
- Geriatric syndromes, including frailty, are common in older people with diabetes.
- Physical and mental dysfunction are consequences of diabetes complications in old age, which may lead to disability.
- Owing to their complex needs, care delivery in older people with diabetes (both type 1 and type 2) should be structured, cover all clinical and non-clinical settings and involve families and carers.

Introduction

With increasing life expectancy and urbanisation of lifestyle, the prevalence of diabetes is increasing, particularly in older people. From the age of 60 years, the lifetime risk of developing diabetes is around 22.4% for women and 18.9% for men [1]. In addition to the traditional micro- and macrovascular complications of diabetes, in old age, diabetes is associated with a high comorbidity burden and increased prevalence of geriatric syndromes, including cognitive and physical dysfunction. Sarcopenia and frailty are emerging as new complications in older people with diabetes. Risk factors that lead to this morbidity burden include shared factors that predispose to diabetes (such as obesity and insulin resistance), diabetes-related factors (such as persistent hyperglycaemia and repeated episodes of hypoglycaemia) and diabetes-associated factors, such as cardiovascular complications.

Diabetes in old age, whether type 1 or type 2, is a disabling disease because of its multimorbidity burden, which increases the risk of premature mortality, increases the risk of disability and care-home admission, and places a substantial burden on individuals and healthcare systems. This chapter reviews the characteristics of older people with diabetes and the care needs that reflect their complex condition (Figure 1). It is meant to be read as applying to type 1 and type 2 diabetes and may also be applicable in parts to type 3c diabetes, where other diseases may affect the pancreas and lead to diabetes such as haemochromatosis.

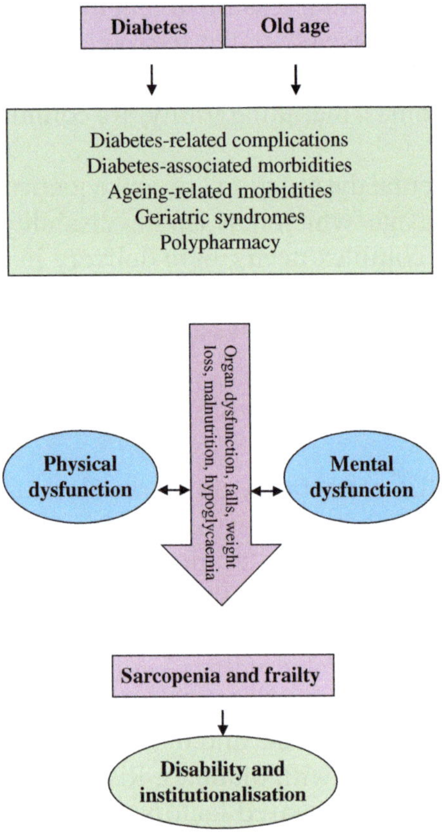

Figure 1: The impact of old age and diabetes on the characteristics of older people with diabetes and the relevant consequences.

Characteristics

Older people with diabetes are likely to have long duration of the disease, which leads to complications, associated morbidities, multiple organ dysfunction and polypharmacy. The prevalent conditions and their consequences in older people with diabetes are summarised in Box 1. Geriatric syndromes are prevalent, including physical and cognitive dysfunction leading to frailty and eventually disability. Furthermore, diabetes is associated with accelerated loss of muscle strength and muscle quality that directly lead to sarcopenia [2]. Diabetes-related complications, such as renal impairment, and diabetes-associated

Box 1: Characteristics of Older People with Diabetes

Prevalent Conditions

- Long duration of diabetes
- Multiple morbidities
- Polypharmacy
- Vascular complications
- Geriatric syndromes
- Physical dysfunction
- Cognitive dysfunction
- Organ dysfunction
- Frailty
- Disability

Consequences

- Frequent falls
- Weight loss
- Malnutrition
- Weakness
- Fatigability
- Recurrent hypoglycaemia
- Hypoglycaemia unawareness
- Atypical presentation of hypoglycaemia
- Increased self-care needs
- Institutionalisation

comorbidities, such as hypertension, increase the likelihood of frailty. Diabetes increases the risk of dementia by at least twofold [3].Frailty is also associated with increased risk of cognitive dysfunction [4] and a functional decline that leads to increased risk of falls, hospitalisation, dependency, disability and institutionalisation [5]. In addition to the physical and cognitive consequences, frailty affects the metabolic characteristics of older people with diabetes, which may influence diabetes trajectory, choice of hypoglycaemic agents and goals of therapy. Frail older people with diabetes can be metabolically different with a spectrum that starts from a sarcopenic obese (SO) phenotype at one end to an anorexic malnourished (AM) phenotype at the other end. These two phenotypes will have different metabolic characteristics as detailed in Table 1. The SO phenotype is characterised by unfavourable metabolic profile of increased insulin resistance, persistent hyperglycaemia and dyslipidaemia. The AM phenotype is characterised by anorexia of

Table 1: Frailty metabolic phenotypes in older people with diabetes.

Factor	Sarcopenic obese	Anorexic malnourished
Dominance	Obesity and sarcopenia	Anorexia and malnutrition
Energy intake	Increased	Reduced
Weight	Continuous gain	Continuous loss
Visceral fat	Increased	Reduced
Insulin resistance	Increased	Reduced
Cholesterol levels	High	Low
Albumin levels	Normal	Low
Hyperglycaemia	More likely	Less likely
Diabetes trajectory	Progressive	Regressive
Hypoglycaemic therapy	Likely intensification	Likely deintensification
Weight-limiting hypoglycaemic agents	More suitable	Not suitable
Important goal of therapy	Reduction of cardiovascular risk	Maintenance of quality of life

ageing, malnutrition and significant weight loss, which reduce insulin resistance [6].

Care Needs

The care of older people with diabetes is challenging because of their complex needs. Care needs should consider the heterogeneous nature of this group of patients. Care plans should, therefore, be individualised and should cover both physical and mental health and goals of therapy are appropriately tailored for each individual taking into account his views and wishes.

Physical Function

In older people, diabetes is associated with increased loss of muscle mass, strength and reduced muscle quality, which leads to the development of sarcopenia and frailty and, eventually, disability. This functional decline will lead to impairment in executing activities of daily living and diabetes-related self-care. Sarcopenia and frailty should therefore be regularly screened for in these patients. Progressive resistance training exercise programmes, together with diet rich in proteins and vitamin D may improve muscle strength and function [7]. Diet should not be too restrictive but shold be healthy and tailored to reflect personal choices. Hypoglycaemic therapy can then be adjusted accordingly to avoid unnecessarily weight loss and malnutrition and to maintain quality of life.

Mental Function

The ability for self-care in older people declines with the development of cognitive dysfunction. Therefore, screening for dementia is important if poor compliance with self-care tasks or repeated hypoglycaemia is observed. Depressive illness is common in older people with diabetes and is associated with worse outcomes. The relationship of depression and diabetes is bidirectional; the presence of one increasing the risk of the other. Healthcare professionals should therefore be actively screening for depression in older people with diabetes. Screening for physical and mental function is summarised in Box 2.

Box 2: Screening for Physical and Mental Dysfunction in Older People with Diabetes

Sarcopenia: SARC-F Scale

- Strength (difficulty lifting a weight of 4.5 kg/10 lb)
- Assistance in walking (difficulty walking across a room)
- Rising from a chair (difficulty in transferring from chair to bed)
- Climbing stairs (difficulty in climbing a flight of stairs)
- Falls (number of falls in past year)

Scoring

Score 0 if no difficulty, 1 if some difficulty, 2 if unable to carry out task, no falls = 0, 1–3 falls = 1, ≥4 falls = 2.

A total score of ≥4 indicates a high risk of adverse outcomes from sarcopenia.

Frailty: FRAIL Scale

- Fatigued (self-reported)
- Resistance (unable to climb a flight of stairs)
- Ambulation (unable to walk a block)
- Illness (has >5 comorbidities)
- Loss of weight (>5 kg in past six months)

Scoring

The presence of ≥3 indicators is diagnostic of frailty.

Clinical Frailty Scale

A nine-point scale based on function and description of characteristics of older people. Varying degrees of frailty are covered between points 4 and 8, with 8 being very severe frailty. Developed from the Frailty Index.

Dementia: Mini-cog

Ask patient to repeat three items (e.g. lemon, key and balloon) then provide a clock face:

- Ask patient to draw the numbers on the clock face
- Ask patient to draw the hands of the clock to show time as 10 minutes to 3 o'clock
- Ask patient to recall the three items they repeated

Scoring

Give one mark for each task performed and each item remembered. A score of ≤ 3 from a maximum of 5 defines cognitive impairment.

Depression: Patient Health Questionnaire (PHQ) 2

- Ask whether patient has little interest in doing things
- Ask whether patient is feeling down, depressed or hopeless

Scoring

Any positive answer triggers assessment using the detailed PHQ-9 assessment.

References

Clinical Frailty Scale: Geriatric Medicine Research, Dalhousie University. (2009). *Clinical Frailty Scale*. http://bgs.org.uk.

Frail Scale:Gleason, L.J., Benton, E.A., Alvarez-Nebreda, M.L. et al. (2017). FRAIL questionnaire screening tool and short-term outcomes in geriatric fracture patients. *J. Am. Med. Dir. Assoc.* 18: 1082–1086. https://doi.org/10.1016/j.jamda.2017.07.005.

Mini-Cog: Mini-Cog© Quick Screening for Early Dementia Detection. (2024). https://mini-cog.com.

PHQs 2 and 9:Anand, P., Bhurji, N., Williams, N., and Desai, N. (2021). Comparison of PHQ-9 and PHQ-2 as screening tools for depression and school related stress in inner city adolescents. *J. Prim. Care Community Health* 12: https://doi.org/10.1177/21501327211053750.

Sarc-F:Malmstrom, T.K. and Morley, J.E. (2013). SARC-F: a simple questionnaire to rapidly diagnose sarcopenia. *J. Am. Med. Dir. Assoc.* 14: 531–532. https://doi.org/10.1016/j.jamda.2013.05.018.

Care Delivery

Care should be holistic and multidisciplinary to cover the complex needs of older people with diabetes. Family involvement is vital for care success. In addition, care should be structured, organised and delivered in all settings (Box 3).

Family Support

Families should be involved in the care of older people with diabetes, especially when they develop cognitive or physical dysfunction and having difficulties in performing day-to-day self-care tasks. Family support may bridge the gap between the deficit in cognitive function and achieving good glycaemic control. Older people with comorbid diabetes and cognitive impairment and low family support had increased odds of poor glycaemic control [8]. This has also been shown in the Health and Retirement Study, where respondents in the lowest quartile of cognitive scores and low levels of social support had significantly higher

Box 3: Care Delivery in Older People with Diabetes – Use of Acronyms to Simplify

Care

- Coordination between primary and secondary care
- Assessing risk of hypoglycaemia especially in patients with cognitive dysfunction
- Regular review of self-care ability
- Education of patients, family and carers

Delivery

- Deintensification of therapy when hypoglycaemia occurs
- Erratic eating monitoring in patients with dementia
- Level of care sensitive to patients' function
- Insulin regimen simplification
- Vision for a personalised care plans
- Ensure adequate hydration, especially in patients with dementia
- Reassess care plans when patient condition changes
- Yearly holistic reviews

haemoglobin A1c levels than those in the highest quartile of cognition or those with high social support [9]. Educational programmes for patients and carers should be available. Assessment of older people with diabetes is needed to tailor educational programmes suitable to their cognitive abilities. Carers should be part of education to assist in the implementation of self-care tasks.

Care Organisation

Poor communication between different professionals, less awareness of holistic assessment in non-specialist settings and lack of coordinated working between practitioners in different areas are barriers to the delivery of good care for people with complex health needs [10]. Increasing awareness of the links between geriatric syndromes and diabetes will help to support the development of targeted treatment. Development of shared care protocols between primary and secondary care is important to help organise care for patients and to reduce unnecessary hospital admissions. Outpatient appointments for patients need to be long enough to allow individualised care planning. In the British qualitative analysis of people living with comorbid conditions, including diabetes, it has been suggested that a partnership is necessary between patients, their carers and professionals. [11] Recognition of the way in which a patient's diagnosis of physical or cognitive disability affects the management of diabetes, flexibility in services to ensure that they are sensitive to the changing needs of patients and their carers over time, and improved collaboration across specialties and organisations are necessary [11].

Continuity of Care

Continuity of care is important, as healthcare professionals can notice the subtle changes in patients function before disability develops and can help in reduction of hospitalisation. In a retrospective cohort study of administrative health databases including 305 patients ≥65 years old with diabetes to examine the relationship between continuity of family physician care and acute hospitalisations, patient groups with higher continuity of care were found to have lower rates of hospitalisation (53.5% vs 68.2%) compared with those who have lower continuity of care [12]. Discharge plans from hospital should include a problem list and a management plan that is communicated appropriately to the community care team for the patient to prevent readmission. A nurse case manager devoted to diabetes could be very efficient in the general follow-up care for patients in the community. A systematic and multidisciplinary team approach to care plans with a focus on providing patients with support to cope with their disease will help in improving the outcome. Long-term telephone support for disease management has been shown to reduce hospitalisations and to improve quality of life of older patients with diabetes living in the community [13].

Care Homes

Older people with diabetes who reside in a care home are likely to have multiple comorbidities, advanced dementia, behavioural problems with erratic eating patterns and higher risk of hypoglycaemia than patients living in the community. Therefore, careful attention to their hypoglycaemic regimen is required. For example, high-hypoglycaemia risk therapies such as sulfonylureas should be avoided or used with caution in these settings. Long-acting insulin analogues may be a good option than insulin analogues as they have less risk of hypoglycaemia and can be conveniently injected once daily. In a cross-sectional study of 2258 patients, mean age 82 years (standard deviation 8 years), with type 2 diabetes, of whom 1138 patients had dementia across 150 nursing homes in Italy, insulin analogues were associated with reduced odds, whereas sulfonylureas monotherapy or combined with metformin were associated with increased odds of severe hypoglycaemia in patients with dementia but not in those without dementia. These results may be due to the ability of adjusting insulin dosages according to irregular eating habits [14]. Introducing advanced nurse practitioners in care homes has a positive impact on improving staff confidence and in reducing hospital admissions. Care homes should have a policy for diabetes care including diabetes screening on admission and individualised care plans for residents and these care plans should be tailored to patient needs. Additionally, a protocol for diabetes management and treatment of hypoglycaemia should be established and care home staff should be associated with a local diabetes team (primary care/community diabetes specialist nurses) for managing the complex problems of older patients with diabetes and multiple morbidities [15].

Conclusion

Diabetes is common in older people and the prevalence is likely to increase due to increased life expectancy. Diabetes in old age is associated with multiple morbidities and geriatric syndromes that lead to physical and mental dysfunction. Therefore, care needs of this age group is challenging and should be adequately organised, and should include multidisciplinary team, involves the family and focuses on maintenance of the quality of life of these vulnerable patients.

Clinical Practice Question

Q1. An 83-year-old woman known to have type 2 diabetes mellitus for the past 36 years. Diabetes is reasonably controlled on a combination of oral hypoglycaemic therapy and insulin. She also suffers from hypertension, ischaemic heart disease, osteoarthritis, osteoporosis and chronic kidney disease. She had a recent cerebrovascular stroke from which she made a good recovery but remains slightly forgetful. She is mobile with a stick but had occasional falls. Her body mass index (BMI) is 21 kg/m^2, her appetite is variable and she recalls some weight loss. What best describes the characteristic of this patient and what are her needs. Choose those that apply.

A. Long duration of diabetes with multimorbidities.
B. Has underlying physical dysfunction.
C. Does not have underlying cognitive dysfunction.
D. Has geriatric syndromes.
E. At risk of disability.

References

Key references only are listed here. For a full list of references visit: `https://www.wiley.com/go/sinclair/1e`.

1. Whiting, D., Guairquata, L., and Shaw, J. (2013). International Diabetes Federation (IDF) Global estimates of prevalence of diabetes for 2011–2030. *Diabetes Res. Clin. Pract.* 44: 311–321.
2. Jang, H.C. (2019). Diabetes and muscle dysfunction in older adults. *Ann. Geriatr. Med. Res.* 23: 160–164.

3. Dove, A., Shang, Y., Xu, W. et al. (2021). The impact of diabetes on cognitive impairment and its progression to dementia. *Alzheimers Dement.* 17: 1769–1778.
4. Kulmala, J., Nykanen, I., Manty, M. et al. (2014). Association between frailty and dementia: a population-based study. *Gerontology* 60: 16–21.
5. Volpato, S., Bianchi, L., Lauretani, F. et al. (2012). Role of muscle mass and muscle quality in the association between diabetes and gait speed. *Diabetes Care* 35: 1672–1679.
6. Abdelhafiz, A.H., Keegan, G.L., and Sinclair, A.J. (2023). Metabolic characteristics of frail older people with diabetes mellitus – a systematic search for phenotypes. *Metabolites* 13: 705.
7. Verdijk, L.B. (2021). Nutritional supplementation to enhance the efficacy of exercise training in older adults: what is the evidence from the latest randomized controlled trials? *Curr. Opin. Clin. Nutr. Metab. Care* 24: 504–510.
8. Strizich, G., Kaplan, R.C., Gonzalez, H.M. et al. (2016). Glycemic control, cognitive function, and family support among middle-aged and older Hispanics with diabetes: the Hispanic community health study/study of Latinos. *Diabetes Res. Clin. Pract.* 117: 6473.
9. Okura, T., Heisler, M., and Langa, K.M. (2009). Association between cognitive function and social support with glycemic control in adults with diabetes mellitus. *J. Am. Geriatr. Soc.* 57: 1816–1824.
10. Bunn, F., Burn, A.M., Goodman, C. et al. (2014). Comorbidity and dementia: a scoping review of the literature. *BMC Med.* 12: 192.

1 Epidemiology and Pathophysiology

Sarah L. Sy
Division of Geriatric Medicine, Department of Medicine, University of British Columbia, Vancouver, BC, Canada

Key Points

- Diabetes is common in older adults (age ≥ 65 years).
- The development of type 2 diabetes in older adults is multifactorial.
- Lifestyle and environmental factors are strong diabetes risk factors.
- Older adults with diabetes are at risk of hypoglycaemia due to changes in glucose counter-regulation. Hypoglycaemia should be avoided in this population.

Introduction

Diabetes mellitus is a chronic medical condition and a major global public health issue that affects millions of people worldwide. It can lead to micro- and macrovascular complications, increased morbidity, reduced life expectancy and significant healthcare expenditure [1]. There is an association between increasing age and the development of diabetes, and its prevalence is highest for older adults (age ≥ 65 years) [1]. This population is heterogenous with varying levels of complexity, geriatric syndromes, functional status and life expectancy. In this chapter, the epidemiology and pathophysiology of diabetes in older adults are discussed.

Care of Older People with Diabetes: A Manual for Healthcare Practice, First Edition.
Edited by Alan J. Sinclair and Ahmed H. Abdelhafiz.

Companion website: www.wiley.com/go/sinclair/1e

Epidemiology

In 2019, there were nearly 136 million people worldwide between the ages of 65 and 99 years living with diabetes. This number is anticipated to rise to 195 million by 2030 and 276 million by 2045, based on projections from the International Diabetes Federation (IDF) Diabetes Atlas [2].

The IDF has organised the world map into seven regions for epidemiology research: North America and the Caribbean, South and Central America, Middle East and North Africa, Europe, Western Pacific, South-East Asia and Africa. In 2019, the highest diabetes prevalences in older adults were in the North America and the Caribbean, and Middle East and North Africa regions, at 27.0% and 24.2%, respectively. The Africa and South-East Asia regions had the lowest diabetes prevalence in older adults [2].

Diabetes prevalences among older men and women were similar across the regions, apart from a few exceptions. In North America and the Caribbean, men had higher rates of diabetes (31.0%) compared with women (23.6%). In contrast, in South and Central America, rates of diabetes in women were higher (24.6%) compared with men (20.3%) [2]. In terms of socioeconomic status, high-income countries tended to have a higher diabetes prevalence in older adults compared with middle- and lower-income countries [1, 2]. This trend is likely driven by urbanisation. China, the United States of America and India are countries with the largest populations of older adults with diabetes [2].

Recent studies have shown that diabetes prevalence tends to peak between the ages of 75 and 79 years and that type 2 diabetes is the most common type, accounting for approximately 96% of cases [3]. Several risk factors have been identified as strong contributors to the development of type 2 diabetes, in order of highest risk: obesity, diet, environmental and occupational exposures, and tobacco use [3].

With respect to cost, diabetes care has significant healthcare expenditure. In 2021, it is estimated that US$966 billion were spent globally for the management of diabetes in individuals between the ages of 20 and 79 years [1]. A large proportion of the cost was incurred in the North America and the Caribbean region (US$415 billion) and the greatest amount of spending was for men between ages 60 and 69 years (US$132.5 billion) [1]. Unfortunately, there are limited amounts of health expenditure data on individuals above the age of 80 years.

Pathophysiology of Diabetes in Older Adults

The majority of older adults with diabetes will have type 2 diabetes. In contrast, type 1 diabetes is an autoimmune disease that presents in younger patients due to destruction of beta islet cells and lack of insulin secretion [4]. There is a small subgroup of patients who share overlapping characteristics between type 1 and type 2 diabetes and present later in adulthood (age $\geq$ 30 years). These individuals have latent autoimmune diabetes in adults (LADA) or type 1.5 diabetes, and have diabetes-associated antibodies. They usually do not require insulin until six months after diagnosis [5].

The development of type 2 diabetes in older adults is a result of age-related alterations in glucose metabolism [4]. There are several other factors, such as genetics, lifestyle and environmental changes, inflammation and comorbidities, that contribute to the development of diabetes (Figure 1.1).

There are several contributing factors to hyperglycaemia in older adults, which leads to an imbalance of insulin secretion and insulin resistance and, ultimately, the development of type 2 diabetes. Age-related decreased beta cell mass and function results in reduced insulin secretion in response to glucose. Genetic predisposition increases an individual's risk of developing diabetes. Lifestyle factors such as diets high in simple sugars and saturated fats lead to increased adiposity, which further increases insulin resistance. A lack of physical activity contributes to a loss of lean muscle mass and decreased insulin sensitivity. Chronic inflammation interferes with insulin signalling pathways thereby increasing insulin resistance. Finally, there are comorbidities and medications that will alter insulin secretion and/or increase insulin resistance.

Age-related Alterations in Glucose Metabolism

With ageing, hyperglycaemia primarily stems from impaired beta cell function and poor adaptation to insulin resistance [6]. Beta cell mass and proliferation decrease with age, and there is reduced beta cell sensitivity to glucose [7, 8]. Studies have demonstrated that insulin secretion in response to glucose is diminished in older individuals compared with

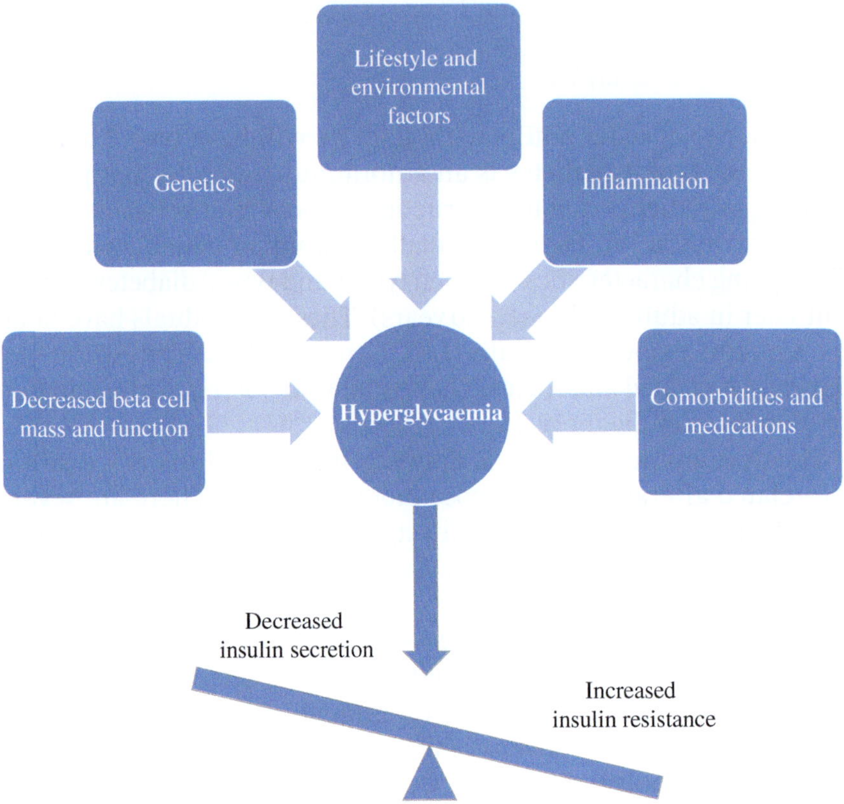

Figure 1.1: Development of type 2 diabetes in older adults.

younger individuals with similar insulin resistance [7]. There was previously a debate as to whether increased insulin resistance and decreased insulin sensitivity were due to the ageing process. However, recent studies have shown that age alone does not increase insulin resistance and that factors such as lifestyle, obesity, lean body mass and sarcopenia are major contributors. Similarly, insulin sensitivity worsens due to increased adiposity and loss of lean muscle mass rather than age alone [6].

There are significant age-related physiological changes that occur in response to hypoglycaemia. In normal and younger individuals, glucagon is secreted by pancreatic alpha cells in response to hypoglycaemia to stimulate liver gluconeogenesis. If the glucagon response is decreased, then the epinephrine response becomes important. When a hypoglycaemia episode becomes prolonged, growth hormone and cortisol are subsequently secreted [9]. In older adults, the response of both glucagon and growth hormone are impaired during hypoglycaemia. Studies have revealed that the glucagon response is dampened in older adults with diabetes for decreasing blood glucose levels whereas epinephrine and cortisol responses increase [10]. As a result, older adults with diabetes will often have little warning of autonomic and neuroglycopenic symptoms at levels of glucose that would usually elicit symptoms in younger patients. It has also been shown that reaction time is slower in older adults during hypoglycaemia, so they may not be able to act quickly to correct their low blood sugar to the normal level [10].

Genetics

There is a strong genetic component to the development of type 2 diabetes [7]. Older adults with a family history of diabetes are at higher likelihood of developing the condition as they age [8]. However, specific genes leading to the development of diabetes in older age have not been identified. There are also certain ethnic groups that have a higher predisposition to developing diabetes [1].

Lifestyle and Environmental Factors

A diet high in saturated fats and simple sugars, and low in complex carbohydrates and fibre increases the risk of developing diabetes [11, 12]. In addition, diets that incorporate ultra-processed foods (e.g. foods that contain food additives, or undergo multiple physical, biological or chemical processing) have been shown to increase the risk of diabetes [13]. There have been small studies investigating supplementation of vitamins C and E, magnesium and zinc in improving glycaemic control; however, the benefits are not entirely clear [4].

It is not uncommon for older adults to become more sedentary as they age, because of increasing frailty, the presence of geriatric syndromes and multiple comorbidities. These individuals subsequently experience a loss of lean muscle mass and develop sarcopenia, which leads to decreased insulin sensitivity [6]. Physical activity that includes both aerobic and resistance training has been shown to be the most helpful in improving glycaemic levels by increasing insulin sensitivity and decreasing insulin resistance. Given the varying levels of frailty and health complexity, exercise programmes will need to be individualised for each patient [6].

In certain regions, obesity is becoming more prevalent because of poor diet, lack of physical activity and urbanisation [3]. Increased adiposity particularly central adiposity contributes to increased insulin resistance [3, 6]. It has been shown in a large study that individuals who implement healthy lifestyle changes (e.g. body mass index $<25\,kg/^{m2}$, diet with low glycaemic load and trans-unsaturated fatty acids, 30 minutes of moderate to vigorous activity per day, no smoking and low alcoholic intake) significantly reduced their risk of developing type 2 diabetes [13].

Other Factors

Inflammation and stress are associated with an increased risk of diabetes in older adults. Proinflammatory cytokines such as C-reactive protein, tumour necrosis factor-α and interleukin-6 inhibit insulin signalling and increase insulin resistance [6]. It has also been suggested that older adults have decreased mitochondrial function and phosphorylation activity, which may contribute to insulin resistance [6]. Furthermore, low levels of sex hormones such as testosterone in men and higher in women have been shown to be associated with increased risk of diabetes [4].

Coexisting comorbidities such as hypertension and obesity increase the risk of developing diabetes in older adults [6]. In addition, acute illness leads to stress-related catecholamine response, thereby inhibiting insulin secretion and increasing insulin resistance. Another contributing factor to hyperglycaemia is medication. Glucocorticoids can cause drug-induced hyperglycaemia by increasing hepatic gluconeogenesis and adipose tissue lipolysis, which in turn leads to increased insulin resistance [6, 14]. Other medications that have been associated with hyperglycaemia include antipsychotics, protease inhibitors, calcineurin inhibitors, thiazide diuretics, fluoroquinolones and some beta blockers [14].

What Are the Key Issues?

Prevention of Diabetes in Older Adults

The number of older adults with diabetes is increasing each year. The complications, morbidity and associated costs have significant implications on the individual, their family and the healthcare system.

Unfortunately, factors such as genetics and age-related changes in glucose metabolism are non-modifiable. However, lifestyle and environmental factors are modifiable diabetes risk factors. Interventions focusing on nutrition and physical activity are important to implement throughout an individual's lifespan. The Diabetes Prevention Program study revealed that lifestyle interventions (diet, physical activity and education) reduced the incidence of diabetes by 58% and was significantly more effective than metformin [15]. Identifying individuals at risk of developing diabetes or with prediabetes will be critical in providing them with management strategies to reduce the risk of progression as they age.

Hypoglycaemia

Older adults with diabetes are at risk of severe and fatal hypoglycaemia due to age-related physiological changes [4]. Hypoglycaemia unawareness is common in older adults. Hypoglycaemic episodes can result in emergency department visits or hospitalisations with falls, cardiac arrhythmias, seizures, delirium, coma and even death. Severe episodes of hypoglycaemia can also increase the risk of developing dementia [16]. Therefore, it is imperative to prevent hypoglycaemia in older adults.

Management

The management of diabetes in older adults requires careful clinical considerations given the age-related physiological changes described earlier (Table 1.1). A collaboration between the primary care physician, endocrinologist, diabetes nurse educator, dietitian and social worker is essential to provide tailored care for older adults with diabetes. Diabetes management strategies for older adults are discussed in later chapters.

Summary

Diabetes is a common chronic medical condition in older adults. The prevalence of diabetes tends to increase with age and is highest in high income countries. The development of diabetes in older adults is due to age-related changes in glucose metabolism along with genetic, lifestyle and environmental factors. Changes in glucose counter-regulation predispose older adults with diabetes to severe and fatal hypoglycaemia,

Table 1.1: Clinical considerations given the physiological changes associated with ageing and diabetes.

Age-related physiological changes	Clinical considerations
Glucose counter-regulation (increased risk of hypoglycaemia)	Education should be provided with respect to signs and symptoms of hypoglycaemia, and how to correct accordingly.
	Management strategies should include efforts to prevent hypoglycaemia episodes. Avoid medications with high risk of hypoglycaemia such as sulfonylureas, meglitinides and insulin if possible. If patients require the use of these medications, then increased monitoring of blood glucose (glucometer or continuous glucose monitor) is needed and close follow-up.
	For patients who are on basal insulin, consider prescribing the insulin in the morning so the effect of the medication wears off overnight when the patient is sleeping and unable to recognise hypoglycaemic symptoms.
Increased adiposity	Nutritional education and counselling should be provided, focusing on decreasing intake of foods with high glycaemic load and saturated fats and avoiding ultra-processed foods. In circumstances of obesity, reduced caloric intake should be considered.
	Prescribe individualised exercise programs focusing on aerobic and resistance training and encourage less time spent in daily sedentary behaviour.
	In select patients, consider using GLP-1 receptor agonists to improve glycaemic control and reduce weight.
Loss of lean muscle mass	Prescribe individualised exercise programmes focusing on resistance training. Balance exercises should also be incorporated to reduce the risk of falls in the setting of sarcopenia.
	Nutritional counselling to be provided to increase protein intake to 1.0–1.5 mg/kg/day if patients do not have contraindications.

GLP-1, glucagon-like peptide-1.

so careful attention is required to avoid hypoglycaemia. Prevention of diabetes and individualised diabetes management strategies are important as this heterogenous population continues to grow and age.

Clinical Practice Question

Q1. Mrs Smith is an 86-year-old woman living alone who was diagnosed with type 2 diabetes approximately 20 years ago. She also has hypertension, dyslipidaemia and chronic kidney disease (estimated glomerular filtration rate 25). Her most recent haemoglobin A1c (HbA1c) was 9.0%. She has been losing weight despite eating three meals per day (primarily simple carbohydrates). Mrs Smith does not exercise but can mobilise short distances using a four-wheeled walker in her apartment. Her diabetes medications include insulin glargine 24 units at bedtime and linagliptin 5 mg daily. She checks her blood sugars fasting and the range is between 7.8 and 11.0 mmol/l (140–198 mg/dl). What is the next step?
Choose one option:

A. Increase insulin glargine to 26 units at bedtime
B. Stop linagliptin and start mealtime insulin.
C. Increase the frequency of glucose monitoring over the next two weeks for glucose pattern analysis and follow-up.
D. Refer for dietitian consultation.
E. Encourage physical activity (walking and resistance bands) 10 minutes after each of her meals.
F. All the above.
G. A, C, D and E.
H. C, D and E.

References

Key references only are listed here. For a full list of references visit: https://www.wiley.com/go/sinclair/1e.

1. Sun, H., Saeedi, P., Karuranga, S. et al. (2022). IDF Diabetes Atlas: global, regional, and country-level diabetes prevalence estimates for 2021 and projections for 2045. *Diabetes Res. Clin. Pract.* 183: 109119.

2. Sinclair, A.S., Saeedi, P., Kaundal, A. et al. (2020). Diabetes and global ageing among 65–99-year-old adults: findings from the International Diabetes Federation Diabetes Atlas, 9th edition. *Diabetes Res. Clin. Pract.* 162: 108078.
4. Meneilly, G.S. and Tessier, D. (2001). Diabetes in elderly adults. *J. Gerontol. A Biol. Sci. Med. Sci.* 56 (1): M5–M13.
5. Buzzetti, R., Tuomi, T., Mauricio, D. et al. (2020). Management of latent autoimmune diabetes in adults: a consensus statement from an international expert panel. *Diabetes* 69 (10): 2037–2047.
6. Lee, P.G. and Halter, J.B. (2017). The pathophysiology of hyperglycemia in older adults: clinical considerations. *Diabetes Care* 40: 444–452.
9. Service, F.J. (1995). Hypoglycemic disorders. *N. Engl. J. Med.* 332 (17): 1144–1152.
10. Meneilly, G.S., Cheung, E., and Tuokko, H. (1994). Counterregulatory hormone responses to hypoglycemia in the elderly patient with diabetes. *Diabetes* 43: 403–410.
12. Hu, F.B., Manson, J.E., Stampfer, M.J. et al. (2001). Diet, lifestyle, and the risk of type 2 diabetes mellitus in women. *N. Engl. J. Med.* 345: 790–797.
15. Knowler, W.C., Barrett-Connor, E., Fowler, S.E. et al. (2002). Reduction in the incidence of type 2 diabetes with lifestyle intervention or metformin. *N. Engl. J. Med.* 346 (6): 393–403.
16. Whitmer, R.A., Karter, A.J., Yaffe, K. et al. (2009). Hypoglycemic episodes and risk of dementia in older patients with type 2 diabetes mellitus. *JAMA* 301 (15): 1565–1572.

2 Screening and Diagnosis

Isabelle Bourdel-Marchasson[1,2]

[1] *Center for Magnetic Resonance of Biological Systems, University of Bordeaux, Bordeaux, France*
[2] *Gerontological Department, University Hospital of Bordeaux, Bordeaux, France*

Key Points

- Population-based screening of diabetes mellitus should be performed in older people every five years due to low rate of symptoms and efficiency of early diabetes control.
- In older people, incident type 1 diabetes mellitus (latent autoimmune diabetes in the adult) or pancreatic cancer should be searched in case of rapidly increase in blood glucose levels.
- In the community, diagnosis of type 2 diabetes mellitus is based on at least two fasting blood glucose measures ≥7 mmol/l. A haemoglobin A1c value of ≥48 mmol/mol (6.5%) may also be used to diagnose type 2 diabetes mellitus but fasting glycaemia should always be determined (World Health Organization).
- High blood glucose levels may be accompanied by symptoms and syndromes requiring immediate blood sugar measurement.
- During corticosteroid treatment, infectious diseases, dehydration and immune checkpoint inhibitor therapy in cancer, blood glucose should be monitored.

Introduction

Diabetes mellitus (DM) is a long-duration chronic disease resulting in frailty, disability, increased rate of adverse events, hospitalisations and premature death. It is recognised that early control of blood glucose

Care of Older People with Diabetes: A Manual for Healthcare Practice, First Edition.
Edited by Alan J. Sinclair and Ahmed H. Abdelhafiz.

Companion website: www.wiley.com/go/sinclair/1e

levels is the most effective preventive measure after prevention of DM itself. Early diagnosis is thus of major importance, including in older people.

Background

Moderate hyperglycaemia or a slow rise in blood glucose levels induces few symptoms. As a result, diabetes mellitus is largely a silent disease. Polydipsia–polyuria occurs mainly in the event of sudden onset of hyperglycaemia. Some people may be unaware of these symptoms. The rate of non-diagnosed diabetes maybe high in low-income countries. In a French community-based study the proportion of diagnosed diabetes and undiagnosed diabetes in older people was, respectively, 8.2% and 1.4%. People with diabetes were less likely to have a high income and more likely to have a lower educational level with no relation to the knowledge of diabetes status. One in five of those undiagnosed had a haemoglobin A1c (HbA1c) level above 8% [1]. In Greece, older age or poor health literacy was associated with higher rate of unknown diabetes [2].

Complications of diabetes may be present at the moment of diagnosis, hindering efficiency of blood glucose control. Given the fact that, in most countries, peak incidence of diabetes occurs in the age range 65–70 years [3], screening of diabetes is a critical point in the promotion of better ageing.

In older people, HbA1c tends to increase, even with a normal fasting blood glucose [4]. Indeed, postprandial or post glucose challenge increase in blood glucose level is a feature of normal ageing [5]. An association with increased cardiovascular risk was, however, found in older subjects with increased post-challenge hyperglycaemia as compared with other older adults [6]. On the other hand, increase in fasting glycemia below the threshold of diabetes diagnosis and hyperinsulinemia are known risk factors for cognitive difficulties [7]. The determination of HbA1c may be of interest in elderly subjects, with the aim of implementing measures for better ageing. Monitoring glucose homeostasis disorders in older people should therefore be included in the preventive plan in any health system.

In older people without specific symptoms, risk factors for developing DM are overweight and obesity and low physical activity. Low quality of life is also associated in older people to increased risk to develop

DM [8]. Alteration in body composition, such as increased trunk fat and thinning of the limbs, are hallmarks of insulin resistance. Hypertension may also precede type 2 DM (T2DM) and shares similar risk factors [9]. DM diagnosis includes heterogeneous phenotypes. A Swedish epidemiological study in newly diagnosed diabetes of all age groups identified five different clusters, depending on body mass index (BMI), the presence of insulin resistance (homeostasis model assessment estimated insulin resistance, HOMA-IR), insulinopenia (HOMA2-B), glutamate decarboxylase (GAD) antibodies and HbA1c levels [10]. The two first include younger subjects with low or normal BMI, with high or very high HbA1c, low HOMA2-B and normal HOMA-IR. The third includes mid-age subjects, with high BMI, normal or high HOMA2-B and high HOMA-IR. The fourth also includes mid-age subjects with high BMI, but with low HbA1c and subnormal HOMA-IR and HOMA2-B. In the fifth cluster, subjects were older, with normal BMI, HbA1c moderately elevated, normal HOMA-IR but slightly decreased HOMA2-B. It was suggested that complications profile may differ according to cluster [10]. Findings in other studies have found conflicting results. However, this first step in precision medicine opens a new approach in the care of DM. Asymptomatic diabetes more often leads to a diagnosis of T2DM.

DM may be suspected after the finding of microvascular complications such as retinopathy, nephropathy or lower-limb neuropathy, or macrovascular complications such as myocardial infarction, lower-limb occlusive arterial disease or cerebral vascular disease.

Symptoms of high blood glucose are polyuria due to high urine glucose output and subsequent polydipsia. Polyuria and polydipsia are more often associated with the presence of rapidly increasing glycaemia. Delirium may be observed following intracellular dehydration or rheological abnormalities of the blood due to high blood glucose levels. Asthaenia and weight loss may occur, particularly in cases of insulinopoenia. High blood glucose favours infections, mostly mycosis infections, including cutaneous, oral or urinary infections. Unknown type 1 DM (T1DM) can be diagnosed after inaugural ketoacidosis. However, in the elderly this situation remains anecdotal. In the case of sudden rise in blood glucose, an autoimmune form of DM, latent autoimmune diabetes in the adult (LADA) should be suspected and confirmed with measure of GAD antibodies. However, as evidenced above, it is possible to observe severe insulinopoenia without GAD antibodies. In the case of sudden hyperglycaemia with or without asthaenia, anorexia and weight loss, a diagnosis of pancreatic cancer should be sought with echography or computed tomography.

Several clinical situations may induce alterations in blood glucose homeostasis, most frequently in older people as a consequence of corticosteroid use, in particular by the general route. Fasting blood glucose levels may be mildly modified, but daytime blood glucose levels rise and remain so until the middle of the night. After cessation of corticosteroid therapy, diabetes may disappear or may persist. Other drugs are known to increase blood glucose such as atypic antipsychotic inducing insulin resistance [11]. One of the severe adverse events of immune checkpoint inhibitor therapy in cancer can be T1DM with inaugural ketoacidosis [12].

In very frail subjects, severe intracellular dehydration may be associated with hyperglycaemia in patients not diagnosed with diabetes. After recovery, hyperglycaemia may persist or decrease to the pre-event level.

Finally, infections may induce diabetes, such as COVID-19, during the course of the infection and afterwards [13].

Key Issues

Screening

In the community, in asymptomatic older people, screening for diabetes should be carried out every five years. In the case of risk factors for diabetes, such as overweight or obesity, sedentary life style, hypertension or deprived conditions, frequency of screening may be increased to every three years. However, a screening strategy based only on a risk-factor profile has not been shown to be more efficient than in the general population [14], and risk factors profile may vary according to population [15]. Furthermore, patients older than 75 years were not included in any of these reports. Before and after the start of treatment known to induce glucose homeostasis disorders (Table 2.1), particularly corticosteroid therapy and some anti-cancer treatment, blood glucose determination must be planned. At diagnosis of any micro- or macrovascular conditions, screening for diabetes should be done, considering the possibility of unknown diabetes. Screening for diabetes should also be carried out immediately in the case of specific symptoms or in the conditions listed in Table 2.1.

Table 2.1: Spectrum of symptoms and conditions suggesting possible high blood glucose levels or diabetes mellitus.

Symptoms/ conditions	Suggested type of glucose homeostasis disorder	Action
Polyuria–polydipsia	Any DM	Measure blood glucose immediately; follow-up for diagnosis
Asthenia	T1DM, cancer	
Weight loss	T1DM, cancer	
Repeated infections	Any	
Mycosis infections (skin, oral, urinary)	Any, corticoids	
Delirium	Any	
Dehydration (intracellular)	Any	
Myocardial infarction	T2DM	
Stroke	T2DM	
Ketoacidosis	T1DM	
Frailty	T2DM	Comprehensive diabetes diagnosis procedure
Microvascular complications	T2DM	Comprehensive diabetes diagnosis procedure
Retinopathy		
Nephropathy		
Neuropathy		
Macrovascular complication		
Ischaemic heart disease		
Occlusive arterial disease		
Cerebral vascular disease		
COVID-19	Any	Glucose monitoring and follow-up for diagnosis

(*Continued*)

Table 2.1: Continued

Symptoms/ conditions	Suggested type of glucose homeostasis disorder	Action
Therapy:		
Corticosteroid	Corticoid-induced DM	Glucose monitoring and follow-up for diagnosis
Atypical antipsychotic	T2DM	Glucose monitoring and symptoms awareness
Immune checkpoint inhibitor therapy	T1DM	

DM, diabetes mellitus; T1DM, type 1 diabetes mellitus; T2DM, type 2 diabetes mellitus.

Diagnosis

A diagnosis of T2DM is based on at least two fasting blood glucose measures ≥7 mmol/l or whenever blood glucose ≥11.1 mmol/l. A HbA1c value ≥48 mmol/mol (6.5%) may also be used to diagnose T2DM but fasting glycaemia should always be determined [16]. A blood glucose level of ≥11.1 mmol/l strongly suggests diabetes, but formal diagnosis is based on fasting blood glucose levels. If a high blood glucose level is measured during an acute event, diabetes will be confirmed one month after recovery and lifestyle interventions will be proposed in the interim.

The characteristics of the diabetes are best recorded before any drug treatment is started (Table 2.2). The minimum necessary is to describe the phenotype of the patient: search for general symptoms (asthenia, exhaustion, anorexia), BMI and waist circumference, history of weight loss or recent weight gain, any evidence of sarcopenia and HbA1c. If the clinical presentation is in favour of insulin deficiency (sudden rise in blood glucose, BMI in the normal range or recent weight loss,) and if GAD antibodies are not detected, cancer of the pancreas should be considered. However, T1DM may be diagnosed later, if insulin is necessary for control within the first two years. Presentations of T2DM is highly heterogeneous and an individualised care plan should rely on biomarkers.

Together with the comprehensive gerontological assessment (see Chapter 16K), vascular risk factors must be assessed (blood pressure, tobacco use and lipid profile) as a preventive strategy. Screening for frailty, using any clinical scale (see Chapter 16a) is carried out at diagnosis, as frailty may precede diabetes.

Table 2.2: Main Differences in Presentation of New-onset Diabetes Mellitus.

Type	Clinical presentation	Biological presentation
1 Latent autoimmune diabetes in the adult	■ Polyuria/polydipsia ■ Normal or low BMI ■ Possibly weight loss ■ Exhaustion or asthenia ■ Repeated infections (mycosis) ■ Insulin needed for blood glucose control within two years after diagnosis ■ (inaugural ketoacidosis) ■ Differential diagnosis: pancreatic cancer	■ Sudden rise in blood glucose ■ Various level at diagnosis of HbA1c ■ GAD antibodies at diagnosis (may not be present) ■ HOMA2-B decreased
2 Type 2 Diabetes Mellitus	■ Often asymptomatic ■ Heterogeneous presentation ■ Resistance to insulin frequent (high BMI), trunk fat deposition (increased waist circumference) ■ Complications are possibly present at diagnosis ■ In the very old (≥ 85 years), normal or decreased BMI	■ Long term increase in blood glucose ■ Various levels at diagnosis of HbA1c ■ HOMA-IR increased or normal ■ In the very old, HOMA2-B slightly decreased

BMI, body mass index; GAD, glutamate decarboxylase; HbA1c, haemoglobin A1c; HOMA2-B, homeostasis model assessment beta cell function; HOMA-IR, homeostasis model assessment estimated insulin resistance.

Clinical Practice Questions

Q1. In older patients a sudden rise in blood glucose levels over 11 mmol/l indicates:

A. Diagnosis of diabetes
B. A pancreatic cancer
C. Type 1 diabetes mellitus
D. Further clinical investigations are necessary
E. The presence of an infection

Q2. In older patients, screening of diabetes should be made:
- **A.** On the basis of risk factors profile for diabetes
- **B.** In overall population each five years
- **C.** In case of frailty
- **D.** After weight gain of 5% of body weight
- **E.** In all patients younger than 80 years

Q3. The most important elements of making a diagnosis of type 2 diabetes in older people are:
- **A.** Ensuring that you use age-specific cut-offs for glucose levels
- **B.** A raised haemoglobin A1c above 42 mmol/mol
- **C.** having microvascular complications at diagnosis
- **D.** a raised random level of glucose above 7.8 mmol/l
- **E.** fasting glucose levels above 7 mmol/l on two separate occasions

References

Key references only are listed here. For a full list of references visit: `https://www.wiley.com/go/sinclair/1e`.

1. Bourdel-Marchasson, I., Helmer, C., Barberger-Gateau, P. et al. (2007). Characteristics of undiagnosed diabetes in community-dwelling French elderly: the 3C study. *Diabetes Res. Clin. Pract.* 76 (2): 257–264.
2. Makrilakis, K., Kalpourtzi, N., Ioannidis, I. et al. (2021). Prevalence of diabetes and pre-diabetes in Greece. Results of the first national survey of morbidity and risk factors (EMENO) study. *Diabetes Res. Clin. Pract.* 172: 108646.
3. Sun, P., Wen, H., Liu, X. et al. (2022). Time trends in type 2 diabetes mellitus incidence across the BRICS from 1990 to 2019: an age-period-cohort analysis. *BMC Public Health* 22 (1): 65.
4. Rhee, M.K., Ziemer, D.C., Kolm, P., and Phillips, L.S. (2006). Postchallenge glucose rises with increasing age even when glucose tolerance is normal. *Diabet. Med.* 23 (11): 1174–1179.
5. Jackson, R.A., Blix, P.M., Matthews, J.A. et al. (1982). Influence of ageing on glucose homeostasis. *J. Clin. Endocrinol. Metab.* 55 (5): 840–848.
6. Crandall, J.P., Shamoon, H., Cohen, H.W. et al. (2009). Post-challenge hyperglycemia in older adults is associated with increased cardiovascular risk profile. *J. Clin. Endocrinol. Metab.* 94 (5): 1595–1601.
7. Bourdel-Marchasson, I., Lapre, E., Laksir, H., and Puget, E. (2010). Insulin resistance, diabetes and cognitive function: consequences for preventative strategies. *Diabetes Metab.* 36 (3): 173–181.

8. Bourdel-Marchasson, I., Dubroca, B., Letenneur, L. et al. (2000). Incidence and predictors of drug-treated diabetes in elderly French subjects. The PAQUID Epidemiological Survey. *Diabet. Med.* 17 (9): 675–681.
9. Gress, T.W., Nieto, F.J., Shahar, E. et al. (2000). Hypertension and antihypertensive therapy as risk factors for type 2 diabetes mellitus. Atherosclerosis Risk in Communities Study. *N. Engl. J. Med.* 342 (13): 905–912.
10. Ahlqvist, E., Storm, P., Käräjämäki, A. et al. (2018). Novel subgroups of adult-onset diabetes and their association with outcomes: a data-driven cluster analysis of six variables. *Lancet Diabetes Endocrinol.* 6 (5): 361–369.

3 Lifestyle Interventions

Abdiazizi Yusuf and
Ahmed H. Abdelhafiz
Department of Geriatric Medicine, Rotherham General Hospital, Rotherham, UK

Key Points

- Diabetes in old age is associated with increased visceral fat and reduced muscle mass, which increases insulin resistance.
- Regular physical activity of at least 150 minutes per week and reducing weight by at least 7% reduces the incidence of diabetes in high-risk patients.
- A combination of resistance exercise training and protein-rich diet maintains muscle mass, improves glycaemic control and enhances overall function.
- Exercise training is feasible in older patients, including those with comorbidities or resident in care homes.
- Educational programmes in lifestyle changes should be tailored to suit patients' preference and cultural backgrounds.

Introduction

The prevalence of diabetes increases with advancing age and is associated with low physical activity and increasing weight [1]. A sedentary lifestyle in older people may lead to obesity and low muscle mass or sarcopenia, which increases insulin resistance and worsens diabetes control. Therefore, weight loss therapy, although it will reduce body fat, it will also reduce muscle mass, which may exacerbate the underlying sarcopenia and increases the risk of frailty. Frail older people with

Care of Older People with Diabetes: A Manual for Healthcare Practice, First Edition.
Edited by Alan J. Sinclair and Ahmed H. Abdelhafiz.

Companion website: www.wiley.com/go/sinclair/1e

diabetes are heterogeneous with different phenotypes such as anorexic malnourished (AM) individuals requiring weight gain and sarcopenic obese (SO) individuals requiring weight loss. In both phenotypes, the main aim of lifestyle interventions is to achieve an ideal body weight and at the same time preserve lean muscle mass [2]. Good nutritional status and good functional capacity through maintenance of a healthy lifestyle may maintain good glycaemic control and a good quality of life in older people with diabetes. Lifestyle intervention programmes may be difficult in older people due to associated comorbidities and difficulties in compliance with diet and exercise. This chapter reviews ways and benefits of lifestyle intervention suitable for older people with diabetes.

Impact of Lifestyle Changes

Lifestyle changes may reduce the incidence of diabetes in high-risk groups and may improve the burden of diabetes in patients who already have the disease. The Diabetes Prevention Program study randomly assigned 3234 subjects without, but at risk of, diabetes to placebo, metformin (850 mg twice daily) or an intensive lifestyle intervention programme [3]. This included weight loss of at least 7% of body weight and physical activity of at least 150 minutes per week. The mean (standard deviation, SD) age of the participants was 50.6 years (10.7 years) and the mean body mass index (BMI) was 34 kg/m^2 (6.7 kg/m^2). After 2.8 years of follow up, the incidence of diabetes was lowest in intensive lifestyle intervention group (4.8%) compared with the metformin (7.8%) or placebo (11%) groups. Intensive lifestyle intervention reduced the risk of diabetes by 58%, while metformin reduced the risk by only 31% compared with placebo. In other words, 6.9 patients need to participate in intensive lifestyle intervention and 13.9 need to take metformin to prevent one case of diabetes [3]. Non-pharmacological lifestyle intervention is the first line of management, before pharmacological interventions. The Look AHEAD (Action for Health in Diabetes) randomised controlled study, which included 5145 subjects, mean (SD) age 58.7 years (6.8 years), BMI 36 kg/m^2 (5.9 kg/m^2) demonstrated the efficacy of intensive lifestyle interventions, which included caloric restriction, physical activity and weight loss of 7% of body weight in overweight or obese participants compared with a usual care control group. The intensive interventions improved fitness, glycaemic control,

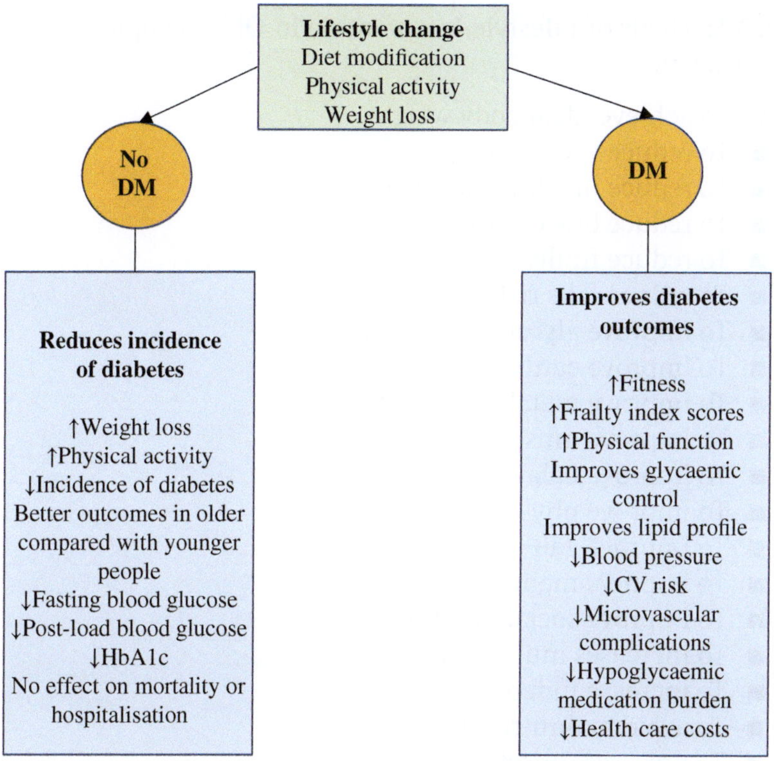

Figure 3.1: Impact of lifestyle changes on high-risk patients with no diabetes and those with diabetes. Lifestyle interventions reduce the incidence of diabetes and improve diabetes-related outcomes. DM, diabetes mellitus; CV, cardiovascular; HbA1c, haemoglobin A1c.

blood pressure, lipid profile and cardiovascular risk [4]. In addition, the regimen reduced microvascular complications, physical dysfunction, hypoglycaemic medication burden, healthcare costs and frailty index scores over 8–11 years of follow-up (Figure 3.1).

Lifestyle Intervention

The main aims of lifestyle intervention are to achieve ideal body weight, reduce visceral fat and maintain muscle mass. This will not only improve metabolic profile and glycaemic control, but will also improve the overall function and reduce adverse events. Goals should be set at the outset, taking into account the patient's potential and wishes (Box 3.1).

Box 3.1: Goals of Lifestyle Intervention in Older People with Diabetes

- To achieve ideal body weight
- To reduce visceral fat
- To reduce insulin resistance
- To reduce blood pressure
- To reduce frailty
- To reduce falls risk
- To improve glycaemic control
- To improve cardiovascular risk
- To improve metabolic profile
- To improve muscle quality
- To improve balance
- To improve physical function
- To improve gait speed
- To improve mental function
- To improve social function
- To increases muscle strength
- To increase independence
- To avoid malnutrition
- To preserve muscle mass
- To maintain good quality of life

Nutrition

A high-fibre diet rich in potassium, vitamin D and micronutrients, such as phosphate, zinc and chromium, but low in saturated fat, salt and refined carbohydrates will have a positive effect on metabolism and improve insulin action and cardiovascular risk profile. An example is the Mediterranean diet, which includes a high intake of vegetables and fruit. Excessive alcohol consumption should be discouraged, as it inhibits gluconeogenesis, causes hypoglycaemia and results in neglecting diabetes self-care. Smoking has negative effects on general health as well as increasing insulin resistance and atherosclerosis. Low glycaemic index carbohydrates with avoidance of concentrated sweet foods will reduce postprandial surges in blood glucose levels. Maintenance of muscle mass will maintain glucose homeostasis and insulin sensitivity. Muscle mass is dependent on the balance between muscle protein synthesis and breakdown. In older people, there is diminished muscle protein synthesis in response to anabolic stimuli such as protein ingestion. Thus, older people need more dietary proteins to compensate for this age-related anabolic resistance. They may also need more protein to offset inflammatory and catabolic conditions associated with chronic morbidities. An average daily intake of protein in the range of 1.0–1.2 g/kg may help to maintain lean body mass and function. This amount may need to be increased to 2.0 g/kg in people with severe malnutrition [5]. Older people with diabetes and no kidney disease can safely have up to 20% of their total energy as protein. Higher protein intake up to 30% of total calorie intake may also be beneficial in reducing the need of hypoglycaemic medications [6]. Anabolic resistance in older people could be overcome by providing sufficient amounts of rapidly digested proteins rich in the essential amino acid leucine, such as whey protein, which may offset muscle loss and reduce sarcopenia [7]. Essential amino acids, in particular leucine, are primarily responsible for stimulation of muscle protein anabolism and positive muscle protein balance [8]. Intake of omega-3 fatty acids may help to preserve muscle mass by relieving the anabolic resistance [9].

Exercise

Exercise is an important part of diabetes prevention and diabetes management to improve body composition, insulin resistance, glycaemic control and overall function. The two common types of exercise are aerobic exercise, such as walking, cycling, swimming or jogging, which require contraction of large groups of muscles, and resistance exercise, which uses muscular strength to lift a weight or to move a load, causing isolated and brief activity of a single muscle group (Table 3.1). Aerobic exercise may not be suitable for all older people due to a high prevalence of comorbidities such as arthritis, cardiovascular disease, peripheral vascular disease, neuropathy or poor mobility. Resistance exercise may be a safer alternative for these patients. Resistance training improves muscle quality, insulin sensitivity and results in skeletal muscle-fibre hypertrophy [10]. Progressive resistance training, defined as exercise in which the resistance against which a muscle generates force is progressively increased over time, can improve glycaemic control. A combination of both exercise modalities may be optimal.

Table 3.1: Differences between resistance and aerobic exercise.

Parameter	Resistance	Aerobic
Example	Weightlifting, resistance bands	Walking, running, swimming, cycling
Muscles involved	Small group	Large group
Muscle contraction	Continuous	Intermittent
Period of activity	Short duration	Long duration
Patient group	Patients with poor mobility	Patients with good mobility
Major effects	Increases muscle mass, strength and bone mass	Increases aerobic capacity and reduces body fat
Effects on metabolism	Positive effect on insulin resistance, glucose uptake and lipid profile	Positive effect on insulin resistance, glucose uptake and lipid profile
Effects on blood pressure	Mild reduction	Moderate reduction
Specific outcome	Improves strength	Improves stamina
General outcomes	Improves gait, balance, risk of falling, coordination, agility	Improves gait, balance, risk of falling, coordination, agility

The combination of resistance (60 minutes) and aerobic (90 minutes) exercise, performed over three days per week, is the optimal exercise strategy for simultaneous reduction in insulin resistance and improvement in physical function. Improvement in insulin resistance is mainly driven by the aerobic exercise, while improvement in physical function is driven mainly by resistance exercise. Reduction of visceral fat and increase in muscle mass may respectively explain the improvement in insulin resistance and in physical function [11]. The choice of exercise type for older people with diabetes may be decided according to the level of comorbidities, personal preferences or the available resources. However, using one or the other type of exercise may be less important than doing some form of physical activity.

Synergy Between Nutrition and Exercise

Exercise training, combined with adequate protein intake, synergistically increases skeletal muscle mass. Exercise maintains a positive balance between muscle protein synthesis and breakdown. Intake of essential amino acids, especially leucine, will promote a net inward gradient for amino acid transport into the intracellular free amino acid pool and providing the building blocks for muscle protein synthesis. Intermittent feeding induces shifts in the net protein balance from negative during fasting state to positive in the fed state. The combination of exercise and feeding induces rise in muscle protein synthesis, an increase in the accretion of proteins and, eventually, an increase in muscle mass. The ingestion of proteins intermittently over 24 hours post exercise, as opposed to one large protein meal, may elicit a potent anabolic response in older people with anabolic resistance and may promote muscle protein accretion and muscle hypertrophy [12]. It has been shown that protein supplementation combined with resistance training has resulted in muscle hypertrophy, increase in muscle strength, muscle mass and performance [13]. Diet quality alone was not associated with preservation of muscle strength but the combination of physical activity with good-quality diet maintained muscle strength, as reported in the NuAge study, which included older Australian men (aged 67–84 years) with diabetes [14].

Care Homes

Exercise in care homes is feasible despite the frail nature of residents. In a systematic review of 13 studies of progressive resistance training for nursing-home residents aged 80–89 years, significant improvements occurred in muscle strength and functional performance outcomes, including chair to stand time, stair climbing, gait speed, balance and functional capacity [15]. Aquatic exercise may be a useful exercise modality to help compliance and adherence and is also suitable for patients with arthritis. Other exercise modalities that may be suitable for people with reduced mobility, such as whole-body electromyostimulation, vibration, yoga and tai chi, may have some benefits and can be considered as an alternative for these patients. The combination of nutrition with resistance exercise in very old (mean age 87.1 years, SD 0.6 years) care-home residents preserved muscle mass and improved physical function [16]. However, the imposition of carbohydrate restrictions on care-home residents is not warranted to avoid malnutrition and dehydration. A liberalised diet for diabetes management to improve nutritional status without affecting glycaemic control is suitable in this population.

Summary

Diabetes in old age is associated with increased visceral fat and reduced muscle mass, which increase insulin resistance. Lifestyle intervention that aim at achieving ideal body weight and maintaining muscle mass may result in reduced insulin resistance, better glycaemic control and improved overall function. Adequate nutrition with good protein supplement combined with exercise training will have a synergistic effect on reducing muscle loss. Exercise is feasible for older people, even those living in care homes. The choice of exercise modality or nutrition is decided according to the patients' prevalent comorbidities and their choices. Appropriately tailored lifestyle educational programmes are the cornerstone in diabetes care in old age and should take into consideration individual preferences, cultural and ethnic backgrounds.

Clinical Practice Question

Q1. A 73-year-old woman known to have type 2 diabetes mellitus is on insulin glargine 30 units once daily and metformin 1 g twice a day. Past medical history includes ischaemic heart disease and hypertension. Her haemoglobin A1c is 63 mmol/mol and total cholesterol is 6.3 mmol/l. Her BMI is 37 kg/m^2 and she recently visited the emergency department due to a fall and was found to have a weak handgrip and difficulty rising from chair. What is the most appropriate lifestyle intervention for this patient:
Choose one option.

A. She should start a low-calorie diet to achieve weight loss.
B. She should start walking at least 150 minutes per week.
C. She should reduce her saturated fat intake.
D. In addition to an adequate diet, she should join a walking and weightlifting exercise programme.
E. She should increase her protein intake to increase her muscle mass.

References

Key references only are listed here. For a full list of references visit: `https://www.wiley.com/go/sinclair/1e`.

1. Amati, F., Dubé, J.J., Coen, P.M. et al. (2009). Physical inactivity and obesity underlie the insulin resistance of aging. *Diabetes Care* 32: 1547–1549.
2. Villareal, D.T., Apovian, C.M., and Kushner, R.F. (2005). Obesity in older adults: technical review and position statement of the American Society for Nutrition and NAASO, the Obesity Society. *Am. J. Clin. Nutr.* 82: 923–934.
3. Knowler, W.C., Barrett-Connor, E., Fowler, S.E. et al. (2002). Reduction in the incidence of type 2 diabetes with lifestyle intervention or metformin. *N. Engl. J. Med.* 346: 393–403.
4. Wing, R.R. (2010). Long-term effects of a lifestyle intervention on weight and cardiovascular risk factors in individuals with type 2 diabetes mellitus: four-year results of the look AHEAD trial. *Arch. Intern. Med.* 170: 1566–1575.
5. Bauer, J., Biolo, G., Cederholm, T. et al. (2013). Evidence-based recommendations for optimal dietary protein intake in older people: a position paper from the PROT-AGE study group. *J Am. Med. Dir. Assoc.* 14: 542–559.
6. Larsen, R.N., Mann, N.J., Maclean, E. et al. (2011). The effect of high-protein, low carbohydrate diets in the treatment of type 2 diabetes: a 12 month randomised controlled trial. *Diabetologia* 54: 731–740.
7. Yang, Y., Breen, L., Burd, N.A. et al. (2012). Resistance exercise enhances myofibrillar protein synthesis with graded intakes of whey protein in older men. *Br. J. Nutr.* 108: 1780–1788.
8. Fujita, S., Dreyer, H.C., Drummond, M.J. et al. (2007). Nutrient signalling in the regulation of human muscle protein synthesis. *J. Physiol.* 582: 813–823.
9. Smith, G.I., Atherton, P., Reeds, D.N. et al. (2011). Dietary omega-3 fatty acid supplementation increases the rate of muscle protein synthesis in older adults: a randomized controlled trial. *Am. J. Clin. Nutr.* 93: 402–412.
10. Brooks, N., Layne, J.E., Gordon, P.L. et al. (2007). Strength training improves muscle quality and insulin sensitivity in Hispanic older adults with type 2 diabetes. *Int. J. Med. Sci.* 4: 19–27.

4 Oral Hypoglycaemic Therapy

Nahian Kazi and Ahmed H. Abdelhafiz

Department of Geriatric Medicine, Rotherham General Hospital, Rotherham, UK

Key Points

- The aims of oral hypoglycaemic therapy are to control hyperglycaemia and reduce diabetes-related complications without inducing hypoglycaemia.
- Low hypoglycaemia-risk agents with positive impact on cardiovascular outcomes are preferred first choices in older people with diabetes.
- Because of their unfavourable metabolic profile, frail individuals who are the sarcopenic and obese stand to benefit most from sodium glucose transporter-2 inhibitor and glucagon like peptide-1 receptor agonist therapies.
- Insulin secretagogues are better avoided in older people with diabetes because of their high risk of hypoglycaemia.
- Novel agents with positive effects on outcomes relevant to older people with diabetes, such as frailty and cognitive function, are still required.

Introduction

The prevalence of diabetes is increasing in older people due to increased life expectancy. Type 2 diabetes mellitus (T2DM) may present asymptomatically; the diagnosis can be made during routine blood testing. T2DM can be treated with non-pharmacological intervention

Care of Older People with Diabetes: A Manual for Healthcare Practice, First Edition.
Edited by Alan J. Sinclair and Ahmed H. Abdelhafiz.

Companion website: www.wiley.com/go/sinclair/1e

of diet and lifestyle alone for a number of years. However, most older people with T2DM will require pharmacological therapy with oral hypoglycaemic agents at some stage in their disease. There are currently available several classes of oral hypoglycaemic therapy with different modes of action, tolerability and adverse effects. This requirement is most relevant in older people, as they tend to have multiple morbidities and organ dysfunctions, which may increase the risk of drug interactions and adverse effects, which may affect their compliance with medications. This chapter reviews different classes of oral hypoglycaemic therapy and their suitability in older people with diabetes and considers their efficacy and safety.

Hypoglycaemic Agents

Traditionally, oral hypoglycaemic therapy aims to reduce blood glucose levels, so the main adverse effect is hypoglycaemia. However, new hypoglycaemic agents with a lower risk of hypoglycaemia have been developed. The currently available hypoglycaemic medications can be divided into low-hypoglycaemia-risk and high hypoglycaemia-risk agents (Table 4.1).

Low Hypoglycaemia-Risk Agents

Metformin

Metformin works by reducing hepatic gluconeogenesis and increasing insulin-mediated uptake of glucose in muscles, so it is an insulin sensitiser with a low risk of hypoglycaemia. The main adverse effects of metformin are gastrointestinal, such as nausea, vomiting, flatulence and diarrhoea. Lactic acidosis is a recognised and serious, but rare, complication of metformin. Lactic acidosis is usually precipitated by conditions that cause dehydration, hypoxia, sepsis and hypotension. Metformin therapy should be temporarily withheld in these conditions. Metformin is weight neutral, but it may promote some weight loss, probably through its anorectic effect. In addition to glucose lowering, metformin has other prognostic benefits such as reducing cardiovascular events and mortality in older people with diabetes and chonic comorbidities [1]. The cardiovascular protection of metformin is independent of glycaemic control and could be related to its favourable

Table 4.1: Advantages and disadvantages of oral hypoglycaemic therapy in older people with diabetes.

Agent	Advantages	Disadvantages
Low hypoglycaemia-risk		
Metformin	Low risk of hypoglycaemia, CV protection, weight neutral; pleiotropic properties	GI adverse effects; lactic acidosis in patients with sepsis; organ dysfunction or dehydration; may cause vitamin B_{12} deficiency
Dipeptidyl peptidase-4 inhibitors	Low risk of hypoglycaemia, neutral CV effects, weight neutral, well tolerated	GI adverse effects; some agents need dose adjustment in CKD; other agents may increase hospitalisation due to heart failure; rare cause of pancreatitis
Sodium glucose transporter-2 inhibitors	Cardiorenal protection, weight loss, low risk of hypoglycaemia	Risk of UTI, dehydration, hypotension and candidiasis; may be associated risk of fractures and DKA; not suitable in anorexic malnourished frail individuals
Glucagon like peptide-1 receptor agonists	Cardiorenal protection, weight loss, low risk of hypoglycaemia	Injectable route, GI adverse effects; rare cause of pancreatitis; may be associated with thyroid C-cell tumours; not suitable in anorexic malnourished frail individuals
Thiazolidinediones	Cardiac protection, low risk of hypoglycaemia, suitable in patients with CKD	Increased fluid retention; exacerbation of heart failure; possible increased risk of fracture and bladder cancer
Alpha-glucosidase inhibitors	May have some CV benefits, low risk of hypoglycaemia	GI adverse effects; less tolerated; weak hypoglycaemic effect
High hypoglycaemia-risk		
Sulfonylureas	Neutral CV effect, suitable in patients with CKD	Weight gain; high risk of hypoglycaemia; may need blood glucose monitoring; some may increase mortality
Meglitinides	Neutral CV effect, suitable in patients with CKD	Weight gain; high risk of hypoglycaemia; may need blood glucose monitoring

CKD, chronic kidney disease; CV, cardiovascular; DKA, diabetic ketoacidosis; GI, gastrointestinal; UTI, urinary tract infection.

effects on cardiometabolic profile, such as lipids, body weight, blood pressure, fibrinolysis and platelet aggregation [2]. Metformin may also delay physical and mental health decline by reducing the risk of frailty, dementia and depression [3, 4]. However, metformin may induce vitamin B_{12} deficiency and the addition of vitamin B_{12} supplements to metformin therapy may have a cognitive protective effect [5].

Dipeptidyl Peptidase-4 Inhibitors

These agents inhibit the enzyme dipeptidyl peptidase-4 (DPP-4), decreasing glucagon release and increasing glucose-dependent insulin release. They also decrease gastric emptying and increase satiety. DPP-4 inhibitors have low risk of hypoglycaemia, are weight neutral and well tolerated, although they lack the cardiovascular benefits of metformin [6]. DPP-4 inhibitors do not increase the risk of composite end points of cardiovascular death, non-fatal myocardial infarction and non-fatal stroke, but the risk of hospitalisation due to congestive heart failure is inconsistent. A meta-analysis of DPP-4 inhibitors trials has shown overall cardiovascular safety but non-significant increases in heart failure, especially with saxagliptin [7]. Because of the controversy over the risk of hospitalisation from heart failure observed with some DPP-4 inhibitors apart from linagliptin and sitagliptin, caution should be considered when using such agents in patients with heart failure. DPP-4 inhibitors may reduce the risk of all-cause dementia [8].

Sodium Glucose Transporter-2 Inhibitors

Sodium glucose transporter-2 (SGLT-2) inhibitors reduce renal glucose reabsorption leading to increased glucosuria, attenuation of hyperglycaemia and reduction in body weight. This diuretic and natriuretic effect reduces plasma volume and cardiac preload, which lowers blood pressure leading to cardiac benefits. In addition, their effects on salt and water homeostasis and reduction of renin–angiotensin–aldosterone system and sympathetic activation reduce renal glomerular hyperfiltration, which is the initial step in the pathogenesis of diabetic kidney disease leading to renal benefits. In the age-stratified meta-analysis of the SGLT-2 inhibitors clinical trials, the hazard ratios for major adverse cardiovascular events were 0.95 (95% confidence interval, CI, 0.86–1.05) in people <65 years old and 0.83

(95% CI 0.71–0.96) for people ≥ 65 years, with no subgroup differences ($P = 0.15$), suggesting that the effect was consistent across all age groups [9]. Although, SGLT-2 inhibitors, owing to their weight-loss properties, may reduce skeletal muscle mass and increase the risk of sarcopenia and frailty, it has been reported that they improve muscle quality, which may have an overall positive effect [10].

Glucagon-like Peptide-1 Receptor Agonists

The gut-derived hormone glucagon-like peptide-1 (GLP-1) maintains blood glucose levels by stimulating postprandial insulin secretion but is rapidly degraded, so its glucose-lowering effect is short lived. GLP-1 receptor agonist (GLP-1RA) is resistant to degradation and have a prolonged glucose lowering effect. The GLP-1RA also have extra-glycaemic beneficial effects reducing blood pressure, low-grade inflammation, visceral fat and body weight, which improve insulin sensitivity [11]. These agents have demonstrated a consistent and significant cardiorenal protective effect and the associated risk of hypoglycaemia is comparable to that of placebo [12]. GLP-1RA may have the potential to improve neurodegenerative conditions, such as Alzheimer's and Parkinson's diseases, as well as bone density in older people with diabetes. These agents also improve liver function and reduce liver fat content in patients with metabolic dysfunction-associated fatty liver disease, thus improving metabolic profile and cardiovascular risk. Precautions for the use of SGLT-2 inhibitors and GLP-1RA in older people with diabetes are summarised in Box 4.1.

Thiazolidinediones

The thiazolidinediones (TZD) activate the nuclear peroxisome proliferator-activated receptor gamma, which increases insulin sensitivity and enhances peripheral glucose uptake. The TZDs are associated with low risk of hypoglycaemia but increased weight gain, probably related to fluid retention. The TZD pioglitazone reduces the risk of major cardiovascular events but is associated with increased risk of heart failure and peripheral oedema. TZDs, through their insulin sensitising properties, may have beneficial effects on reducing the loss of lean muscle mass but may be associated with bone loss and an increased risk of fractures [13].

Box 4.1: Precautions with the Use of SGLT-2 Inhibitors and GLP-1RA in Older People with Diabetes

- Monitor renal function.
- Predisposing factors for acute kidney injury, such as concomitant initiation of loop diuretics or non-steroidal anti-inflammatory drugs, must be avoided or closely monitored.
- Antihypertensive medications may need to be reduced or stopped.
- Monitor for genitourinary infections, especially in female patients with poorly controlled diabetes.
- Due to increased gastrointestinal adverse effects with GLP-1RA, lowering the dose, use of a longer-acting preparation or avoiding of other diarrhoea or nausea-promoting medications may help to reduce the incidence of these adverse events.
- Temporary withhold SGLT-2 inhibitors if patients are unwell, fasting, suffer acute severe illness, dehydration due to, for example, diarrhoea and/or vomiting or requiring a major surgery.
- Owing to increased weight loss with these agents, resistance exercise training should be offered to avoid the loss of muscle mass.

Alpha-glucosidase Inhibitors

Alpha-glucosidase inhibitors work by competitively inhibiting the alpha-glucosidase enzymes in the intestinal brush border cells, thus inhibiting carbohydrate reabsorption and the breakdown of sucrose into glucose and fructose. They have a low risk of hypoglycaemia but are associated with increased gastrointestinal adverse effects such as flatulence, diarrhoea and abdominal pain. The alpha-glucosidase inhibitor acarabose is associated with a low risk of hypoglycaemia and weight loss, and many have some cardiovascular benefits.

High Hypoglycaemia Risk Agents

Sulfonylureas

Sulfonylureas bind to adenosine triphosphate-sensitive potassium (K-ATP) channels in the beta cells of the pancreas, leading to influx of calcium and the stimulation of insulin secretion. Because they are insulin secretagogues, the main adverse effects are weight gain and increased risk of hypoglycaemia. Sulfonylureas such as gliclazide appeared to have neutral effects on cardiovascular events, although other sulfonylureas, such as glimepiride, glibenclamide, glipizide and tolbutamide, were associated with increased all-cause mortality [14].

Meglitinides

Meglitinides, similar to sulfonylureas, exert their effects by regulating K-ATP channels in the pancreatic beta cells, causing an increase in insulin secretion. Their adverse effects include weight gain and increased risk of hypoglycaemia. Meglitinides appear to have neutral effects on cardiovascular outcomes, although few data are available.

Therapeutic Approach

The main aim of oral hypoglycaemic therapy is to control hyperglycaemia and reduce diabetes-related complications, especially cardiovascular complications, and to avoid hypoglycaemia. Therefore, the initiation of oral hypoglycaemic therapy should start with agents that either have cardioprotective properties or at least do not have cardiovascular adverse effects and have a low risk of hypoglycaemia. Metformin remains the first line therapy in older people with diabetes due to its various pleiotropic properties including anti-frailty and anti-ageing effects, as well as its low risk of hypoglycaemia. The new therapy of SGLT-2 inhibitors and the GLP-1RA should be considered early on, because of their cardiorenal protection especially in patients with high cardiovascular risk. Older people who are sarcopenic, obese and frail with diabetes are likely to benefit most from such therapy because of their unfavourable metabolic profile. The cardioprotective properties of these agents appear early on therapy and independent of tight glycaemic control, which make it advantageous in frail older people who have multimorbidities and at risk of hypoglycaemia. DPP-4 inhibitors are adjuvant therapy and although they have no clear cardiovascular protection they are well tolerated. Pioglitazone is another add on therapy with cardiovascular protection but should be avoided in patients with congestive cardiac failure at risk of decompensation. Alpha-glucosidase inhibitors are less tolerated due to their gastrointestinal adverse effects. Sulfonylureas and meglitinides are better avoided in older people due to

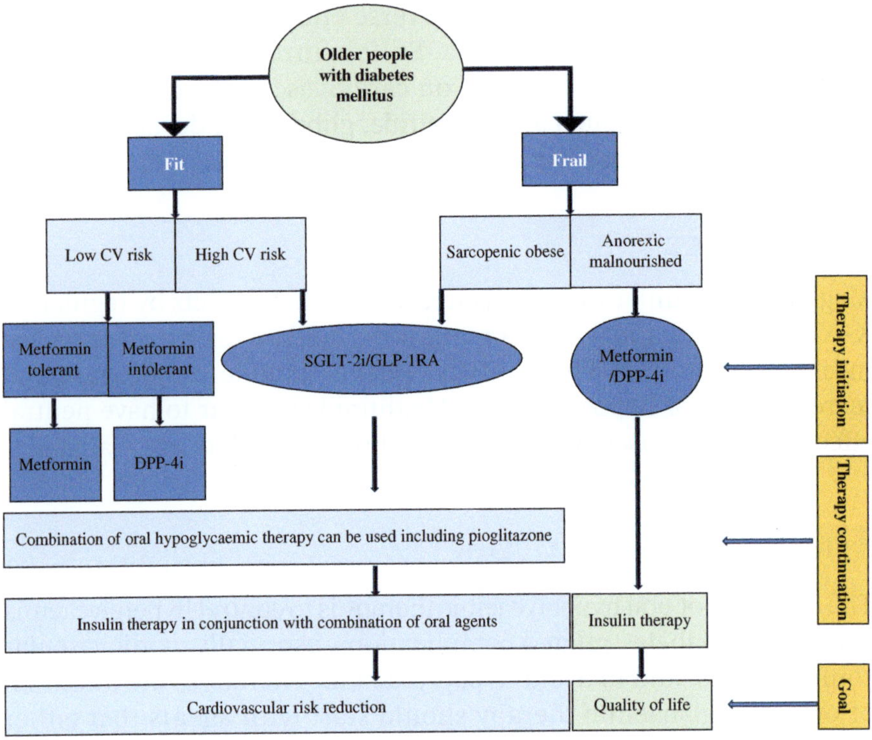

Figure 4.1: Suggested therapeutic approach of oral hypoglycaemic agents in older people with diabetes mellitus. Agents with low hypoglycaemia-risk and cardiovascular (CV) benefits are the preferred first choice for people with high cardiovascular risk followed by other agents. Insulin can be considered earlier in malnourished frail individuals. DPP-4i, dipeptidyl peptidase-4 inhibitor; GLP-1RA, glucagon-like peptide-1 receptor analyst; SGLT-2i, sodium glucose transporter-2 inhibitor.

their high risk of hypoglycaemia. A suggested therapeutic approach of oral hypoglycaemic therapy in older people with diabetes is illustrated in Figure 4.1.

Summary

Oral hypoglycaemic therapy aims to control hyperglycaemia and reduce diabetes-related complications without inducing hypoglycaemia. Therefore, in older people with diabetes, low hypoglycaemia-risk agents with positive impact on cardiovascular outcomes are the preferred first-line choices. Individuals who are sarcopenic, obese and frail stand to benefit most from the new therapies of SGLT-2 inhibitors and GLP-1RA due to the unfavourable metabolic profile of these therapies. Insulin secretagogues are better avoided in older people with diabetes because of the high risk of hypoglycaemia with tese drugs.

Future Perspectives

The effects of most oral hypoglycaemic agents, apart from metformin, on outcomes relevant to older people with diabetes, such as frailty and cognitive function, are still not clear. The current evidence is inconclusive and needs future studies. In addition, the outcomes of frailty or cognitive function are not commonly addressed in the current clinical trials, which normally focus on glycaemic control and cardiovascular or renal outcomes. Frailty is linked to cardiovascular and renal diseases. Therefore, the cardiorenal protective effects of SGLT-2 inhibitors and GLP-1RA and their positive impact on frailty should be explored. Similarly, repeated episodes of hypoglycaemia are associated with the development of cognitive impairment and whether these new therapies with low risk of hypoglycaemia will have a positive impact on cognitive function also needs to be investigated.

Clinical Practice Question

Q1. A 76-year-old woman with type 2 diabetes mellitus for 11 years, who is on metformin 1 g twice a day. She has a past medical history of hypertension, heart failure and hypercholesteraemia, and she is an ex-smoker. She usually mobilises with a stick for short distances and her body mass index is 36 kg/m^2. Her last haemoglobin A1c level was 53 mmol/mol. What is the next course of action? Choose the options that apply.

- **A.** Continue current therapy of metformin, which gives her good glycaemic control.
- **B.** Continue metformin and add an SGLT-2 inhibitor.
- **C.** Continue metformin and add DPP-4 inhibitors for their safety.
- **D.** Refer her for a diet and weight reduction programme.
- **E.** Recommend resistance exercise training.

References

Key references only are listed here. For a full list of references visit: https://www.wiley.com/go/sinclair/1e.

1. Crowley, M.J., Diamantidis, C.J., McDuffie, J.R. et al. (2017). Clinical outcomes of metformin use in populations with chronic kidney disease, congestive heart failure, or chronic liver disease: a systematic review. *Ann. Intern. Med.* 166: 191–200.
2. Grant, P.J. (2003). Beneficial effects of metformin on haemostasis and vascular function in man. *Diabetes Metab.* 29 (4 Pt 2): 6S44–6S52.
3. Wang, C.P., Lorenzo, C., and Espinoza, S.E. (2014). Frailty attenuates the impact of metformin on reducing mortality in older adults with type 2 diabetes. *J Endocrinol. Diabetes Obes.* 2: 1031.
4. Wang, C.P., Lorenzo, C., Habib, S.L. et al. (2017). Differential effects of metformin on age related comorbidities in older men with type 2 diabetes. *J. Diabetes Complications* 31: 679–686.
5. Moore, E.M., Mander, A.G., Ames, D. et al. (2013). AIBL investigators. Increased risk of cognitive impairment in patients with diabetes is associated with metformin. *Diabetes Care* 36: 2981–2987.
6. Lozano-Ortega, G., Goring, S., Bennett, H.A. et al. (2016). Network meta-analysis of treatments for type 2 diabetes mellitus following failure with metformin plus sulfonylurea. *Curr. Med. Res. Opin.* 32: 807–816.
7. Secrest, M.H., Udell, J.A., and Filion, K.B. (2017). The cardiovascular safety trials of DPP-4 inhibitors, GLP-1 agonists, and SGLT2 inhibitors. *Trends Cardiovasc. Med.* 27: 194–202.
8. Kim, Y.G., Jeon, J.Y., Kim, H.J. et al. (2019). Risk of dementia in older patients with type 2 diabetes on dipeptidyl-peptidase IV inhibitors versus sulfonylureas: a real-world population-based cohort study. *J. Clin. Med.* 8: 28.
9. Giugliano, D., Longo, M., Ida Maiorino, M. et al. (2020). Efficacy of SGLT-2 inhibitors in older adults with diabetes: systematic review with meta-analysis of cardiovascular outcome trials. *Diabetes Res. Clin. Pract.* 162: 108114.
10. Sano, M., Meguro, S., Kawai, T., and Suzuki, Y. (2016). Increased grip strength with sodium-glucose cotransporter 2. *J. Diabetes* 8: 736–737.

5 Insulin Therapy

Giuseppe Maltese[1,2]

[1] School of Cardiovascular Medicine and Sciences, King's College London, London, UK
[2] Department of Diabetes and Endocrinology, Epsom and St Helier University Hospitals, Surrey, UK

Key Points

- Insulin is a life-maintaining treatment in people with type 1 diabetes, even in old age.
- Insulin may be required in older people with type 2 diabetes, when oral therapy is not sufficient to meet personalised glycaemic targets.
- A long-acting analogue once daily in combination with oral agents often guarantees a satisfactory glycaemic control in most older people with type 2 diabetes and is associated with a low risk of hypoglycaemia.
- A basal bolus regimen is usually essential in older people with type 1 diabetes and in some individuals with type 2 diabetes; however, alternative regimens can be considered.
- The insulin regimen should be chosen based on patient's preferences, health status and comorbidities, cognitive capacities, hypoglycaemia risk, living situation, presence and severity of frailty and life expectancy.

Introduction

Insulin therapy is a life-maintaining treatment in people with type 1 diabetes (T1DM) and may be needed in type 2 diabetes (T2DM) as well, at onset or several years after the diagnosis, when oral antidiabetic

Care of Older People with Diabetes: A Manual for Healthcare Practice, First Edition.
Edited by Alan J. Sinclair and Ahmed H. Abdelhafiz.

Companion website: www.wiley.com/go/sinclair/1e

agents fail to ensure satisfactory glucose levels. Because of progressive beta cell function decline, a large number of older individuals with T2DM may require insulin at some point in life.

Insulin is the most effective glucose-lowering treatment and should not be regarded as the last resort, even though it is associated with the burden of frequent injections, finger-prick glucose testing and increased risk of hypoglycaemia.

The use of basal insulin in combination with non-insulin glucose-lowering agents is an effective option and is well tolerated in the older population [1]. Continuing some antidiabetic agents, such as metformin, and/or one of the gliptins and/or a sodium glucose transporter-2 inhibitor, has several advantages: reduced insulin requirement, improved insulin resistance and attenuated weight gain [1]. Insulin can also improve muscle mass and function independent of glycaemic control.

Basal Insulin Analogues

For decades, the intermediate human insulin neutral protamine Hagedorn (NPH), also called isophane, was the main basal insulin. However, NPH has relevant pharmacological limitations, including variable onset and absorption, a limited duration of action (14–16 hours) and a peak of action within a few hours of administration, which can potentially lead to hypoglycaemia, particularly overnight if the insulin is used in the evening [1]. For this reason, since 1996, basal insulin analogues have been progressively preferred to NPH.

Basal insulin analogues are characterised by more stable action profiles, slower and more prolonged absorption rates and constant pharmacokinetic/pharmacodynamic. All these characteristics ensure steady glucose levels over a period of 24 hours or more and reduce the potential risk of hypoglycaemia, when compared with NPH insulin [1].

A basal insulin analogue is usually the first choice for insulin therapy in older adults because of its efficacy and the once-daily dosing; it can also be prescribed as a single treatment or as an add-on [1]. See Table 5.1 for a description of all insulins discussed.

Four basal insulin analogues have been approved for the management of diabetes: glargine U-100 (Gla-100), detemir, and the second-generation (ultra-long-acting) insulins degludec and glargine U-300 (Gla-300).

Table 5.1: Type of rapid acting and long-acting insulin for use in older people with diabetes.

Insulin type	Onset	Peak time	Duration	Dose timing
Rapid acting (aspart, lispro, glulisine)	15 minutes	1 hour	2–4 hours	Usually taken 15–20 minutes before a meal, but in frail older people with variable appetite it can be administered soon after
Regular acting (Actrapid®, Novo Nordisk)	30 minutes	2–3 hours	3–6 hours	30 minutes before a meal
Intermediate acting (neutral protamine Hagedorn insulin–isophane)	2–4 hours	4–12 hours	12–18 hours	Can be given in the morning or at night
Long-acting analogues (glargine U-100, detemir)	2 hours	No peak	Up to 24 hours	Can be given in the morning or at night
Ultra-long-acting (degludec, glargine U-300)	6 hours	No peak	36 hours or longer	Can be given in the morning or at night
Premixed (30/70, 25/75)	5–60 minutes	Peak varies	10–16 hours	Administered before breakfast and dinner

The efficacy and safety of Gla-100 has been demonstrated in numerous trials involving even older people. In older patients, when compared with NPH, Gla-100 is superior in terms of glycaemic control and hypoglycaemia frequency [2].

Detemir and Gla-100 have similar glucose-lowering efficacy and comparable incidence of hypoglycaemia. Detemir typically necessitates a twice-daily dosing regimen to achieve therapeutic goals, which can be inconvenient for older people.

Insulin degludec is an ultra-long-acting basal insulin with a half-life of >25 hours and a duration of action of >42 hours [3]. In comparison with other insulins, degludec is characterised by a reduced intra- and interindividual variability and can ensure a more stable glucose-lowering action and improved pharmacodynamic and pharmacokinetic activity, translating into reduced risk of hypoglycaemia across different age groups, including older people [4].

When compared with Gla-100, degludec has a lower pharmacodynamic variability and a more predictable glucose-lowering effect. Degludec is comparable to Gla-100 in terms of cardiovascular safety [4].

In a meta-analysis of data from patients aged 65 and above, the use of degludec was associated with a 24% lower estimated rate of hypoglycaemia and 36% lower risk of nocturnal hypoglycaemia when compared with Gla-100 [5].

The long duration of action of degludec provides dosing time flexibility, especially for those older people who have their insulin administered by a caregiver or district nurses. Gla-300, the other ultra-long-acting analogue, has a more stable and prolonged duration of action than Gla-100 and can last up to 36 hours [6]. Findings from clinical trials have shown that Gla-100 and Gla-300 provide similar haemoglobin A1c reduction in younger and older adults. However, in older people, Gla-300 is associated with a lower risk of daytime and nocturnal hypoglycaemia and less weight gain [6].

The superiority of Gla-300 over Gla-100 in terms of hypoglycaemia risk reduction has been demonstrated in other studies. The risk of nocturnal hypoglycaemia is lower when the insulin is given before breakfast [6].

In clinical trials, the ultra-long-acting insulin degludec and Gla-300 have been shown to ensure similar glycaemic control, with lower rates of hypoglycaemia when compared with the first generations insulin [3, 7].

Rapid-acting Analogues

Rapid-acting analogues (lispro, aspart, glulisine) or regular insulin (Actrapid®, Novo Nordisk, Gatwick, UK) are used to counteract the postprandial rise in glucose levels. Rapid-acting analogues are more expensive than regular insulin but have some advantages. Fast-acting analogues are preferred to human regular insulin as they have a short duration of action and are therefore associated with a lower risk of hypoglycaemia and can be administered immediately after a meal. In contrast, regular insulin should be given at least 30 minutes before meals. Rapid-acting insulin is usually used before or with meals and snacks; however, if appetite and oral intake are variable or the mealtime is not predictable, a bolus can be given after food and a dose reduction can be considered if the person does not finish their meal.

There are also two ultra-rapid acting analogues: aspart with the addition of niacinamide and l-arginine, and lispro, containing treprostinil and citrate. Both are characterised by faster absorption compared to traditional rapid-acting insulin analogues.

Treatment Regimens

In individuals using oral antidiabetic agents, adding a basal insulin is an effective strategy to achieve the desired glycaemic targets. The addition of glargine to non-insulin glucose-lowering agents results in improved control and a reduced frequency of hypoglycaemia when compared with up-titration of the oral agents [8]. The basal insulin is commonly given in the morning, as postprandial glucose levels contribute more than fasting glucose levels to hyperglycaemia in older people. The basal insulin can be titrated against fasting glucose levels and is associated with a lower risk of early morning hypoglycaemia.

The basal bolus therapy is certainly the best treatment option, even for older people with T2DM when appropriate, but it may not be easily accepted or feasible in frail individuals, due to the living setting and the high level of dependence. The use of boluses permits matching of the insulin dose to the meal carbohydrate content and can more precisely counteract the postprandial rise in glucose levels and reduce the risk of hypoglycaemia. Nonetheless, there are downsides, including the higher number of insulin injections and the need for more frequent glucose testing.

In older people with T1DM the basal bolus regimen remains the gold standard treatment. Older people with autoimmune diabetes with onset in adult age (latent autoimmune diabetes of adults) frequently require basal-bolus therapy at the time of diagnosis. These individuals can be started on a total daily dose of 0.2–0.5 units/kg, with 50% of this total given as basal insulin and the remaining 50% given as rapid acting insulin before meals [8].

Insulin therapy is needed in older people with T1DM to avoid hyperglycaemia and diabetic ketoacidosis. Insulin treatment strategies should be personalised based on health status, presence and severity of frailty and life expectancy.

For older people with T1DM and a good health status, a basal bolus regimen with twice daily detemir or once daily ultra-long-acting analogue, is the gold standard.

Adults with T1DM use an insulin to carbohydrate ratio to calculate the dose of rapid acting insulin for their meals. The insulin to carbohydrate ratio is estimated dividing 500 by the total daily dose [9]. A correction dose estimated using a correction factor is added, if premeal glucose levels are above the recommended targets. The correction factor is calculated dividing 100 by the total daily dose.

This mathematical approach for the estimation of the premeal insulin dose may be complex for older people, particularly if they are affected by any degree of cognitive impairment and may require the involvement of a caregiver.

Over the years people living with diabetes may lose their numeracy skills and/or dexterity due to concomitant morbidities and might not be able to manage a basal bolus regimen. If a person with T1DM loses their self-care capabilities due to cognitive impairment or altered dexterity, the insulin is usually administered either by a relative or by nursing staff if a care home is the living setting.

For frail older people, regardless of the living setting, degludec or Gla-300 is the first choice, and a rapid-acting analogue is given according to needs.

For individuals with moderate frailty who rely on a district nurse for the insulin administration, degludec or Gla-300 can be used in combination with a rapid-acting analogue at breakfast and dinner or at breakfast only. The choice depends very much on diet and oral intake, so a standard treatment cannot be recommended.

Simplified regimens (e.g. twice-daily NPH insulin or premixed 30/70 or 25/75 insulin before breakfast and dinner) are not recommended unless the patient is unwilling to have multiple injections or relies on a district nurse for administration of insulin. With a premixed insulin, snacks-between main meals and nocturnal glucose testing are often needed to reduce the hypoglycaemia risk.

Summary

Insulin therapy is essential in older people with T1DM and may be required for some individuals with T2DM. In both T1DM and T2DM in old age, the type of insulin and insulin regimen should be chosen according to patient's preferences, health status and comorbidities, cognitive capacities, hypoglycaemia risk, living situation, presence and severity of frailty and life expectancy.

Clinical Practice Question

Q1. An 86-year-old man is known to have a longstanding history of type 2 diabetes and other comorbidities, including heart failure and chronic disease stage 4. He has lost his self-care skills and his Clinical Frailty Scale score is 7. His diabetes is managed with a twice-daily premixed insulin 30/70 which is given at a dose of 24 units before breakfast and 18 units before dinner. The insulin is administered by district nurses. His latest haemoglobin A1c was 72 mmol/mol. His fasting and pre-dinner glucose levels have ranged between 8 and 12 mmol/l but lately he has experienced episodes of hypoglycaemia around mid-morning and early in the afternoon due to reducing appetite. One of these episodes of hypoglycaemia required paramedic assistance. Which treatment change would you consider in his case?
Choose one option.

A. Discontinue the premixed insulin and start metformin.
B. Replace the current insulin with gliclazide before breakfast and dinner.
C. Prescribe an ultra-long-acting analogue in place the premixed insulin.
D. Reduce the premixed insulin dose.

References

1. Cersosimo, E., Lee, P.G., and Pandya, N. (2019). Challenges of diabetes care in older people with type 2 diabetes and the role of basal insulin. *Clin. Diabetes* 37 (4): 357–367.
2. Lee, P., Chang, A., Blaum, C. et al. (2012). Comparison of safety and efficacy of insulin glargine and neutral protamine Hagedorn insulin in older

adults with type 2 diabetes mellitus: results from a pooled analysis. *J. Am. Geriatr. Soc.* 60 (1): 51–59.
3. Vora, J., Cariou, B., Evans, M. et al. (2015). Clinical use of insulin degludec. *Diabetes Res. Clin. Pract.* 109 (1): 19–31.
4. Haahr, H. and Heise, T. (2014). A review of the pharmacological properties of insulin degludec and their clinical relevance. *Clin. Pharmacokinet.* 53 (9): 787–800.
5. Sorli, C., Warren, M., Oyer, D. et al. (2013). Elderly patients with diabetes experience a lower rate of nocturnal hypoglycaemia with insulin degludec than with insulin glargine: a meta-analysis of phase IIIa trials. *Drugs Aging* 30 (12): 1009–1018.
6. Becker, R.H., Dahmen, R., Bergmann, K. et al. (2015). New insulin glargine 300 units ml^{-1} provides a more even activity profile and prolonged glycemic control at steady state compared with insulin glargine 100 units mL^{-1}. *Diabetes Care* 38 (4): 637–643.
7. Lau, I.T., Lee, K.F., So, W.Y. et al. (2017). Insulin glargine 300 U/mL for basal insulin therapy in type 1 and type 2 diabetes mellitus. *Diabetes Metab. Syndr. Obes.* 10: 273–284.
8. ElSayed, N.A., Aleppo, G., Aroda, V.R. et al. (2023). 13. Older adults: standards of care in diabetes 2023. *Diabetes Care* 46 (Suppl 1): S216–S229.
9. King, A.B. and Armstrong, D.U. (2007). A prospective evaluation of insulin dosing recommendations in patients with type 1 diabetes at near normal glucose control: bolus dosing. *J. Diabetes Sci. Technol.* 1 (1): 42–46.

6 Use of Continuous Glucose Monitoring in Older People with Diabetes

Giuseppe Maltese[1,2]

[1] School of Cardiovascular Medicine & Sciences, King's College London, London, UK
[2] Department of Diabetes and Endocrinology, Epsom and St Helier University Hospitals, Surrey, UK

Key Points

- Finger-prick glucose testing is associated with a considerable burden and provides a static view of the glucose control, which may not unveil excursions and asymptomatic hypoglycaemia.
- Older people with type 1 diabetes and those with type 2 diabetes on sulfonylurea or insulin are at risk of hypoglycaemia, often requiring third-party assistance (severe hypoglycaemia).
- Hypoglycaemia in older people can have short- and long-term disastrous consequences (falls and fractures, myocardial infarction, arrhythmias, progression of cognitive impairment, accident and emergency department attendances and hospitalisations).
- The use of continuous glucose monitoring is associated with a reduced diabetes-related burden and other benefits, including prevention and early detection of hypoglycaemia and lower rates of related negative outcomes.

Care of Older People with Diabetes: A Manual for Healthcare Practice, First Edition.
Edited by Alan J. Sinclair and Ahmed H. Abdelhafiz.

Companion website: www.wiley.com/go/sinclair/1e

Introduction

Self-monitoring blood glucose monitoring (SBGM) has represented a key element of diabetes self-management since 1950 and still guides insulin dose adjustments and confirms hypoglycaemia. However, finger-prick glucose testing provides only a static view of the glucose profile of a person with diabetes and may not unveil glucose excursions and episodes of asymptomatic hypoglycaemia.

Impairment of hypo-awareness and the occurrence and recurrence of symptomatic or asymptomatic hypoglycaemia have a considerable impact on quality of life and both diabetes, and non-diabetes-related health outcomes in older people [1]. In older people, hypoglycaemia can lead to disastrous consequences, including falls and fractures, myocardial infarction, arrhythmias, progression of cognitive impairment, accident and emergency department attendances and hospitalisations [1]. Furthermore, individuals experiencing frequent hypoglycaemia or fear of hypoglycaemia tend to avoid certain daily activities; this contributes to worsened anxiety and social isolation, which have a deleterious impact on health-related outcomes and quality of life [2].

Since the 2000s, the use of technology has become more common among young adults with type 1 diabetes mellitus (T1DM) and is progressively increasing in older people [3].

Continuous Glucose Monitoring

Continuous glucose monitoring (CGM), either flash or real time, reveal glucose levels and trends [2]. CGM systems measure the interstitial glucose levels every one to five minutes and have customisable alarms for high and low readings [2]. Some devices can also predict when glucose levels will reach a set threshold and provide the user with a warning. A reader or a mobile application displays the glucose readings [2].

The identification of glucose patterns is extremely valuable in older people, given the high prevalence of impaired or absent hypo-awareness and the high likelihood of unrecognised hypoglycaemic events, particularly during the night. Older individuals with high glucose variability are more likely to spend more time below range (< 3.9 and < 3.0 mmol/l), compared with those with limited glucose variability [2].

In older adults with T1DM and type 2 diabetes mellitus (T2DM) on multiple daily injections, the use of CGM can lead to a significant reduction in haemoglobin A1c (HbA1c) and glucose variability, and to a high patient satisfaction. More importantly, the use of CGM is associated with a lower incidence of severe hypoglycaemia, and the number of call outs and emergency department attendances [2]. CGM has also been shown to have a positive impact on general wellbeing and feelings of safety [2].

There is a paucity of research on CGM in older people with diabetes, but those very few milestone trials reported in the published literature have demonstrated remarkable benefits for this patient group (Table 6.1).

In a sub-analysis of the DIAMOND trial, 116 individuals aged above 60, with T1DM or T2DM managed with multiple daily injections were randomised to either SBGM or CGM [4]. After 24 weeks, people using CGM achieved a statistically significant reduction in HbA1c (estimated 0.4%), a reduction in glycaemic variability and time spent above range (TAR, > 13.9 mmol/l) and an improved time in range (TIR, 3.9–10.0 mmol/l) [4].

Another study in the field of diabetes technology in old age, the WISDM (Wireless Innovation for Seniors with Diabetes Mellitus) trial, randomised a larger number of individuals ($n = 203$) with T1DM aged over 60 years to either SBGM or CGM. At baseline, it was found that more than half of patients included in the trial spent at least 4% of time with glucose levels < 3.9 mmol/l and 37% of time with values > 10 mmol/l [5]. After six months, trial data revealed a 90% reduction in

Table 6.1: Continuous glucose monitoring in older people with diabetes.

Advantages	Disadvantages
Improved haemoglobin A1c	Maintenance (changing sensor)
Lower risk of hypoglycaemia	Need for dexterity, and preserved sight and hearing
Reduced burden related to finger prick testing	High cost
Availability of alarm/alerts	Feeling overwhelmed due to amount of CGM data
'Share' feature for remote monitoring of CGM data by relatives and carers	Errors in insulin dose estimation due to anxiety triggered by CGM data

CGM, continuous glucose monitoring.

the rate of severe hypoglycaemia. The authors also reported a reduction in time below range (< 3.9 and < 3.0 mmol/l) and a greater TIR [5]. Other smaller trials involving older individuals with T2DM have demonstrated a statistically significant reduction in HbA1c between 0.3% and 0.5% [6].

Most studies on CGM in older people have been conducted in T1DM but the evidence demonstrating the clinical benefits of CGM even for individuals with T2DM on insulin is progressively growing [2]. There is certainly need for well-designed clinical trials including individuals older then 70 years, with or without cognitive impairment and/or physical disability and looking at outcomes of interest to the older population.

Patient Assessment

Because of the heterogeneity of diabetes in older people related to clinical, psychological and functional characteristics, clinicians are expected to carry out a comprehensive assessment to establish whether a person can use a device and the best device for that person [3]. Some individuals are relatively healthy and independent, and live in their own homes; others may present various degrees of frailty and may require assistance from a carer or a relative or may live in a care home. Level of function and the living environment influence the feasibility of use of any technological device [3].

Older people with diabetes are often affected by comorbidities, namely geriatric syndromes, which might represent a barrier to technology use [2]. For instance, impaired dexterity and sight and cognitive impairment affecting numeracy skills and literacy, often preclude the use of CGM devices and insulin pumps [2].

Clinical practice guidelines from various diabetes societies stress the importance of carrying out periodic assessment of cognition and physical function in older individuals with diabetes, particularly in those ones who use technological devices [7].

CGM can be used via a smartphone and the specific application allows to benefit from the ‘share’ feature. Relatives of frail older people can review glucose levels remotely on compatible smartphones and provide instructions on actions to take. The ‘share’ feature allows the users to share their glucose data with up to five people.

When the ‘share’ feature is used, a carer or relative can be trained to upload CGM data to the platform and may be asked to assist healthcare professionals during a consultation with a remote review of the data. The latest American Diabetes Association clinical guidelines recommend HbA1c target < 53 mmol/mol for older adults who are relatively healthy with a preserved cognitive function and no or a few comorbidities [8]. More relaxed HbA1c targets are proposed for individuals with comorbidities and physical and/or cognitive impairment. For older people with severe frailty and limited life expectancy, the HbA1c target is set < 69 mmol/mol [8]. All three groups may benefit from the use of CGM, but the main indication is certainly the inability to sense episodes of hypoglycaemia.

The American Diabetes Association standards of care highlight that CGM should be considered to prevent hypoglycaemia particularly for those older people with cognitive and physical disabilities, who rely on a caregiver for glucose monitoring [8]. The American Association of Clinical Endocrinology guidelines recommend the use of CGM in older people to reduce HbA1c levels, improve quality of life and decrease the rate of hypoglycaemia [9].

With regard to CGM metrics, an international consensus recommends a TIR above 50% and time below range < 1% for older adults aged 65 years and older, regardless of comorbidities, health status and life expectancy (Table 6.2) [10]. Future research is needed to identify CGM metrics targets for older people with diabetes, tailored to health status and severe of frailty.

Some CGM devices can be integrated with insulin pumps, which deliver small doses of rapid-acting insulin (as small as 0.1 unit/hour) throughout the day. A bolus calculator estimates the insulin to be delivered prior to meals, based on preprogrammed or inserted insulin to carbohydrate ratio, sensitivity factor and glucose levels target. The

Table 6.2: International consensus on time in range.

Time	**In range**	**Below range**		**Above range**	
Range (mmol/l)	**3.9–10**	**3.0–3.9**	**<3.0**	**>10**	**>13.9**
Older adults/high risk with T1DM or T2DM (%)	>50	<1	~0	<50	<10
Young adults with T1DM or T2DM (%)	>70	<4	<1	<25	<5

T1DM, type 1 diabetes mellitus; T2DM, type 2 diabetes mellitus.
Source: Battelino et al. [19].

insulin is delivered through a tube connected to the pump containing the reservoir and a cannula inserted into the skin. The infusion set is to be changed every three days. Pump data can be downloaded and reviewed by the diabetes team responsible for the patient's care. There is a body of evidence showing that the benefits of insulin pumps in young and older people are very similar [11]. Connecting GCM to an insulin pump enables the use of sensor-augmented pumps or hybrid closed loops that suspend the insulin delivery whenever hypoglycaemia occurs or is predicted.

Challenges

The use of CGM in older people is not only associated with benefits but also presents some challenges. For example, replacing the sensor every 10–14 days may be a complicated procedure for an older person with impaired dexterity and sight, and may require the support of a caregiver [2]. Review of the CGM data can be psychologically overwhelming for an older person. Problem-solving skills decline with age and the acquisition of the CGM data can trigger distress, leading to hurried and inappropriate actions, such as overcorrection or hypoglycaemia over-treatment [2]. Finally, in the presence of hearing loss, the alarms for low and high readings may not be heard, which compromises patient safety [2]. In these circumstances, the use of technology is feasible only if a relative or a caregiver is involved in the diabetes management and adequately trained.

A comprehensive assessment of each single patient is therefore crucial to identify factors preventing the achievement of benefits related to the use of technology and to develop strategies for overcoming these challenges.

Clinical Practice Question

Q1. An 81-year-old woman with a 51-year history of type 1 diabetes is on multiple daily injections and uses continuous glucose monitoring. Her basal bolus regimen includes degludec 18 units in morning and aspart at a dose between 4 and 6 units before each meal. She is known to have mild cognitive impairment and her Clinical Frailty Scale score is 5. Her husband assists in some daily activities. Her glucose metrics show time in range 78%, time below range 3%, glucose management indicator 47 mmol/mol and a pattern of nocturnal hypoglycaemia. Which treatment change and continuous glucose monitoring metrics targets would you consider for this patient?

Choose the most appropriate statement.

A. Reduce the dose of degludec and aim for time in range between 50% and 60% and time below range < 1%.

B. Reduce the aspart dose at dinner and aim for time in range 60–70% and time below range < 4%.

C. No treatment changes are need as CGM metrics are appropriate for this lady

D. Reduce the dose of degludec and aim for time in range < 50% and time below range < 1%.

References

1. Shah, V.N., Wu, M., Foster, N. et al. (2018). Severe hypoglycemia is associated with high risk for falls in adults with type 1 diabetes. *Arch. Osteoporos.* 13 (1): 66.
2. Prasad-Reddy, L., Godina, A., Chetty, A., and Isaacs, D. (2022). Use of continuous glucose monitoring in older adults: a review of benefits challenges and future directions. *touchREV Endocrinol.* 18 (2): 116–121.
3. Huang, E.S., Sinclair, A., Conlin, P.R. et al. (2023). The growing role of technology in the care of older adults with diabetes. *Diabetes Care* 46 (8): 1455–1463.
4. Ruedy, K.J., Parkin, C.G., Riddlesworth, T.D. et al. (2017). *J. Diabetes Sci. Technol.* 11 (6): 1138–1146.
5. Carlson, A.L., Kanapka, L.G., Miller, K.M. et al. (2021). Hypoglycemia and glycemic control in older adults with type 1 diabetes: baseline results from the WISDM study. *J. Diabetes Sci. Technol.* 15 (3): 582–592.
6. Beck, R.W., Riddlesworth, T.D., Ruedy, K. et al. (2017). Continuous glucose monitoring versus usual care in patients with type 2 diabetes receiving multiple daily insulin injections: a randomized trial. *Ann. Intern. Med.* 167 (6): 365–374.
7. Sinclair, A., Morley, J.E., Rodriguez-Manas, L. et al. (2012). Diabetes mellitus in older people: position statement on behalf of the International Association of Gerontology and Geriatrics (IAGG), the European Diabetes Working Party for Older People (EDWPOP), and the International Task Force of Experts in Diabetes. *J. Am. Med. Dir. Assoc.* 13 (6): 497–502.

8. ElSayed, N.A., Aleppo, G., Aroda, V.R. et al. (2023). 13. Older adults: standards of care in diabetes-2023. *Diabetes Care* 46 (Suppl 1): S216–S229.
9. Grunberger, G., Sherr, J., Allende, M. et al. (2021). American Association of Clinical Endocrinology Clinical Practice Guideline: the use of advanced technology in the management of persons with diabetes mellitus. *Endocr. Pract.* 27 (6): 505–537.
10. Battelino, T., Danne, T., Bergenstal, R.M. et al. (2019). Clinical targets for continuous glucose monitoring data interpretation: recommendations from the international consensus on time in range. *Diabetes Care* 42 (8): 1593–1603.
11. Matejko, B., Cyganek, K., Katra, B. et al. (2011). Insulin pump therapy is equally effective and safe in elderly and young type 1 diabetes patients. *Rev. Diabet. Stud.* 8 (2): 254–258.

7 Education: Key Features for Achieving Success

Kirsty Winkley and Angus Forbes

Florence Nightingale Faculty of Nursing and Midwifery, King's College London, London, UK

Key Points

- Age increases the risk of diabetes and the risks of morbidity and mortality associated with it.
- Frailty assessment (mental and physical) is essential, as frailty impacts on diabetes self-management capacity and the support needed.
- Personalised glycaemic targets are important for older adults with diabetes.
- Technology such as continuous glucose monitoring should be considered for older people with diabetes who are treated with insulin.

Introduction

Ageing impacts a range of physiological processes that have a deleterious effect on health, with all bodily systems being affected. Risk of diabetes in older adults occurs in combination with genetic predisposition, lifestyle factors and the ageing process. Insulin resistance, atherosclerosis, chronic inflammation, oxidative stress and mitochondrial dysfunction are common to ageing and diabetes. These changes alter metabolic functioning and contribute to the complications of diabetes and treatment-related hazards such as hypoglycaemia.

Care of Older People with Diabetes: A Manual for Healthcare Practice, First Edition.
Edited by Alan J. Sinclair and Ahmed H. Abdelhafiz.

Companion website: www.wiley.com/go/sinclair/1e

Frailty, which does not occur because of ageing but is more common in advancing years, can add further complexity to diabetes management, as it affects metabolic function as well as functional status and self-management capacity.

People with diabetes have high rates of mortality and this is especially so in older adults, who may have additional risk factors related to diabetes, including diabetes complications, polypharmacy, increased risk of hypoglycaemia and cognitive impairment [1, 2]. With an ageing population in many countries, there is an increased risk for excess mortality and morbidity, as age increases the likelihood of chronic disease such as type 2 diabetes mellitus (T2DM) and it is also true that people with type 1 diabetes mellitus (T1DM) are now living longer into old age [1].

Population data from the United States estimates that there are currently 11.5 million older adults with diabetes (aged 65 years or more) [3]. The majority of older people living with diabetes have T2DM and this brings some additional challenges that impact on some of the key elements of diabetes management, such as lifestyle advice and treatment choices. As the proportion of people with T1DM advancing to older age increases, it is also important to consider whether adjustments are needed to ensure safe glucose levels and capacity for self-management. This chapter outlines some of the key issues to consider and some common clinical dilemmas and potential solutions.

Key Issues

Key issues are outlined in Box 7.1.

Box 7.1: Key Issues to be Considered

- Diabetes complications
- Other comorbidities not specific to diabetes
- Polypharmacy
- Antidiabetes oral and injectable agents
- Hypoglycaemia
- Risk of falls and fractures
- Cognitive impairment

Diabetes Complications

The prevalence of diabetes complications is more likely in older adults. Older adults with a long duration of T1DM are more likely to have microvascular complications such as retinopathy, nephropathy and neuropathy [4]. Whereas in older adults with T2DM, the duration of disease exposure is more variable, so the prevalence of microvascular complications will differ between those diagnosed in younger adult life compared with those diagnosed in older age. The mean age for T2DM diagnosis in the UK is around 55 years, with an estimated prevalence for microvascular complications of approximately 30% [5]. Hence, many older adults with T2DM will have diabetes complications. The functional deficits associated with diabetes complications and ageing in respect of vision, cognition, sensation, and digital dexterity changes, can impact on self-management capacity and increase treatment hazards such as hypoglycaemia. In addition, peripheral neuropathy, may affect balance and increase the risk of falls, and chronic kidney disease is more common, which is also associated with cognitive decline [6].

In T2DM, cardiovascular disease (CVD) is the most common complication of diabetes, and is often evident in prediabetes. Dyslipidaemia and hypertension are core features of the altered metabolism associated with excess bodily weight and impaired glucose regulation [7]. CVD is a leading cause of mortality for older people with T2DM, responsible for 50% of deaths [8]. It is also present in 44% of older people with T1DM who have a diabetes duration > 50 years [9]. Hyperglycaemia and hyperlipidaemia increase atherosclerosis risk, affect endothelial function and therefore the vasculature, hypertension and autonomic dysfunction further increase the risk of stroke and myocardial infarction [10]. Heart failure risk also increases with age, presence of diabetes, nephropathy and CVD [11].

Psychological problems such as depression are more common in people with diabetes, although not especially within older age groups, however, comorbidity associated with having depression, diabetes and being older is thought to lead to greater healthcare costs [12].

It is essential that older people with diabetes attend screening for diabetes complications at least annually or more frequently to determine glycaemia. This will involve checks for diabetic eye disease and assessment of sensation and circulation to the feet. Blood pressure, serum cholesterol, and HbA1c will determine management of hypertension, hyperlipidaemia and hyperglycaemia. Finally, kidney function/disease is checked by assessing urine for microalbuminuria and serum for creatinine and to calculate estimated glomerular filtration rate (eGFR).

Other Comorbidities Not Specific to Diabetes

There are other comorbidities not necessarily specific to diabetes, which appear to be impacted by damage to small and large blood vessels generally. For example, in a systematic review and meta-analysis, the risk of hearing loss was doubled in people with diabetes compared with those without diabetes [13]. Many other comorbidities are also more prevalent in people with diabetes including respiratory conditions (chronic obstructive pulmonary disease, asthma and pneumonia) [14], cancer [15], chronic pain [16], urinary incontinence and urinary tract infection, particularly for postmenopausal women [17]. It is therefore important to consider these problems during clinical consultations with the person with diabetes.

Polypharmacy

Diabetes therapies are key in managing glucose levels but can introduce additional hazards in older people, the risk of hypoglycaemia increases in older adults with T1DM and T2DM. While the risk of hypoglycaemia is greatest in those treated with insulin, in people with T2DM there is also a risk from sulfonylureas. Hypoglycaemia in older adults with T2DM increases cardiovascular distress and has been associated with fatality in cardiovascular outcome studies [18, 19]. Polypharmacy is common in older adults and diabetes-specific polypharmacy is an important consideration for older adults with T2DM who are likely to have been prescribed accumulative hypoglycaemic therapies over the duration of their disease. Some of the advantages and disadvantages of diabetes therapies in older age are outlined below.

Anti-diabetes Oral and Injectable Agents

Biguanides such as metformin are useful as they improve insulin sensitivity, do not cause hypoglycaemia and can protect against CVD. The main issues are the adverse gastric effects and need to be reduced if the individual has impaired renal function (eGFR $< 30\,\text{ml/minute}/1.73\,\text{m}^2$). There can be an increased risk of lactic acidosis usually attributed to dehydration or intercurrent illness, so it important for older people to stop this drug if not eating and drinking normally [20].

Sulfonylureas stimulate the pancreas to increase insulin production and can be problematic for older people with T2DM because of the increased risk of hypoglycaemia caused by mistiming of food/carbohydrate intake or failure to eat. Sulfonylureas have also been associated with sarcopenia (loss of muscle tissue), which has additional metabolic consequences. Caution is also needed in older people with hepatic or renal impairment as clearance is reduced increasing the risk of hypoglycaemia. Meglitinides, such as repaglinide, also stimulate beta cells to produce insulin and, like sulfonylureas, can increase the risk of hypoglycaemia if not taken before food.

Thiazolidinedione therapies act by altering gene transcription involved in carbohydrate and lipid metabolism and improve insulin sensitivity. These drugs should be used with caution in older people as adverse effects include reduced bone density increasing the risk of fractures. They have also been associated with increased risk of infection, bladder cancer, heart failure and myocardial infarction.

Drugs targeting the incretin pathway are increasingly common in diabetes. Dipeptidyl peptidase-4 (DPP-4) inhibitors increase insulin and lower glucagon secretion. They do not cause any significant drug interactions or hypoglycaemia and are weight neutral. Most are appropriate for older people with diabetes although in individuals with renal impairment linagliptin is indicated. Glucagon-like peptide 1 (GLP-1) receptor agonists, augment insulin secretion in response to blood glucose and slow gastric emptying. They are predominantly administered by injection although oral preparations are now available. GLP-1 may reduce appetite and increase weight-loss, which can be important in older adults as attenuating appetite may lead to deficits in nutrient intake and could increase the risk of sarcopenia. The most common adverse effects are gastrointestinal; pancreatitis is also a risk, so older people (and their carers) should be advised to report symptoms such as abdominal pain, nausea or vomiting.

Sodium-glucose co-transporter-2 (SGLT2) inhibitors prevent the reuptake of glucose at the renal proximal convoluted tubule and thereby increase glucose excretion in the urine. One of the main adverse effects of these drugs are increased genitourinary excretion and infection, this can be problematic in older people with continence problems. As with GLP-1, they can also cause weight loss which needs to be considered in relation to the nutritional status of the older person. Dizziness is an additional adverse effect that may increase the falls risk in older people. There is a risk of atypical diabetic ketoacidosis, which can develop with normal or slightly elevated blood glucose levels. Therefore, older people need to understand the signs and symptoms of diabetic ketoacidosis and how to check their blood/urine for ketones.

Insulin treatment is essential for older adults with T1DM and important for many with T2DM. The main adverse effect is hypoglycaemia, which is a significant risk for older people as hypoglycaemia awareness can be blunted in older age. Older people with T1DM will be using multiple daily injections or an insulin pump, together with either capillary or continuous glucose monitoring (CGM). Some older people will have a sensor-enabled pump, which can suspend insulin delivery when the glucose level if falling or hybrid closed loop system. Insulin pumps may introduce complexity for some older or frail people with diabetes, although they can also potentially be protective if there is an automated suspension or alarm function when used with CGM. Pumps can cause problems in the context of hospitalisation, as hospital inpatient teams may have variable experience and training with these devices [21]. Connected pens that are linked to a CGM device and indicate when the last injection was taken may be useful for older adults with T1DM or T2DM who may have some memory decline to avoid accidental overdose. For older adults with T2DM, it may only be necessary to supplement oral agents with one injection of basal insulin, depending on the degree of beta-cell loss/hyperglycaemia. It is important to bear in mind that insulin requirements and responses may change with ageing and hence regular review and adjustment may be needed as established dose assumptions may need changing. Safety should be an important consideration and this needs to include a capacity assessment to ensure that the older person will be safe to self-administer insulin or whether third party administration is required.

Hypoglycaemia

In older adults with diabetes, risk of hypoglycaemia is complicated by altered physiological response to the hypoglycaemic state. There is ageing of the counter-regulatory response and the usual autonomic response to hypoglycaemia, which includes pancreatic glucagon production triggering hepatic glycogenolysis and gluconeogenesis, adrenal gland release of epinephrine and norepinephrine producing hunger and tremor, the autonomic response and adaptive cardiac perfusion

[22]. Together, these processes can deprive the brain of glucose, which means that cognitive tasks become impaired and increase risk of life-threatening cardiovascular events such as ventricular arrhythmias [22]. There can be multiple factors that contribute to the risk of hypoglycaemia. One of the main factors is polypharmacy, but also reduced food or fluid intake, cognitive impairment, CVD, renal impairment and endocrine problems. Therefore, it is essential that older people with support as needed are checking their blood glucose levels so that hypoglycaemia can be prevented.

Risk of Falls and Fractures

Falls and fractures related to hypoglycaemia are a significant issue for older adults with diabetes. Falls are a major hazard for older people with diabetes and can result in hospitalisation. Compared with people without diabetes, the odds of fracture following a fall in older people with diabetes are 78% higher and there is a twofold increased risk death [23], comorbid dementia increases these risks further. Reducing risk of hypoglycaemia will reduce the risk to the older person with diabetes.

Cognitive Impairment

Hypoglycaemia and hyperglycaemia are risk factors for cognitive dysfunction and relationships are bidirectional. Older adults with T2DM have a two-fold increased risk of dementia [24], but there is a less consistent pattern for older adults with T1DM [25]. Cognitive impairment can be mild or more severe and it can be progressive without intervention [25]. The impact of cognitive impairment on people with T2DM versus T1DM is also varied. In T2DM, there can be deficiency in executive function (problem solving, changing habits), memory and learning whereas for people with T1DM there may be deficits in mental flexibility.

As cognitive function often declines gradually it can be difficult to recognise. For example, it could be that there is some failure to fulfil the usual self-management requirements in terms of monitoring glucose levels, timing or administration of insulin or tablets, calculation of insulin doses in respect of carbohydrate intake or planning for exercise or, worryingly, in the recognition of hypoglycaemia and failure to act. Assessment of cognitive status may be conducted formally using screening tests, but not all clinicians or diabetes professionals are familiar with these tests. Clinical guidance indicates when cognitive deficits are identified someone who knows the person well or a carer needs to be given appropriate information so that they can support the older person and reduce hazards such as accidental overdosing or omitting medication. In the case of insulin in more severe cognitive impairment, third-party insulin administration or remote access CGM may be indicated, although this needs to be negotiated sensitively with the older person.

Nutrition

Adequate nutrition is needed to promote glycaemia and prevent sarcopenia and frailty in older adults with diabetes [26]. However, cognitive impairment increases the risk of malnutrition by 50% in older adults with T2DM [27], particularly among those with a low body mass index (BMI). Obesity and high BMI are often more prevalent in older adults with diabetes. This poses the risk of functional disability, indicating that a balanced approach to nutrition is needed ensuring adequate nutrition, maintaining quality of life and, where necessary, supporting weight loss in the case of obesity. Sarcopenic obesity (high body fat in proportion to muscle due to atrophy) is more prevalent in diabetes [28] compared with those without diabetes and is associated with increased atherosclerosis and mortality in older people with diabetes [29]. An assessment of the older person's diet, ideally from a dietitian, is an essential element of diabetes care.

Management

As has been outlined, the needs of older people with diabetes are heterogeneous. Therefore, managing diabetes in the older person requires a personalised approach sensitive to the needs of the individual. A balanced approach is needed considering both the needs to reduce the metabolic hazards of diabetes and promote quality of life. Outlined below are some important considerations in the management of diabetes in the older person.

Determine Frailty Risk

Frailty can have a significant mediating effect on diabetes, which needs to assessed as part of diabetes management in older age. Frailty should be assessed regularly; at a minimum annually but, as frailty can present or escalate rapidly, more regular review is recommended. There are multiple screening and diagnostic tools for frailty [30], a commonly used method is the Frailty Index [31], which is a cumulative deficit model and has been incorporated into the medical record systems of general practices in the UK. The validated five-item FRAIL (fatigue, resistance, ambulation, illness, and loss of weight) score is another tool that can be used to score a patient during a clinical consultation [32].

In a 2021 consensus statement on the management of older adults with T2DM, three broad categories according to frailty, are suggested [33]: (1) the healthy, pre-fail or those with mild frailty who are a functionally independent; (2) those with moderate frailty who have more than two comorbidities; and (3) those with severe frailty who have significant comorbidity and functional deficits affecting independence. While these frailty groups are specifically for adults with T2DM, they could also be used for adults with T1DM. At each level of frailty, it is important to make appropriate adjustments in therapeutic objectives and treatments for the older person with diabetes to manage any potential risks.

Deprescribing and Optimisation

Most diabetes management plans use HbA1c levels as the basis for planning treatment. Mortality risk is increased at low and high HbA1c levels for older people with diabetes [34], so a target HbA1c for older adults should consider both as equal risks. It has been recommended that the frailty score and life-expectancy should be used to guide the care objectives and therapeutic options in T2DM [33]. It has also been recommended that glucose levels should be deintensified for older frail individuals aiming for a HbA1c of 59–64 mmol/mol without hypoglycaemia [35], and this may necessitate review of current treatment and deprescribing.

In T2DM, treatment can be simplified by using medications with a lower risk of hypoglycaemia, such as metformin, DPP4, SGLT2 inhibitors or incretin therapies. If insulin is necessary, a once-daily basal insulin can be used to target fasting glucose, with the other oral or injectable therapies used to prevent glucose excursions at mealtimes [25]. However, for older adults with T1DM, these strategies may be more challenging, as people with T1DM have been programmed to avoid hyperglycaemia. They may be resistant to these changes and this change will need to be managed sensitively. If cognitive dysfunction is present, supervision with insulin dosing and technology could help patients to maintain their independence for longer (e.g. use of CGM, insulin pump or connected pens) [25]. Connected insulin pens pair with a smartphone, can calculate/track insulin use and provide reminders for injection. In more advanced cognitive decline, third-party insulin administration and remote glucose monitoring (linking glucose data from CGM to a carer's mobile phone), should be considered, again with the consent of the person with diabetes if they have the capacity.

Glucose Monitoring and Insulin Delivery Technologies

For older people with T1DM, CGM-augmented insulin pumps and/or hybrid closed loop systems could help to reduce the risk of hypoglycaemia. CGM can also be useful for older adults with T2DM who are insulin treated, which is around one fifth of the total population of people with T2DM [21]. The primary benefit of CGM is early detection and avoidance of hypoglycaemia. However, most trials have not included older adults or those with cognitive dysfunction. Two recent trials have included adults aged 60+ years (the DIAMOND study of T1DM and T2DM, the WISDM study in adults with T1DM), both of which randomised to either CGM or blood glucose monitoring and demonstrated reduced hypoglycaemia and time in range [36, 37]. CGM should also be considered for people with diabetes who need assistance with monitoring, as carers can view blood glucose readings and there is reduced reliance on finger-prick testing, which is difficult to do with reduced dexterity.

Physical Exercise

As physical inactivity increases risk of frailty and dementia, it is important for older adults to engage in exercise safely [26]. Physical activity counters insulin resistance and inflammation, so it is especially relevant for older adults with diabetes. Weight-bearing exercise, aerobic activities and resistance training have all demonstrated benefits for older adults with diabetes, particularly in strengthening lower limbs, improving gait and balance, and should be discussed as part of the diabetes consultation [38].

Healthy Diet

People with high and low BMI are at risk of cognitive impairment, frailty and mortality, so it is important for older adults with diabetes to have sufficient energy and protein intake to reduce their risk [26]. European guidance suggests 30 kcal/kg body weight/day and 1.0–1.5 g/kg body weight/day of protein for older adults with chronic illness [39]. Protein intake is important to reduce risk of sarcopenia. Other nutrients, such as vitamins, particularly vitamin D, and polyunsaturated fatty acids, which can affect CVD risk, are also important. The Mediterranean diet, which incorporates healthy fats with fish and vegetables, is thought to be of particular benefit for older people and provision of further information for the person with diabetes and their carer may assist them in making healthy choices [40].

Diabetes Self-management Education for Older People

In general, although the population of people with diabetes is essentially an older group, there has been little research focusing on older adults. A systematic review and meta-analysis of 13 randomised controlled trials of diabetes self-management programmes for older adults ($N = 4517$) compared with treatment as usual did demonstrate a positive effect/reduction in HbA1c (−2 mmol/mol, −0.2%, 95% CI −0.3 to −0.1) and a reduction in total cholesterol (−5.81 mg/dl, 95% CI −10.33 to −1.29) [41]. However, none of the included studies were based in the UK; most were conducted in the United States. Older adults are not excluded from participating in diabetes self-management education, but their specific needs may not have been met, such as the potential for a lack of digital skills or access to digital resource, and their individual requirements based on the presence of comorbidity, frailty and psychological or cognitive needs. It is therefore likely that older adults may not have been able to access or fully engage with diabetes education and there is a need for continuing education and self-management discussion and support, with a carer as appropriate, during clinical consultations.

Clinical Practice Question

Q1. A 68-year-old woman with T2DM lives alone and manages diabetes with multiple daily injections of insulin is admitted to hospital with hypoglycaemia. She is discharged home on lower doses of insulin. What, if any, changes to her treatment plan are required and how would you support her?

Choose one or more appropriate options:

A. Make no changes.

B. Change her insulin to twice-daily premixed insulin.

C. Change her insulin to once-daily basal insulin and ask the district nurses to visit.

D. Conduct a full assessment to determine her ability and dexterity in terms of insulin injection, hypoglycaemia treatment, assessment of cognitive ability, nutritional status, frailty and her own worries and concerns in relation to her diabetes treatment.

References

Key references only are listed here. For a full list of references visit: `https://www.wiley.com/go/sinclair/1e`.

1. Livingstone, S.J., Levin, D., Looker, H.C. et al. (2015). Estimated life expectancy in a Scottish cohort with type 1 diabetes, 2008–2010. *JAMA* 313 (1): 37.
2. Nwaneri, C., Cooper, H., and Bowen-Jones, D. (2013). Mortality in type 2 diabetes mellitus: magnitude of the evidence from a systematic review and meta-analysis. *Br. J. Diabetes Vasc. Dis.* 13 (4): 192–207.
6. Yaffe, K., Ackerson, L., Tamura, M.K. et al. (2010). Chronic kidney disease and cognitive function in older adults: findings from the chronic renal insufficiency cohort cognitive study. *J. Am. Geriatr. Soc.* 58 (2): 338–345.
8. Preis, S.R., Hwang, S.J., Coady, S. et al. (2009). Trends in all-cause and cardiovascular disease mortality among women and men with and without diabetes mellitus in the Framingham heart study, 1950 to 2005. *Circulation* 119 (13): 1728–1735.
9. Adamsson Eryd, S., Svensson, A.-M., Franzén, S. et al. (2017). Risk of future microvascular and macrovascular disease in people with type 1 diabetes of very long duration: a national study with 10-year follow-up. *Diabet. Med.* 34 (3): 411–418.

19. Miller, M.E., Williamson, J.D., Gerstein, H.C. et al. (2014). Effects of randomization to intensive glucose control on adverse events, cardiovascular disease, and mortality in older versus younger adults in the ACCORD trial. *Diabetes Care* 37 (3): 634–643.
21. Huang, E.S., Sinclair, A., Conlin, P.R. et al. (2023). The growing role of technology in the care of older adults with diabetes. *Diabetes Care* 46 (8): 1455–1463.
22. Sircar, M., Bhatia, A., and Munshi, M. (2016). Review of hypoglycemia in the older adult: clinical implications and management. *Can. J. Diabetes* 40 (1): 66–72.
24. Ott, A., Stolk, R.P., van Harskamp, F. et al. (1999). Diabetes mellitus and the risk of dementia. *Neurology* 53 (9): 1937–1937.
41. Sherifali, D., Bai, J.-W., Kenny, M. et al. (2015). Diabetes self-management programmes in older adults: a systematic review and meta-analysis. *Diabet. Med.* 32 (11): 1404–1414.

8 Carers and Care Needs

Puja Merwaha and Ahmed H. Abdelhafiz
Department of Geriatric Medicine, Rotherham General Hospital, Rotherham, UK

Key Points

- Diabetes mellitus is a chronic condition that requires regular self-care tasks.
- With increasing age, patients will need additional help with the management of diabetes and self-care.
- The role of carers is vital to improve outcomes for older people with diabetes.
- The burden on carers is increasingly recognised. this burden may have a negative impact on carers' own physical and mental health.
- A structured approach to care, which considers health needs and quality of life, is required to improve outcomes for both patients and carers.

Introduction

The prevalence of diabetes continues to increase in older people, with an increased likelihood of multiple comorbidities, risk of complications and frailty, which lead to increased prevalence of both cognitive and physical disabilities [1]. In addition, diabetes requires a myriad of self-care tasks, which may become more challenging in older age. The role of carers for older people with diabetes is therefore vital. This chapter reviews the detailed aspects of the care needs of older people with diabetes, the role of carers and the support required to maintain their role.

Care of Older People with Diabetes: A Manual for Healthcare Practice, First Edition.
Edited by Alan J. Sinclair and Ahmed H. Abdelhafiz.

Companion website: www.wiley.com/go/sinclair/1e

Care Needs

Care for diabetes in old age is similar to those of a younger age group, but older people may need extra care due to the complex morbidities associated with ageing. This complexity may affect independent self-care tasks, especially if there are comorbid cognitive and physical dysfunctions. For example, older people may need additional aids and assistance in compliance with medications intake, regular exercise, blood glucose monitoring and aspects of personal care. In addition, frailty, characterised by anorexia and weight loss, may need a different approach from younger people, with relaxation of dietary restrictions to maintain weight and reduce muscle loss. Most importantly, routine check by carers help to identify early signs of deterioration and complications, such as hypoglycaemia, and could be life saving. Care requirements may vary significantly between individuals; the general requirements for the carers are summarised in Box 8.1.

Box 8.1: Knowledge Requirement for Carers of Older People with Diabetes

- Symptoms of diabetes mellitus, hypoglycaemia and hyperglycaemia
- Interpretation of blood glucose levels
- Knowledge about insulin regimens and injection site complications
- Understanding of patients' diabetes management, dose and timings of medications, and importance of compliance
- Identification of acute decompensation
- Basic understanding haemoglobin A1c values
- Awareness of comorbidities and impact on diabetes management
- Education about the necessary diet and exercise requirements
- Awareness of mental health complications of diabetes and recognition of early signs of cognitive or mood disturbance
- Education around maintenance of foot care
- Education on key long-term complications of diabetes mellitus
- Knowledge about sick day rules
- Ability to communicate with healthcare providers for advice when needed

Carer Groups

A carer is any person who delivers care to someone who needs additional help to take care of themselves. People may need care because of a decline in their cognitive or functional abilities, which affect their independence in activities of daily living. Care can be formal, delivered by paid professionals, or informal such as voluntarily offered by family members, neighbours or friends. Social organisations such as religious or community groups can also function as sources of care and support for older people. Care can be delivered in various settings, such as patients' homes, hospitals and care homes. Care can even be delivered via remote carers through use of technology. Care setting may also differ by ethnicity; for example, in some ethnic groups, where the extended family lives in the same house, family members may play a more significant role as informal carers.

Role of Carers

Carers' roles range from simple emotional support, providing company, offering general help to taking care of all aspects of activities of daily living such as household chores and personal care. In addition, carers can help in diabetes-specific medical care such as administration of medications, insulin injections, regular blood glucose monitoring and identification of additional needs and concerns. Moreover, carers are of significant help attending appointments with the patient and healthcare providers. Carers can write down concerns and bring them to the appointment and to record any instructions given to patients during the appointment. The carers' role can be direct, through providing the care, or indirect, through management care being delivered. Carers should be aware of and educated about the lifestyle needs of older people with diabetes and their daily routine tasks, and should be able to recognise acute complications of diabetes. They should have easy and quick access to specialised care if it is urgently required. The roles of carers are summarised in Box 8.2.

Box 8.2: Role of Carers in Caring for Older People with Diabetes

- Emotional support
- Providing company
- Offering general help
- Assistance in activities of daily living
- Intimate care, such as bathing and hygiene
- Medication administration, including insulin
- Blood glucose monitoring
- Help compliance with diet and exercise
- Help in attending medical appointments
- Assistance in daily tasks for diabetes care
- Assistance in early recognition of acute diabetes complications
- Help in fast access to medical care in emergencies

Benefit of Care on Outcomes

Care provided by carers has a positive holistic effect on older people with diabetes, including physically, emotionally and socially. This effect will extend to involve the patient's whole family. For example, it helps by taking off the pressure, concerns and worries, giving a sense of assurance and comfort. In addition, carers have a positive impact on diabetes-related parameters. A systematic review of family-based interventions for adults with diabetes and their impact on patients' diabetes outcomes found that the degree of family involvement varied across studies, but there was evidence for improvement in patients' self-efficacy, perceived social support, diabetes knowledge and diabetes self-care [2]. In another systematic review to explore the role of carers in the remote monitoring of patients with type 2 diabetes, the evidence suggested a positive impact of carers on clinical, economic and humanistic outcomes, ranging from diabetes-related parameters to patients' compliance with monitoring [3].

Caring for Carers

Chronic diseases will have effects, not only on patients, but also on their carers. These effects are likely to increase in proportion with the severity of the medical condition and disability of patients. These effects may have negative impacts on carers' health physically, socially and psychologically. It is therefore important to check the carers' burden and its effect on their health to help identify their needs and ability to continue providing the level of care required [4].

Carers' Burden

The carers' burden is the level of multifaceted strain perceived by carers from caring for a patient over time, which may lead to negative consequences [5]. Carers' burden includes negative effects on both mental health, such as increased risk of anxiety and depression, and on physical health, such as musculoskeletal pain and headache [4]. Other factors, such as social isolation, less free time and financial stress, may lead to a term labelled as 'carers' syndrome', which may have negative effects on carers' quality of life [4]. Carers' burden can also put carers at risk of worsening their own medical conditions, developing new conditions or even leading to significant morbidity and risk of mortality [6]. In addition, it may affect patients under their care, increasing the risk of functional deterioration, disability and care home admission [6]. Concerning diabetes, carer' burden increases with poor diabetes control, associated complications and morbidities. For example, in a study that included frail older people, mean age 83.1 years (standard deviation 4.9 years), with diabetes who have high comorbid conditions, median Charlson index 8 (interquartile range 2.3) including advanced dementia, 81.4% of carers reported severe overburden [7]. Despite improving glycaemic control of these patients, simplifying their medications, reducing risk of hypoglycaemia and optimising their nutrition, the carers' burden remains significantly high after six months of follow-up [7]. Another observational study concluded that the lesser the burden on family carers, the better the health status of people with diabetes mellitus, which suggests that reducing carers' burden will have better health outcomes [8]· Carers' burden could be assessed and measures with the use of tools such as the Caregiver Strain Index, which measures multifaceted aspects of carers' burden [9].

Supporting Carers

Carers may feel regularly overwhelmed with lack of adequate support and education. For example, many carers have reported to spend 35 hours or more a week on providing care without adequate support or diabetes-related information from professionals [10]. The carers provided comprehensive care, including diabetes-specific care, general care and personal care, which may increase the level of the carer's burden [10]. Supporting carers is a key consideration from the outset of initiating care for older people with diabetes. Support should be available and provided whenever needed, and escalated in parallel with the progression of patient's condition. Carers may require emotional, social, financial and health-related interventions, which will allow them to continue to look after their patients without compromise of their own wellbeing. General and regular education about diabetes care, suitable to carers' ethnic background and educational level, is required. In addition, instructions and information specific to the patient and their comorbid conditions is important. For example, in patients with comorbid diabetes and dementia, carers should be educated to manage unexpected behavioural or psychological problems as well as the difficulties that may arise with erratic oral intake and compliance with medications. This will ensure that carers are partners in the provision of care for their patients. Carers may also need information in case of unexpected difficulties and know whom to contact if urgently required. It has been demonstrated that carers, when they look after patients with comorbid depression, may suffer from mental health issues themselves and inferior quality of life, so psychological support is suggested for these carers [11]. Healthcare systems should provide respite for carers for short breaks to help relieve some of the carers' burden (Figure 8.1). Support plans, which set out the carers' needs, wishes around providing care and balance with their own life should be developed in partnership with the carer and regularly reviewed (Box 8.3).

Summary

Diabetes mellitus is a unique chronic condition associated with a need for daily self-care tasks. With increasing age, older people with diabetes will have multiple comorbidities and frailty, which may lead to reduced ability on to perform daily self-care. The role of carers in looking after older people with diabetes is thus vital to achieve good outcomes and maintain the quality of life of this group of vulnerable patients. Carers themselves will have their own burden and health-related issues that need to be regularly assessed to maintain their ability

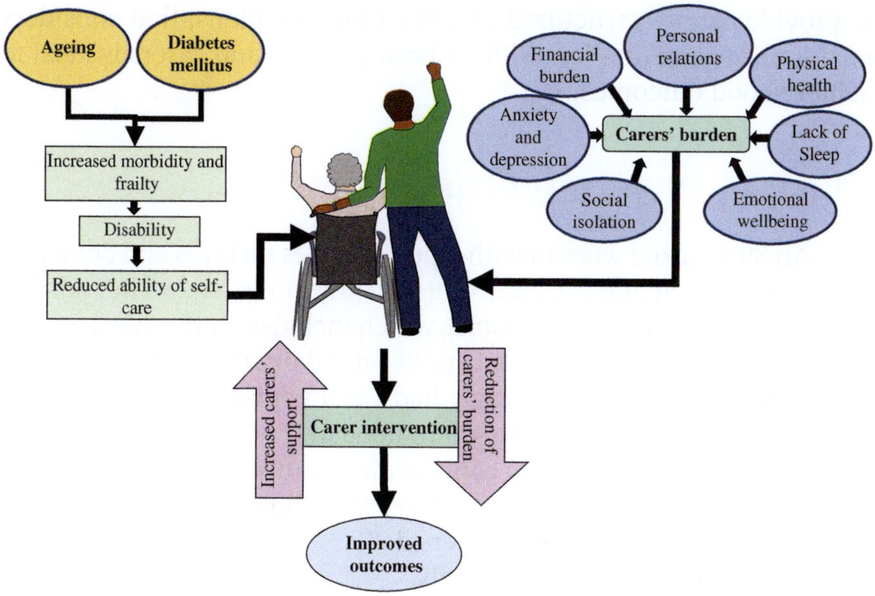

Figure 8.1: Increasing age and diabetes mellitus lead to reduced ability of self-care and the carers' role in improving outcomes.

Box 8.3: Supporting Carers of Older People with Diabetes

- Provide the necessary education sensitive to the carer's level of knowledge and culture
- Help to create a care plan for the the person they care for
- Provide full information relevant to the person they care for
- Offer access to healthcare professionals
- Provide contacts for emergencies when they arise
- Provide regular breaks from care if needed
- Increase awareness to avoid carer burden
- Encouragement to ensure that the carer maintains their own wellbeing
- Offer mental health advice if required
- Emotional and social support
- Negotiate times for regular check on their coping
- Offer help for their tasks when required
- Make sure that the carer feels needed and valued

to provide care. A structured approach for care plans, that considers health needs and quality of life of both patients and carers is ideal to achieve good outcomes.

Clinical Practice Question

Q1. An 89-year-old woman with type 2 diabetes mellitus and dementia lives alone at home. Carers visit her three times a day. They administer her diabetes medications, which includes metformin 1 g twice a day and insulin glargine 18 units once daily. Carers have recently noticed that she increasingly had vacant episodes, which last for a few minutes but resolve spontaneously. They have also reported that she engaging less in conversation compared with previously. She has been eating less and recently has lost two pounds in weight. What should the carers do?
Select all the options that apply:
A. Check her blood glucose when she has vacant episodes.
B. Encourage regular feeds- even small amounts.
C. Seek advice from health care professionals.
D. Admit to hospital.
E. Dietician advice to add food supplements.

References

1. Gregg, E.W., Engelgau, M.M., and Narayan, V. (2002). Complications of diabetes in elderly people: underappreciated problems include cognitive decline and physical disability. *BMJ* 325: 916–917.
2. Baig, A.A., Benitez, A., Quinn, M.T. et al. (2015). Family interventions to improve diabetes outcomes for adults. *Ann. N. Y. Acad. Sci.* 1353: 89–112.
3. Seng, J.J., Gwee, M.F., Yong, M.H. et al. (2023). Role of caregivers in remote management of patients with type 2 diabetes mellitus: systematic review of literature. *J. Med. Internet Res.* 25: e46988.
4. Longacre, M.L., Wong, Y.N., and Fang, C.Y. (2014). Caregiver psychological health and hospitalization characteristics of older adult care recipients: an integrative review of US studies. *Res. Gerontol. Nurs.* 7: 139–147.
5. Liu, Z., Heffernan, C., and Tan, J. (2020). Caregiver burden: a concept analysis. *Int. J. Nursing Sci.* 7: 438–445.
6. Jayani, R. and Hurria, A. (2012). Caregivers of older adults with cancer. *Semin. Oncol. Nurs.* 28 (4): 221–225.

7. Ripoll, J.M., Llinares, V.J., Pérez, M.J. et al. (2018). Caregiver burden in the management of frail elderly patients with diabetes in internal medicine. *Health* 10: 1383.
8. Kristaningrum, N.D., Ramadhani, D.A., Hayati, Y.S. et al. (2021). Correlation between the burden of family caregivers and health status of people with diabetes mellitus. *J. Public Health Res.* 10: 2227.
9. Robinson, B.C. (1983). Validation of a caregiver strain index. *J. Gerontol.* 38: 344–348.
10. Sinclair, A.J., Armes, D.G., Randhawa, G. et al. (2010). Caring for older adults with diabetes mellitus: characteristics of carers and their prime roles and responsibilities. *Diabet. Med.* 27: 1055–1059.
11. Sewitch, M.J., McCusker, J., Dendukuri, N. et al. (2004). Depression in frail elders: impact on family caregivers. *Int. J. Geriatr. Psychiatry* 19: 655–665.

9a Macrovascular Complications: Peripheral Arterial Disease

Leocadio Rodríguez-Mañas, Rubí E. Sandoval-Santoyo and Marta Castro-Rodríguez

Geriatric Medicine Department, University Hospital of Getafe, Madrid, Spain

Key Points

- Lower extremity peripheral arterial disease is a leading cause of vascular mortality and morbidity, only surpassed by coronary artery disease and stroke.
- Since peripheral arterial disease is a treatable condition, early detection and appropriated management can lead to avoid limb loss, ulcers, pain and functional decline and poor quality of life.
- Severe disability that limits the patient's quality of life must be the main reason for revascularisation when medical treatment fails.

Epidemiology

Risk Factors

Atherothrombosis accounts for 70% of all deaths in people older than 70 years. The factors that lead to atherosclerotic disease are multiple, including genetic factors, metabolic diseases, inflammatory diseases, lifestyle and local and systemic conditions of the vascular system [1, 2]. Their major risk factors include age, smoking, hypertension, dyslipidaemia, type 2 diabetes mellitus, physical inactivity and abdominal obesity, which are responsible for 90% of cardiovascular diseases [3].

Care of Older People with Diabetes: A Manual for Healthcare Practice, First Edition.
Edited by Alan J. Sinclair and Ahmed H. Abdelhafiz.

Companion website: www.wiley.com/go/sinclair/1e

However, the weight of each one of these risk factors is different for each clinical expression of atherosclerotic disease. Age and smoking are the main risk factors for developing peripheral arterial disease (PAD). Moreover, smoking is directly associated to the severity of PAD and it affects the prognosis of revascularization interventions. Diabetes mellitus is not only a qualitative risk factor but also a quantitative one. Poor glycaemic control is one of the strongest risk factors for PAD and its main consequence is amputation. Amputation is 10 times more frequent in people with diabetes than in people without diabetes.

Prevalence

The prevalence of PAD in older people in high-income countries increases with age. At 85–89 years, it is 18.38% (95% confidence interval, CI, 11.16–28.76%) in women and 18.83% (95% CI 12.03–28.25%) in men [4]. Patients with PAD and diabetes have nearly twice the cardiovascular mortality than those without diabetes [5]. In addition, the ankle–brachial index (ABI) is a marker of subclinical functional decline [6]. Asymptomatic PAD is associated with markers of functional decline.

Pathogenesis

Factors involved in the pathophysiology of PAD in older people with diabetes are the same than in non-older population, but it is potentiated by the presence of age-associated changes in the vascular bed.

Atherosclerosis is in the centre of the process. It is a universal process, although it shows some pathophysiological differences depending on the anatomical location of the occurrence. Endothelial dysfunction is the starting point of the process, leading to atherosclerosis, jointly to insulin-resistance, oxidative stress and a chronic low-grade inflammatory phenotype that participates in defective endothelial vasodilation. Vascular endothelial dysfunction, oxidative stress and chronic inflammation of the vascular wall form a vicious circle leading to the development of atherosclerosis. Glyco-oxidation contributes to the development of atherosclerosis in the below-the-knee peripheral artery tree in type 2 diabetes. Advanced glycosylation end-products levels increase with ageing and in diabetes, with the highest levels in those with PAD [7]. In addition, lipid oxidation and a low antioxidant capacity are associated with diabetic peripheral angiopathy. The final consequence is the same: an imbalance between the oxygen needs of the tissues and the provided supply. Higher levels of inflammation (which happens in ageing and diabetes mellitus) are associated with greater functional impairment and faster functional decline in persons with PAD.

Consequences of Peripheral Arterial Disease

Peripheral arterial disease increases the risk of cardiovascular morbidity and mortality. There is a higher incidence of stroke (mainly in the elderly), fatal and non-fatal coronary disease, heart failure, and a poor prognosis in all forms of cardiovascular disease have been shown in people with PAD, in both in the short (three to four years) and long term (10 years) [8].

Peripheral arterial disease increases functional decline and produces faster rates of functional decline. Older patients with PAD have lower physical activity levels, slower walking speed, poorer balance, poorer walking endurance, and higher and faster rates of mobility loss [9]. In the Cardiovascular Health Study, severity of PAD significantly increased at each level of frailty (non-frail, pre-frail, frail) [10]. These data reinforce the bidirectional relationship between atherosclerosis and frailty [11].

Current data suggest that PAD detection and treatment are lower than other forms of atherosclerotic disease, although there is evidence to support a prognostic significance and an impact on quality of life comparable to other forms of cardiovascular disease [12].

Investigations

Anamnesis

Older people are often asymptomatic and even when they are not, patients frequently minimise symptoms, attributing them to normal ageing. The 2017 American College of Cardiology and American Heart Association consensus document on the management of PAD recommends investigations including questions related to a history of walking impairment, symptoms of claudication, ischaemic rest pain, or non-healing wounds in patients ≥ 70 years of age [13].

Among symptomatic patients, atypical symptoms are more common than claudication, usually focused on functional issues, physical inactivity and alterations in pain perception. A gradual decline in activity level or a progressive loss of independence in the activities of daily life may mask the symptoms of PAD. A careful history, including a comprehensive geriatric assessment, should reveal a functional impairment when this is the clinical presentation [14].

Physical Examination

The physical assessment should include an examination with shoes and socks off, paying special attention to pulses (femoral, popliteal, posterior tibial and pedal), bruits, hair loss, skin colour, temperature, ulcers and trophic skin changes.

The functional impairment can be measured using several validated tests and scores. The most frequently suggested instruments are the short physical performance battery and the six-metre walking speed.

Comprehensive geriatric assessment should be a routine measure in older people with type 2 diabetes at diagnosis and at regular intervals. At a minimum, an annual inspection of the feet by a healthcare professional is recommended, including a vascular and neurological examination, even if no symptoms are present. When available, an ABI determination should be done. Detection of asymptomatic PAD has value because it identifies patients at increased risk of atherosclerosis at other sites [15].

Non-invasive Tests

A variety of non-invasive examinations are available to assess the presence and degree of PAD. In primary care we strongly recommend ABI (Figure 9a.1). Calculation of the ABI is performed by measuring the systolic blood pressure (by Doppler probe) in the brachial arteries and in posterior tibial or dorsalis pedis arteries. The highest of the four measurements in the ankles and feet is divided by the higher of the two brachial measurements.

Several categories are defined:

- Normal ABI is 1.0–1.3; values > 1.30 suggest a non-compressible calcified vessel.
- ABI < 0.9 has 95% sensitivity (and 100% specificity) for detecting angiogram-positive PAD and is associated with ≥ 50% stenosis in one or more major vessels.
- ABI 0.40–0.90 suggests arterial obstruction often associated with claudication.
- ABI < 0.4 represents advanced ischaemia.

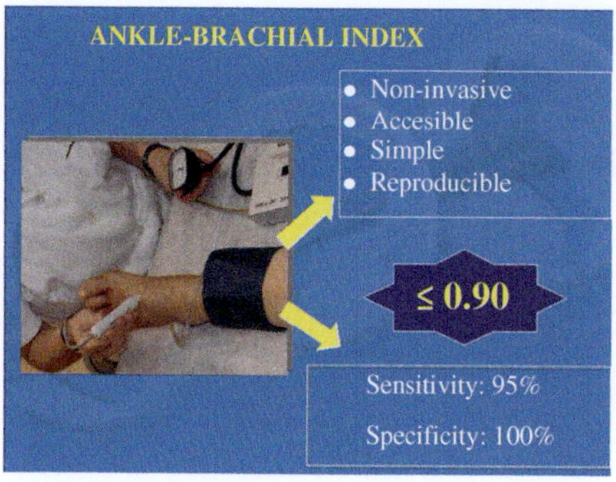

Figure 9a.1: Measurement and diagnostic characteristics of the ankle–brachial index.

Invasive Tests

Contrast angiography is the 'gold standard' for the diagnosis of PAD. It should be performed only in selected patients (surgical patients).

Management

Medical treatment embraces risk factor modification, exercise, foot care and drugs. If the disease progresses and/or the patient meets a few established criteria, percutaneous intervention or surgery should be performed.

Risk Factor Modification

There is no concluding evidence about the relation between the control of risk factors and mortality. The blood pressure goal in these patients should be the same as that in patients with hypertension and established cardiovascular disease. Lipid-lowering therapy reduces disease progression (as measured by angiography) and alleviates symptoms, and improvements in walking distance and pain-free walking time are seen. The goals for lipid levels are not clearly established [16].

Exercise Rehabilitation

Several studies have demonstrated the benefit of exercise rehabilitation programmes in reducing symptoms of claudication. There are available guidelines for exercise prescription.

Foot Care

The use of appropriate footwear to avoid pressure injuries, moisturising cream to prevent dryness and fissuring, daily inspection and cleansing by the patient and chiropody are necessary measures to reduce the risk of skin ulceration, necrosis and amputation. There are no studies evaluating their impact on older patients with diabetes and PAD.

Pharmacological Therapy

Drug therapy of claudication is aimed at symptomatic relief or slowing progression of the natural disease. The evidence of benefit is convincing only for antiplatelet agents, mainly aspirin and cilostazol.

Antiplatelet Therapy

All patients with evidence for atherosclerosis in other vascular beds should be prescribed an antiplatelet drug. Aspirin is the agent of choice; clopidogrel may be used if aspirin cannot be tolerated or in the patients with symptomatic PAD. Anticoagulation is not indicated.

Cilostazol

Cilostazol suppresses platelet aggregation and is a direct arterial vasodilator. Benefit may be noted as early as four weeks. However, its adverse effects, its contraindications (heart failure) and its interaction with other drugs and foods hamper its use in older people.

Revascularisation

There are two important criteria for revascularisation: severe disability that limits the patient's daily life with failure to respond to exercise rehabilitation and pharmacological therapy. These patients and patients with critical and acute limb ischaemia should be referred to a vascular surgeon [17].

Clinical Practice Question

Q1. A 92-year-old man attends his GP driving his own car, which he had to park in front of the main entrance since he is not able to walk along the pavement to access the building. Six months ago, he attended for his follow-up routine appointment for diabetes and he was able to walk that distance. Today, he feels palpitations while he is in the waiting room.

An electrocardiogram showed atrial fibrillation with a ventricular rate of 110 bpm, and an ankle–brachial index test gave a result of 0.4 on the left lower limb and 0.5 on the right.

How would you treat this patient?

Select all the options that apply:

A. Offer him aspirin or direct oral anticoagulants.
B. Offer him statins.
C. Offer bisoprolol for control of the atrial fibrillation rate, if needed.
D. Refer him for vascular surgical advice.
E. All of the above.

References

Key references only are listed here. For a full list of references visit: `https://www.wiley.com/go/sinclair/1e`.

3. Teo, K.K. and Rafiq, T. (2021). Cardiovascular risk factors and prevention: a perspective from developing countries. *Can. J. Cardiol.* 37 (5): 733–743.
4. Eid, M.A., Mehta, K.S., and Goodney, P.P. (2021). Epidemiology of peripheral artery disease. *Semin. Vasc. Surg.* 34 (1): 38–46.
5. Mueller, T., Hinterreiter, F., Luft, C. et al. (2014). Mortality rates and mortality predictors in patients with symptomatic peripheral artery disease stratified according to age and diabetes. *J. Vasc. Surg.* 59: 1291–1299.
6. McDermott, M.M., Liu, K., Greenland, P. et al. (2004). Functional decline in peripheral arterial disease: associations with the ankle brachial index and leg symptoms. *JAMA* 292 (4): 453–461.
7. Aboyans, V., Lacroix, P., and Criqui, M.H. (2007). Large and small vessels atherosclerosis: similarities and differences. *Prog. Cardiovasc. Dis.* 50: 112–125.
8. Criqui, M.H., Ninomiya, J.K., Wingard, D.L. et al. (2008). Progression of peripheral arterial disease predicts cardiovascular disease morbidity and mortality. *J. Am. Coll. Cardiol.* 52: 1736–1742.
11. Soysal, P., Arik, F., Jackson, S.E. et al. (2020). Inflammation, frailty and cardiovascular disease. *Adv. Exp. Med. Biol.* 1216: 55–64.
13. Gerhard-Herman, M.D., Gornik, H.L., Barrett, C. et al. (2017). 2016 AHA/ACC guideline on the management of patients with lower extremity peripheral artery disease: a report of the American College of Cardiology/

American Heart Association Task Force on Clinical Practice Guidelines. *J. Am. Coll. Cardiol.* 69 (11): e71–e126.
14. McDermott, M.M. (2018). Medical management of functional impairment in peripheral artery disease: a review. *Prog. Cardiovasc. Dis.* 60 (6): 586–592.
15. Sinclair, A.J., Paolisso, G., Castro, M. et al. (2011). European diabetes working party for older people 2011 clinical guidelines for type 2 diabetes mellitus. Executive Summary. *Diabetes Metab.* 37: S27–S38.

9b Macrovascular Complications: Coronary Arterial Disease

Leocadio Rodríguez-Mañas, Rubí E., Sandoval-Santoyo and Marta Castro Rodríguez

Geriatric Medicine Department, University Hospital of Getafe, Madrid, Spain

Key Points

- The clinical presentation of coronary artery disease in older patients with type 2 diabetes mellitus is often atypical, requiring a high degree of clinical suspicion and the need for complementary tests.
- Assessment of functional status, cognitive status and frailty may contribute to prognostic estimation and treatment choice in people over 75 years of age with type 2 diabetes and coronary heart disease.
- Optimising medical treatment for patients with coronary artery disease is substantially important. Regardless of conservative treatment or revascularisation, older patients will benefit from revision of treatment.

Epidemiology

Coronary artery disease (CAD) is a major cause of mortality in older adults and, even more relevant, is a leading cause of functional decline. Add to this, age is the strongest factor for developing CAD and the strongest factor for poor results once coronary atherosclerosis manifests. The risk factors are the same as those for peripheral arterial disease (PAD) but their contribution to CAD is different.

Care of Older People with Diabetes: A Manual for Healthcare Practice, First Edition.
Edited by Alan J. Sinclair and Ahmed H. Abdelhafiz.

Companion website: www.wiley.com/go/sinclair/1e

The prevalence of symptomatic CAD increases with age. The National Health and Nutrition Examination Survey and the Cardiovascular Health Study have reported a greater prevalence of coronary heart disease over 80 years of age. Moreover, 60% to over 90% of older individuals may have evidence of subclinical coronary atherosclerosis as assessed by coronary artery calcium, carotid intimal–medial thickness, stenosis and ankle–brachial index and that older patients are more likely to present with left main CAD, multivessel CAD and left ventricular dysfunction, which could contribute to worse outcomes [1].

Pathogenesis

Coronary artery disease has been described in PAD. Some differences appear, depending upon the vascular bed. The atherosclerotic plaques located in the lower limbs are very fibrous and may result in strictures. By contrast, when present at the coronary arteries, the atherosclerotic plaque usually consists of a large extracellular lipid core and a large number of foam cells, coated with a thin cover susceptible to breakage, which is the ultimate cause triggering the acute event.

Medical Treatment

Optimised medical treatment brings substantial benefits to older patients with CAD, whether treated conservatively or after revascularisation [2]. However, some specific recommendations for frail older people include the following:

- Aspirin remains one of the main drugs for secondary prevention of cardiovascular disease [3]. However, it has not shown any benefit for primary prevention in people over 70 years of age with T2DM and may also be harmful even in healthy older people [1].
- It is important to individualise dual antiplatelet therapy after acute coronary syndrome (ACS) or percutaneous coronary intervention, tailoring treatment to account for ischaemic protection and reduce the risk of bleeding, taking into account the risk–benefit ratio of each individual. Frailty is an independent predictor of bleeding.

- Nitrates relieve angina symptoms effectively and improve coronary blood flow by reducing the ischaemic burden on the heart and improving ischaemic symptoms, but caution should be exercised, as these drugs may cause hypotension and, hence, falls and fractures.
- Beta-blockers are prescribed in the early stages of ACS, if not contraindicated. They reduce myocardial oxygen demand and improve long-term outcomes. They should be used with caution in patients with heart failure, where beta-blockers with additional alpha-blocking properties, such as carvedilol, are preferable.
- Angiotensin-converting enzyme inhibitors have been shown to reduce mortality, admissions secondary to heart failure and improve outcomes in patients with ACS [3]. However, these benefits have not been proven in the subgroup of patients over 75 years of age or frail patients.

Indications for Revascularisation

The management of ACS in the older patient with diabetes faces several challenges, including multivessel disease or multiple coronary lesions.

Predictive tools such as Thrombolysis in Myocardial Infarction (TIMI) and the Global Registry of Acute Coronary Events (GRACE) are available for risk assessment and management. The reliability of the TIMI score in geriatric populations has been somewhat restricted [3]. The GRACE score has been validated in older adults, but accuracy decreases in this subgroup. Frailty, as measured by the Clinical Frailty Index, was an independent predictor of mortality and significantly improved the GRACE 12-month mortality estimate [4].

Current guidelines recommend the same invasive approaches in older adults as in younger patients, except those with ST-segment elevation and cardiogenic shock [1]. In ACS, coronary angiography with primary percutaneous coronary intervention is recommended in patients of all ages within two hours of symptom onset [3], although rates of ischaemia and bleeding after reperfusion are higher in older adults.

For non-ST-segment elevation ACS, current guidelines recommend coronary angiography and subsequent revascularisation if indicated but, in older people, the benefits of surgical treatment are controversial [3].

Management of Cardiovascular Risk Factors According to Baseline Functional and Cognitive Status

The use of conventional cardiovascular risk calculators is not appropriate for older adults [5]. Instead, it is recommended to assess functional status, including frailty and cognitive status, which have been shown to independently predict mortality in patients with coronary heart disease. Gait speed and grip strength have been shown to predict future cardiovascular events. These measures are preferable in older people with T2DM and CAD, as they are non-invasive, help to implement functional improvement interventions and to inform the goals and benefits of new interventions in these patients [6].

Effect of Glycaemic Control on Cardiovascular Events

Individualised follow-up after measurement of functional status and multimorbidity in older adults is often the best option: in healthy patients, haemoglobin A1C a target of <7.5%, for those with multimorbidities <8%, and for frail patients or those with a limited short-term life expectancy a target of <8.5% [6].

The use of sodium glucose transporter-2 inhibitors and glucagon-like peptide-1 receptor agonists, has demonstrated positive effects on cardiac (20–30% reduction in the risk of hospitalisation for heart failure) and renal outcomes (slowing of the progression of chronic kidney disease in patients with T2DM and overt nephropathy), in addition to the favourable effect on glycaemic control. Although this benefit has been demonstrated in the older age group (>65 years), it is still reasonable to express caution when using these agents in frail older people with diabetes, because of the high risk of adverse events in this group [7].

Effect of Blood Pressure Control

Lowering blood pressure to a cut-off point of 150 mmHg in older people, even in those over 90 years of age, is beneficial as in frail patients [8].

Lipid Monitoring

Several consensuses highlight that lipid-lowering therapies need a long time to provide benefit. For this reason, the potential risks may outweigh the benefits if they are given for a short period in older patients with a limited life expectancy [3].

Physical Exercise and Diet

The combination of diet and regular physical exercise has been shown to be effective against cardiovascular disease and functional status in older adults.

Frailty Management

Frailty and comprehensive assessment of older patients can guide diagnostic decisions and therapeutic goals. Frailty portends adverse cardiovascular events in older patients. Sometimes these patients benefit from specific interventions. The MID-Frail study, a randomised clinical trial aiming to evaluate the efficacy of a multimodal intervention (education, diet and resistance exercise) in frail and pre-frail subjects >70 years with T2DM has shown a clinically relevant and cost-effective improvement in functional status as measured by the Short Physical Performance Battery [9]. Frail patients with limited cognitive and functional status may not achieve meaningful goals of care with aggressive cardiac intervention, so symptom palliation and end-of-life discussions may be more appropriate.

Management

Older people with T2DM are at high risk for coronary heart disease and often present with atypical symptoms of acute and chronic coronary events, so a high level of suspicion should be maintained. Patients will benefit from complementary tests other than electrocardiography, which are sometimes only offered at second level. If suspicion of ACS is confirmed, the patient should be referred for myocardial enzyme measurement and echocardiogram.

If the patient presents with typical or atypical symptoms of stable CAD, a cardiology specialist should be consulted, and a geriatrician

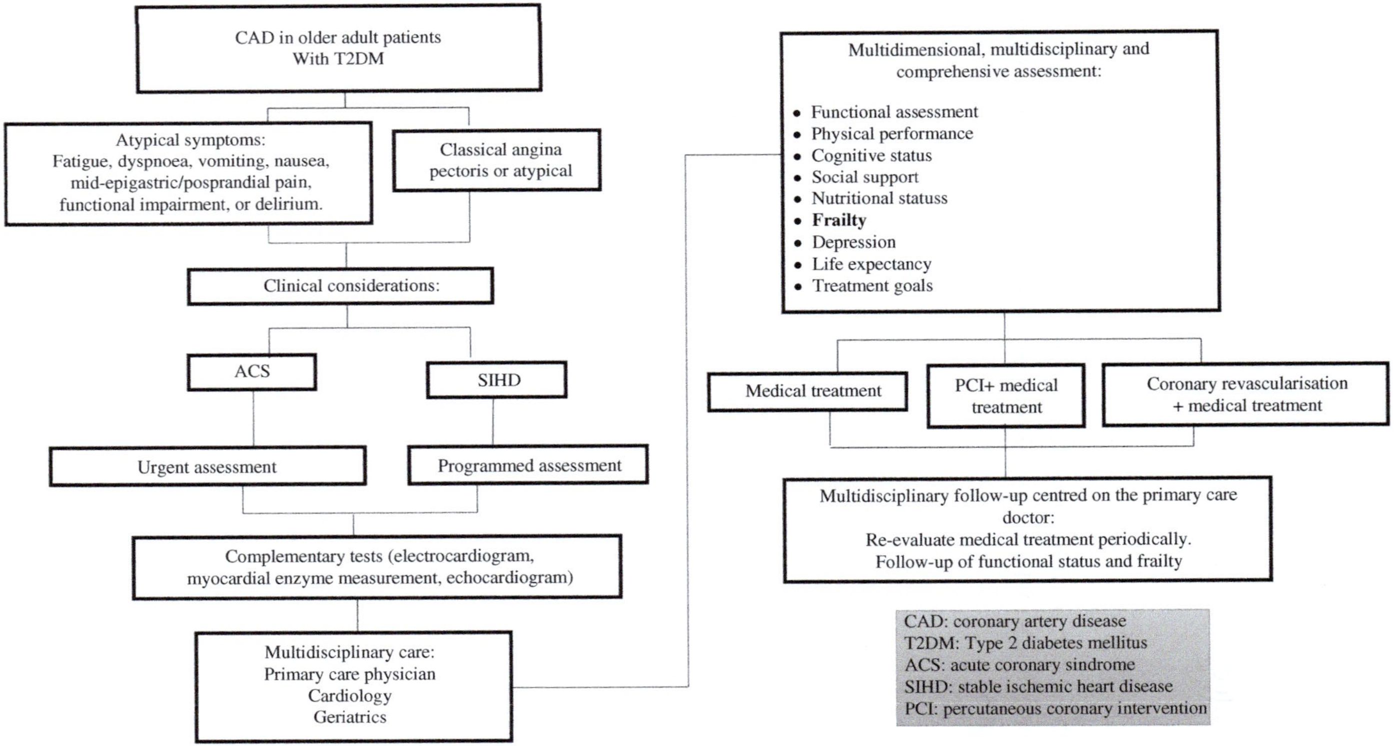

Figure 9b.1: Flowchart for referral to a specialist.

should be consulted if a comprehensive assessment is required, including functional and cognitive status, nutritional status and frailty screening to define therapeutic goals (Figure 9b.1) [10].

Summary

Type 2 diabetes mellitus is an independent risk factor for CAD. Patients with T2DM and CAD have an increased risk of mortality [1]. However, usual cardiovascular risk calculators are not useful in this population [5].

The preventive approach, diagnosis and therapeutic goals of older patients with diabetes mellitus and CAD should be established, taking into account functional status, cognitive status and frailty assessment.

Collaboration between healthcare professionals, including primary care physicians, cardiologists and geriatricians is essential to ensure optimal management of CAD in older adults, promoting both cardiovascular health and general wellbeing [3].

Clinical Practice Question

Q1. An 81-year-old woman who lives with her husband in a second-floor flat used to be independent for basic daily life activities (Barthel 100, Lawton 8, no cognitive impairment) but over the past three months she has had difficulty climbing stairs due to shortness of breath, so she stopped going out (shopping, etc). She has history of type 2 diabetes mellitus for 30 years and currently she is receiving treatment with metformin + linagliptin. She also suffers from hypertension and osteoarthrosis. She consulted her general practitioner with epigastric pain lasting 20 minutes, which had started while she was sitting on her armchair watching television and persisted on arrival, accompanied by a feeling of shortness of breath. What would be the most appropriate steps for her general practitioner to take? Choose one option:

A. Suspect coronary syndrome, perform an electrocardiogram and refer her to an emergency cardiology hospital for further tests to determine whether she is a candidate for a procedure.

B. Refer her to specialist on a scheduled basis for an echocardiogram.

C. Request laboratory tests to check for adequate metabolic control of her type 2 diabetes.

References

1. Madhavan, M.V., Gersh, B.J., Alexander, K.P. et al. (2018). Coronary artery disease in patients ≥80 years of age. *J. Am. Coll. Cardiol.* 71 (18): 2015–2040.
2. Sanchis, J., Bueno, H., Miñana, G. et al. (2023). Effect of routine invasive vs conservative strategy in older adults with frailty and non-ST-segment elevation acute myocardial infarction: a randomized clinical trial. *JAMA Intern. Med.* 183 (5): 407–415.
3. Marx, N., Federici, M., Schütt, K. et al. (2023). 2023 ESC guidelines for the management of cardiovascular disease in patients with diabetes. *Eur. Heart J.* 44 (39): 4043–4140.
4. Anand, A., Cudmore, S., Robertson, S. et al. (2020). Frailty assessment and risk prediction by GRACE score in older patients with acute myocardial infarction. *BMC Geriatr.* 20 (1): 102.
5. Vischer, U.M., Safar, M.E., Safar, H. et al. (2009). Cardiometabolic determinants of mortality in a geriatric population: is there a "reverse metabolic syndrome"? *Diabetes Metab.* 35 (2): 108–114.
6. Soler, P.A., Mañas, L., and Cortés, J.J. (ed.) (2020). *Tratado de medicina geriátrica: fundamentos de la atención sanitaria a los mayores*, 2e. Barcelona: Elsevier.
7. Abdelhafiz, A.H. and Sinclair, A.J. (2020). Cardio-renal protection in older people with diabetes with frailty and medical comorbidities – a focus on the new hypoglycaemic therapy. *J. Diabetes Complications* 34 (9): 107639.
8. Sinclair, A.J. and Abdelhafiz, A.H. (2020). Cardiometabolic disease in the older person: prediction and prevention for the generalist physician. *Cardiovasc. Endocrinol. Metab.* 9 (3): 90–95.
8. Rodriguez-Mañas, L., Laosa, O., Vellas, B. et al. (2019). Effectiveness of a multimodal intervention in functionally impaired older people with type 2 diabetes mellitus. *J. Cachexia. Sarcopenia Muscle* 10 (4): 721–733.
9. Cacciatore, S., Spadafora, L., Bernardi, M. et al. (2023). Management of coronary artery disease in older adults: recent advances and gaps in evidence. *J. Clin. Med.* 12 (16): 5233.

9c

Macrovascular Complications: Cerebrovascular Disease

Abubakhr Subkhan, Arshad Majid and Ali Ali

Department of Geriatrics and Neurosciences, Royal Hallamshire Hospital, Sheffield Teaching Hospitals NHS Foundation Trust, and the University of Sheffield, Sheffield, UK

Key Points

- Cerebrovascular disease is a major cause of death among patients with diabetes.
- The major cerebrovascular complications of diabetes are stroke and dementia.
- Many risk factors for cerebrovascular disease in diabetes are modifiable risk factors, which account for over 90% of the excess cardiovascular death in diabetes.
- Aggressive management of cerebrovascular disease risk factors is a major cornerstone of diabetes care and involves both behavioural and pharmacological approaches.

Introduction

In the complex interplay between diabetes and cardiovascular health, the connection to complications presents a significant challenge for healthcare practitioners. Cerebrovascular disease poses a considerable threat, with individuals contending with diabetes exhibiting an increased risk of experiencing a spectrum of cerebrovascular complications, including stroke (both haemorrhagic and ischaemic subtypes) and cerebral small vessel disease (CSVD). This chapter

Care of Older People with Diabetes: A Manual for Healthcare Practice, First Edition.
Edited by Alan J. Sinclair and Ahmed H. Abdelhafiz.

Companion website: www.wiley.com/go/sinclair/1e

focuses on the essential risk factors intricately wound into the fabric of the association of cerebrovascular disease with diabetes, unearthing novel insights into the molecular and genetic foundations that govern the heightened susceptibility of these individuals. Comprehensive management strategies are reviewed, exploring both pharmacological interventions and the increasingly recognised role of lifestyle modifications as well as prognosis of cerebrovascular events and complications in this population, synthesising recent findings to guide clinicians in prognosticating and mitigating the impact of cerebrovascular disease.

Epidemiology

The prevalence of diabetes has reached alarming proportions, affecting approximately 530 million people worldwide and posing a significant burden on healthcare systems with this number to double by 2050 [1]. This burden of disease has now spread from Western countries to the East and other developing nations, such that China now reports the highest number of adults with diabetes, over 90 million. Further, a substantial proportion of people with diabetes are confronted with an elevated risk of cerebrovascular disease. Notably, individuals with diabetes face a 2.5–3.5 times higher lifetime risk of developing stroke compared with those without diabetes [2]. This association extends beyond type 1 diabetes, with type 2 diabetes accounting for many cases and demonstrating a particularly robust link to cerebrovascular complications. In patients with recognised stroke disease, 20–25% have known diabetes with a further 20% new diagnoses made in the 12 weeks after stroke [3]. Similarly, in people living with dementia, up to 20% are known to have diabetes, thus the burden of diabetes in cerebrovascular disease is great.

Risk Factors

Multiple risk factors have been associated with the development of cardiovascular disease in diabetes and reflect a complex interplay between genetics and environmental factors. Ageing and hypertension are the major risk factors for stroke, together with other traditional cardiovascular factors (Box 9c.1).

Box 9c.1: Recognised Risk Factors for Cerebrovascular Disease in Diabetes

- Hypertension
- Dyslipidaemia
- Smoking
- Physical inactivity
- Obesity
- Chronic kidney disease and albuminuria
- Female gender
- Increasing age
- Family history-stroke in first-degree relative men aged <55 years or women <65 years
- Elevated inflammatory markers (e.g. C-reactive protein)

Aetiology and Pathophysiology

The link between diabetes and cerebrovascular complications is intricate and multifaceted, driven by a convergence of metabolic, inflammatory, and endothelial dysfunction pathways Prolonged exposure to hyperglycaemia triggers the production of advanced glycation end-products and activates multiple pathways, including the polyol, hexosamine and protein kinase C pathways. These pathways lead to oxidative stress, endothelial dysfunction, inflammation and increased deposition of extracellular matrix proteins within blood vessels. Hyperglycaemia-induced oxidative stress and inflammation disrupt the balance between vasodilators and vasoconstrictors promoting vasoconstriction, platelet aggregation and leukocyte adhesion [4]. Consequently, this creates a prothrombotic and proinflammatory milieu conducive to atherosclerosis and vascular complications (Figure 9c.1).

Presentation

The spectrum of cerebrovascular disease in diabetes spans ischaemic and haemorrhagic stroke as well as CSVD, which predisposes to dementia (Figure 9c.2). The clinical presentation of stroke or transient ischaemic attack (TIA) is often acute, while that of CSVD and dementia is indolent and gradual.

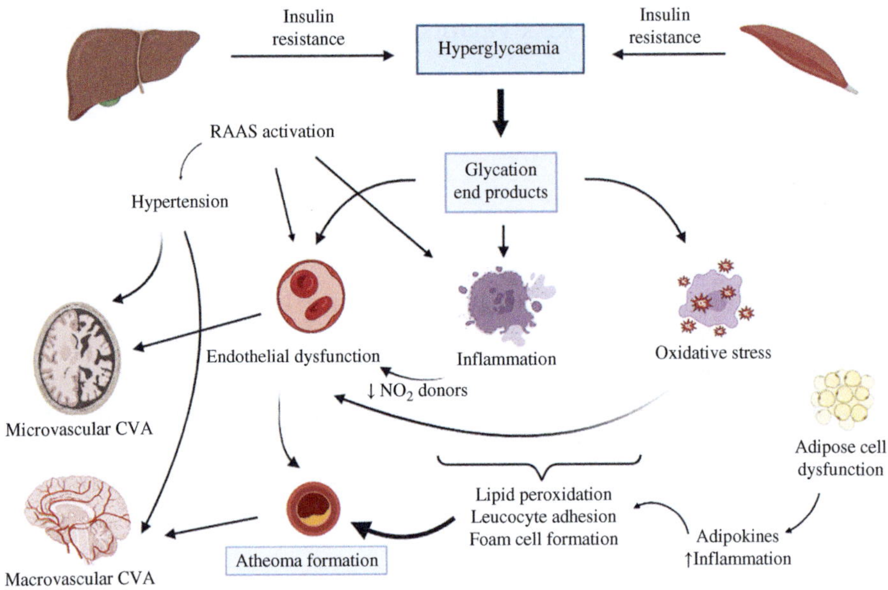

Figure 9c.1: Pathophysiology of cerebrovascular disease in diabetes. RAAS, renin–angiotensin–aldosterone system; NO, nitric oxide; CVA, cerebrovascular accident.

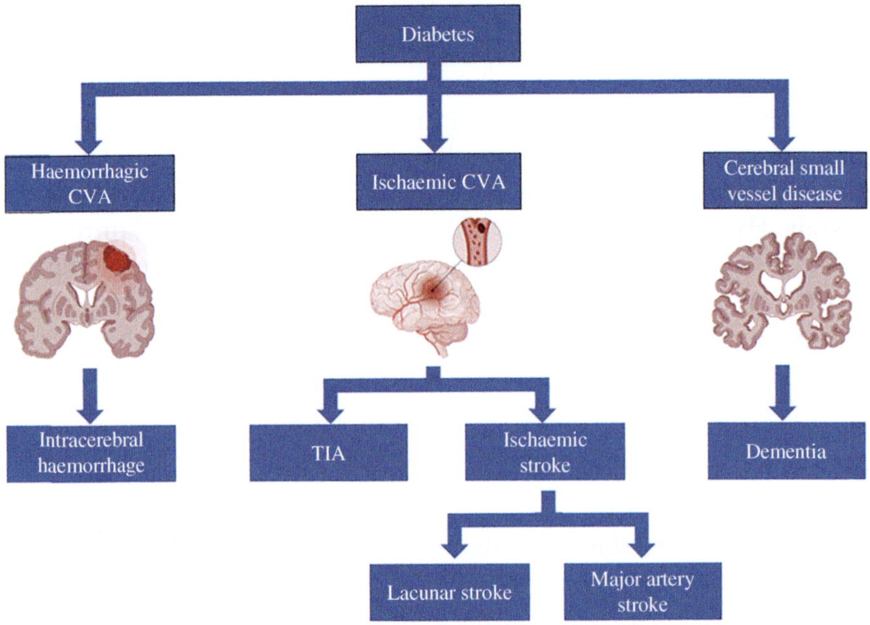

Figure 9c.2: Spectrum of cerebrovascular accident (CVA) presentation. TIA, transient ischaemic attack.

Stroke and Transient Ischaemic Attack

Diabetes increases the risk of first ever stroke up to fourfold and doubles the risk of stroke recurrence in those already affected by stroke. Further, clinical outcomes including mortality are poorer in those with diabetes. Worsening glycaemic control further increases this risk such that in the United Kingdom Prospective Diabetes Study a 1% increase in haemoglobin A1c (HbA1c) was associated with a 37% increased risk of death from stroke [5]. People experiencing both ischaemic and haemorrhagic types of stroke may present with sudden-onset focal neurological symptoms such as facial asymmetry, motor weakness, sensory loss, speech impairment (either aphasia or dysarthria), neglect, visual field defect, diplopia, ataxia or dysphagia depending on arterial territory affected. Approximately 10–15% of patients also present with seizures or altered consciousness. It is not possible to differentiate ischaemic from haemorrhagic types clinically; this requires neuroimaging such as computed tomography and magnetic resonance imaging. Evidence suggests that lacunar infarcts resulting from occlusion of small penetrating arterioles are more common among people with diabetes, however the GRASP (Glucose Regulation in Acute Ischaemic Stroke Patients) study showed that over 70% of all strokes in diabetics were still non-lacunar [6]. By its very nature, symptoms of TIA are transient, with 90% of individuals experiencing symptoms that last less than 60 minutes, with the vast majority less than 10 minutes. It should be noted also that 'silent infarcts', those that do not produce major neurological symptoms, are more common in patients with diabetes and contribute to the incidence of cognitive impairment.

Cerebral Small Vessel Disease and Dementia

Cerebral small vessel disease progresses silently and leads to an accumulation of subcortical white matter damage, which results in a gradual decline in short-term recall, gait, dexterity, executive function, language and, eventually, to the clinical picture of dementia. Often, there are intervals of acute 'stepwise' deterioration that are common in vascular subtypes of dementia. Type 2 diabetes mellitus (T2DM) is a robust predictor of cognitive impairment and decline in older adults. Population based studies show that people with T2DM experience a twofold increased rate of cognitive decline over a five-year period compared with people without diabetes. Further, meta-analytical data demonstrates a 56% increased lifetime risk of developing Alzheimer's disease and a twofold increased risk of vascular dementia among those with T2DM [7]. These associations may be due to the impact that diabetes has on neurogenesis, blood–brain barrier function, central nervous system inflammation, episodes of hyper- and hypoglycaemia and microvascular dysfunction.

Management of Cerebrovascular Disease

Management of cerebrovascular disease in diabetes can be divided into acute management (stroke and TIA) and risk factors management (all cerebrovascular diseases). Overall management strategies are similar whether or not individuals have diabetes; however, there are specific aspects of care that warrant particular consideration in diabetes (Table 9c.1).

Acute Stroke

When patients present with vascular occlusions in acute ischaemic stroke, urgent consideration of reperfusion therapies, thrombolysis or thrombectomy, is required to save the ischaemic penumbra and enhance chances of neurological recovery. It is recognised that both hyperglycaemia and hypoglycaemia can mimic the symptoms of acute stroke and thus ensuring normoglycaemia in a patient that presents to the hyperacute stroke unit is required prior to consideration of reperfusion. While individuals with diabetes who are otherwise eligible will still derive benefit from these therapies, there outcomes following thrombolysis and thrombectomy are worse compared with patients without diabetes, relating mainly to an approximate doubled risk of intracranial bleeding following treatment. It is thought that this risk is raised due to a heightened risk of reperfusion injury in hyperglycaemia, as recanalisation rates are similar [8]. Admission hyperglycaemia is also associated with early neurological deterioration and higher inpatient complication rates, such as pneumonia, in both ischaemic and haemorrhagic strokes. However, attempts to normalise blood glucose acutely after stroke have not improved outcomes. On the contrary, the Glucose Insulin in Stroke

Table 9c.1: Summary of acute stroke management considerations in diabetes.

Aspect of care	Issue	Practical management
Acute stroke diagnosis	Hypo/ hyperglycaemia can mimic acute stroke	Ensure that blood sugar is checked urgently in stroke assessment
Thrombolysis and thrombectomy	Increased risk of intracerebral bleeding with reperfusion therapy	Counsel patient with diabetes that intracerebral haemorrhage rates may be higher (up to twice), but that they are likely to still benefit
Hyperacute and acute phase of care	Higher risk of early neurological deterioration and complications	Close monitoring of blood sugars, 4- to 6-hourly, and aim for levels 5–12 mg/dl
Dysphagia and feeding	Controlling blood sugars in patients who are nil by mouth or have enteral feeding tubes	VRII for those nil by mouth who do not have feeding tubes. Always continue background long-acting insulins during VRII. Match insulin regimen to feeding regimen (e.g. split dose insulin for continuous enteral feeding) 50% at start of feed and then 50% halfway through. Bolus insulin 20 minutes before feed bolus with background insulin for bolus feeding

VRII, variable-rate insulin infusion.

Trial demonstrated that tight glucose control using a variable insulin sliding scale was associated with worsening of neurological outcomes. This is probably because of the total reliance of the brain on glucose for energy substrate and the more frequent occurrence of hypoglycaemic episodes with insulin therapy [9]. Thus, finger-prick glucose levels in the range 5–12 mg/dl are recommended, alongside close monitoring for hypoglycaemia four to six hourly. Dysphagia occurs in up to 60% of individuals with stroke, among whom a significant proportion have such severe dysphagia that they are deemed nil by mouth. For type 1 diabetes, this will necessitate the interim use of a variable rate insulin infusion until an enteral feeding tube is placed. It is important to continue any long-acting insulin analogues during this process if they were previously prescribed. Once feed is established, a subcutaneous insulin regimen can be restarted. The regimen may need to be adjusted initially to account for the total carbohydrate load in the new enteral feed regimen and the way the feed is given (continuous infusion verse bolus feeding), so close liaison with dietetics will be required. However, a common regimen for continuous feeds includes using a premixed (30/70) human insulin spilt into two doses, 50% given at the start of the feed and then the other 50% halfway through (e.g. at 10 hours for a 20-hour feed infusion). For bolus feeding, long-acting insulin can be maintained in the background while single doses of soluble mixed insulin given 20 minutes prior to the feed is a commonly used regimen.

Management of Risk Factors

Management of risk factors remains the cornerstone of reducing risk of recurrence of stroke and TIA and slowing progression of CSVD, and thus reducing the morbidity and mortality associated with diabetes. A large prospective study indicated that cerebrovascular disease risk in people with diabetes who met target ranges of HbA1c, blood pressure, lipid profiles, smoking status and albuminuria was similar or only slightly increased compared with age- and sex-matched controls without diabetes. However, in the United States, only around 7% of individuals meet these targets. Ensuring that these risk factors are aggressively managed is of paramount importance and drive treatment targets (Table 9c.2). Physical activity of at least 150 minutes of moderate to vigorous exercise per week will reduce the risk of cerebrovascular disease [10]. Healthy diet and weight loss improve insulin sensitivity and glycaemic control, and reduce other cardiovascular risk factors such as hypertension and dyslipidaemia. Smoking cessation is a critical component of managing diabetes and cerebrovascular disease risk. A populational Korean study of nearly 350 000 people with T2DM showed that smoking cessation was associated with a 20% reduction in risk of myocardial infarction and stroke over five years compared with those who did not stop [11]. Use of e-cigarettes and vaping is generally not recommended to aid smoking cessation. While the link between poor glycaemic control and cerebrovascular disease risk is clear, evidence supporting interventions to improve glycaemic control are equivocal. However, an HbA1c goal of less than 7% (53 mmol/mol) for most patients with diabetes is reasonable. Blood pressure control and cholesterol-lowering therapy are of great importance in cerebrovascular

Table 9c.2: General targets for cerebrovascular disease risk reduction in diabetes.

Aspect of care	Target
Physical activity	At least 150 minutes of moderate-to-vigorous physical activity per week. At least 75 minutes vigorous physical activity per week in younger more physically able individuals. At least 20 minutes 2–3 times per week of resistance exercises
Glycaemic control	HbA1c < 7% (53 mmol/mol); less stringent in the very old or frail, or for those prone to hypoglycaemic episodes
Blood pressure	Aim for blood pressure < 120/80 mmHg. Consider single antihypertensive if ≥ 130/80 mmHg and two agents if ≥ 160/100 mmHg
Cholesterol	High-intensity statins for all patients presenting with ischaemic stroke or TIA. Consider addition of ezetimibe or PCSK9 inhibition in high-risk individuals where these targets cannot be achieved
Antiplatelet therapy	Aspirin for primary prevention is not routinely recommended. Dual antiplatelets (aspirin in combination with clopidogrel, prasugrel or ticagrelor) for 3 weeks following mild acute stroke and TIA, followed by long-term clopidogrel monotherapy. Consider bleeding risk in individual cases

TIA, transient ischaemic attack.

disease risk reduction. Aspirin is not routinely recommended as a primary prevention but is frequently used for secondary prevention of stroke in diabetes. Following stroke, aspirin in combination with a P2Y12 inhibitor (clopidogrel, prasugrel or ticagrelor) should be used for around three weeks following minor stroke and TIA, following which aspirin can be discontinued. For people with stable coronary, carotid or peripheral vascular disease and low bleeding risk, a combination therapy using aspirin and low-dose rivaroxaban (a direct anticoagulant) supports longer term cerebrovascular disease risk reduction.

Prognosis

Development of cerebrovascular disease in diabetes is accelerated and presents at an earlier age than in patients without diabetes. Outcomes in almost all cerebrovascular disease complications, including ischaemic and haemorrhagic stroke, TIA and CSVD is worse both for types 1 and 2 diabetes, and seems to be related to both severity of illness and response to treatments. For example, studies have demonstrated higher rates of carotid artery restenosis following carotid endarterectomy and carotid artery stenting in patients with diabetes [12]. Overall, individuals with diabetes are nearly 30% less likely to return to independence following thrombolysis and thrombectomy and have a twofold higher 30-day mortality for stroke compared with patients without diabetes [13].

Summary

Cerebrovascular disease is a major burden in people with diabetes compared with those without diabetes. It is clear that optimising vascular risk factors is pivotal to reduce the burden of cerebrovascular disease in diabetes and will involve a coordinated and multidisciplinary approach to managing the multifaceted nature of diabetes-related cerebrovascular disease. Timely and tailored treatment strategies, lifestyle and dietary modifications, patient education, and adherence to medications are integral components in improving outcomes and enhancing prognosis for people with diabetes and cerebrovascular disease.

Clinical Practice Question

Q1. A 58 year-old man with type 1 diabetes and hypertension, not normally on any antithrombotic therapy is brought in by paramedics to the acute stroke unit suspected of having suffered a stroke. Computed tomography radiography of the brain confirms no intracerebral bleeding, his blood pressure is 158/87 mmHg, and they are within the time window for thrombolysis. They are drowsy (Glasgow Coma Scale score 12/15) and it is clear that they will not be able to swallow as a consequence of their presentation. Choose the most appropriate management plan.

- **A.** Administer thrombolysis immediately and then check the blood glucose to decide whether a variable-rate insulin infusion is required.
- **B.** Check the blood glucose first and, if it is normal, administer thrombolysis then institute a variable-rate insulin infusion to ensure tight glycaemic control in the hyperacute period.

C. Check blood glucose first and, if it is normal, administer thrombolysis and monitor blood glucose closely afterwards, aiming for a target of between 5 and 12 mg/dl.
D. Administer thrombolysis and insert an enteral feeding tube so that his regular insulin can be delivered as normal with his enteral feed.

References

Key references only are listed here. For a full list of references visit: `https://www.wiley.com/go/sinclair/1e`.

1. Standl, E., Khunti, K., Hansen, T.B. et al. (2019). The global epidemics of diabetes in the 21st century: current situation and perspectives. *Eur. J. Prev. Cardiol.* 26: 7–14.
2. Bunn, F., Goodman, C., Malone, J.R. et al. (2016). Managing diabetes in people with dementia: protocol for a realist review. *Syst. Rev.* 5: 5.
3. Leon, B.M. and Maddox, T.M. (2015). Diabetes and cardiovascular disease: epidemiology, biological mechanisms, treatment recommendations and future research. *World J. Diabetes* 6: 1246–1258.
6. Johnston, K.C., Hall, C.E., Kissela, B.M. et al. (2009). Glucose regulation in acute stroke patients (GRASP) trial: a randomized pilot trial. *Stroke* 40: 3804–3809.
7. Cholerton, B., Baker, L.D., Montine, T.J. et al. (2016). Type 2 diabetes, cognition, and dementia in older adults: toward a precision health approach. *Diabetes Spectr.* 29: 210–219.
8. Lu, G.D., Ren, Z.Q., Zhang, J.X. et al. (2018). Effects of diabetes mellitus and admission glucose in patients receiving mechanical thrombectomy: a systematic review and meta-analysis. *Neurocrit. Care* 29: 426–434.
10. Colberg, S.R., Sigal, R.J., Yardley, J.E. et al. (2016). Physical activity/exercise and diabetes: a position statement of the American Diabetes Association. *Diabetes Care* 39: 2065–2079.
11. Jeong, S.M., Yoo, J.E., Park, J. et al. (2023). Smoking behavior change and risk of cardiovascular disease incidence and mortality in patients with type 2 diabetes mellitus. *Cardiovasc. Diabetol.* 22: 193.
12. Achim, A., Lackó, D., Hüttl, A. et al. (2022). Impact of diabetes mellitus on early clinical outcome and stent restenosis after carotid artery stenting. *J. Diabetes Res.* 2022: 4196195.
13. Zhou, H., Zhang, X., and Lu, J. (2014). Progress on diabetic cerebrovascular diseases. *Bosn. J. Basic Med. Sci.* 14: 185–190.

10a Microvascular Complications: Diabetic Eye Disease

Archith Kamath[1] *and Nachiketa Acharya*[2]

[1] *Princess Alexandra Eye Pavilion, NHS Lothian, Edinburgh, UK*
[2] *Directorate of Ophthalmology, Royal Hallamshire Hospital, Sheffield Teaching Hospitals NHS Trust, Sheffield, UK*

Key Points

- Chronic hyperglycaemia affects the retina by damaging the microvasculature, causing chronic inflammation and mediating retinal neurodegeneration.
- Diabetic retinopathy is visible on fundoscopy as microaneurysms, dot–blot haemorrhages, lipid exudates, cotton wool spots and, ultimately, neovascularisation.
- Diabetic retinopathy is a progressive and often irreversible cause of visual loss due to neovascularisation and macular oedema, which may be asymptomatic until later stages.
- Specialist treatments include laser, intraocular steroids, intravitreal anti-vascular endothelial growth factor and vitrectomy surgery.
- Primary prevention is the best treatment with tight glycaemic control, management of risk factors and regular screening.

Care of Older People with Diabetes: A Manual for Healthcare Practice, First Edition.
Edited by Alan J. Sinclair and Ahmed H. Abdelhafiz.

Companion website: www.wiley.com/go/sinclair/1e

Introduction

Diabetes mellitus is a leading cause of blindness both in the United Kingdom (UK) and around the world; however, with appropriate recognition and timely intervention, this can often be prevented or slowed [1]. Diabetic retinopathy (DR) and its complications are the main mechanisms of visual loss and are the primary focus of this chapter, but diabetes is also associated with increased incidence of cataract and glaucoma, both of which are also cause of visual loss [2].

Epidemiology

The global prevalence of DR is estimated to be around 35% in patients with diabetes. The prevalence increases with increased duration of disease, poor glycaemic control and is more common in type 1 diabetes mellitus [3]. Older people are more likely to be affected by retinopathy (due to long duration of diabetes) and the resulting visual loss. Many of the treatments to halt the progression of DR to the later stages are initiated by specialists. However, the mainstay of managing DR is primary prevention, by promoting optimum glycaemic control and encouraging patients to enrol in the national screening programme. Controlling other vascular risk factors, such as hypertension and dyslipidaemia, is also crucial in preventing diabetes-related visual loss. An understanding of DR can help non-ophthalmic healthcare professionals to counsel their patients on how best to protect their eyes.

Presentation

Patients with DR may experience a variety of non-specific symptoms, so it is important to be aware of how they may present. An understanding of the clinical and fundoscopic signs described below is helpful; however, identifying potential presenting features of DR in a patient with or without an existing diagnosis of diabetes may save their vision. DR is often asymptomatic until its later stages, but patients may experience features, such as blurred or distorted vision, floaters or complete vision loss. Features may be unilateral or bilateral, and should be urgently investigated with appropriate blood tests and referrals if necessary. If there were any uncertainty, discussion with local ophthalmology team (on-call doctor or triage nurse) for advice on how to proceed would be appropriate.

Pathophysiology

There are two main subtypes of DR recognised, which may be further substratified to help guide urgency of referral. The first is non-proliferative DR, characterised by damage to the retinal vessels without new vessel growth. The second is proliferative DR (PDR), in which hypoxia induces new vessel formation (neovascularisation). Diabetes-related hyperglycaemia damages both the vascular and neural aspects of the retina, which leads visual loss occurring due to two main pathological processes:

1. Retinal neovascularisation leading to haemorrhage and detachment.
2. Oedema of the macula (the sensitive part of the retina responsible for central vision).

Diabetic retinopathy is a microvascular complication of diabetes. Microvascular damage is predominantly mediated by chronic hyperglycaemia and the resultant activation of alternative pathways of glucose metabolism [4]. On fundoscopic examination, microvascular damage presents with microaneurysms, dot–blot haemorrhages, lipid exudates, cottonwool spots (focal areas of ischaemia) and, ultimately, neovascularisation (Table 10a.1) [5]. Circulatory damage and resultant hypoxia induce the production of vascular endothelial growth factor (VEGF), which is a driver of retinal neovascularisation and oedema. For colour photographs of the fundoscopic abnormalities in DR, we recommend consulting the standard photographs from the Early Treatment of Diabetic Retinopathy Study (ETDRS), the historical gold standard for grading DR. We have also included some example fundus photographs in Figure 10a.1.

Many of the existing therapeutic options available for established DR target the microvascular pathology, including anti-VEGF therapies and laser photocoagulation. The role of chronic hyperglycaemia in inducing microvascular changes reinforces the importance of primary prevention of diabetic retinopathy by tightly controlling blood glucose and other vascular risk factors. Chronic low-grade inflammation and retinal

Table 10a.1: United Kingdom national screening guidelines for diabetic retinopathy [5].

Stage	Findings	Appearance	Action
Diabetic retinopathy			
R0	No retinopathy	None	Annual screening
R1	Mild/moderate NPDR	Microaneurysms, dot-blot haemorrhages, exudates	Frequent screening
R2	Severe NPDR	Intraretinal microvascular abnormality, cotton wool spots ± the above	Frequent screening ophthalmology referral
R3	PDR	New vessels on disc, haemorrhage, fibrous proliferation ± the above	Urgent ophthalmology referral
Macular disease			
M0	Criteria in M1 not met		Annual screening
M1	Maculopathy	Exudates/ thickening/ haemorrhage or microaneurysms near the macula	Ophthalmology referral
Non-specific findings			
Unclassifiable	Any uncertainty		Refer for further examination

NPDR, non-proliferative diabetic retinopathy; PDR, proliferative diabetic retinopathy.

neurodegeneration by apoptosis are proposed additional pathophysiological mechanisms in DR, independently from microvascular changes, but also due to hyperglycaemia and oxidative stress [6]. These may prove to be attractive targets for future trials in the prevention and/or treatment of DR.

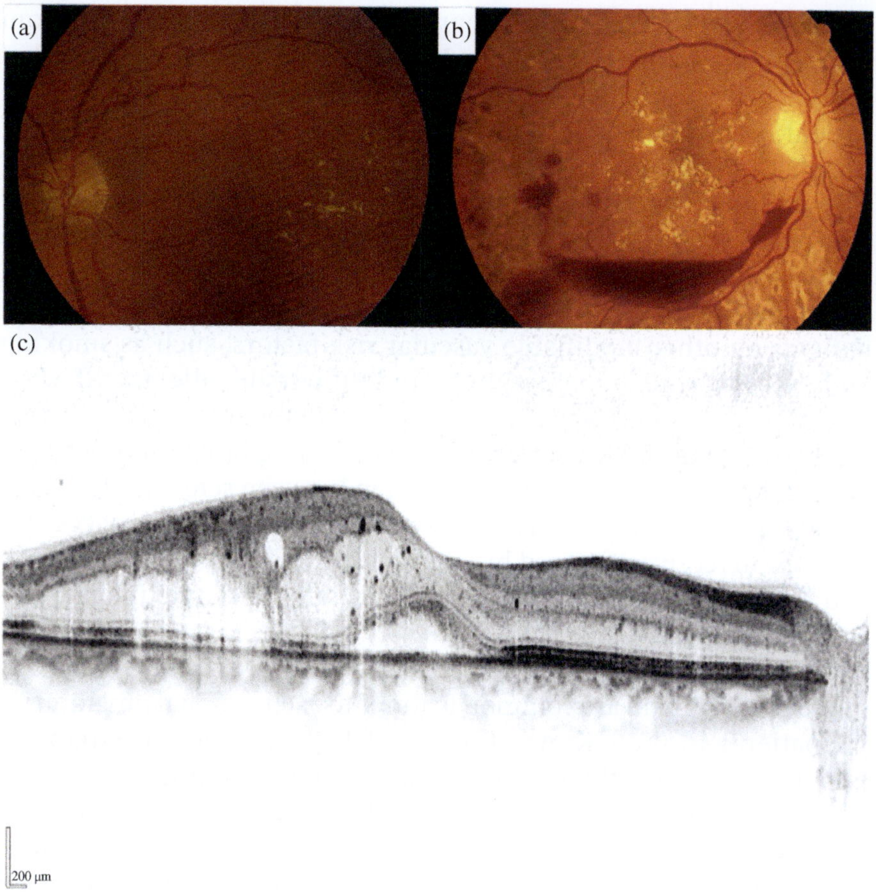

Figure 10a.1: Fundus photographs showing: (a) non-proliferative diabetic retinopathy with diabetic maculopathy; (b) proliferative diabetic retinopathy with preretinal haemorrhage; (c) Optical coherence tomography scan showing macular oedema.

Management

Primary Care

We have alluded many times so far to the importance of preventing DR from developing, as this is the best way to ensure that vision is protected. While this may be considered to be under the remit of public health specialists, we feel that it is the responsibility of all healthcare professionals involved in the care of patients with diabetes, from primary care to ophthalmology. Measures must be implemented at every level: nationally, regionally and at the level of the individual patient. Controlling risk factors also helps to slow the progression of established DR [7].

In addition to controlling blood glucose levels (crucial as much of the damage is mediated directly by hyperglycaemia), DR progression can also be slowed by controlling blood pressure and serum lipid levels. Due to the microvascular pathophysiology, it is also valuable to counsel patients on other modifiable vascular risk factors, such as smoking and excess alcohol consumption, and on possible dietary/lifestyle modifications. Finally, it is vital to ensure that patients are enrolled on the National Health Service retinal screening programme and are vigilant for any changes in their vision in between screening appointments. When receiving a referral to secondary diabetic eye services, it is essential to receive a focused history to help guide further investigation and management. A summary of helpful information to include can be seen in Figure 10a.2.

Diabetic retinopathy screening varies slightly across different regions in the UK, but there are common features to each regional programme. All patients in the UK over the age of 12 years who have diabetes mellitus are currently offered annual retinal screening, although a risk-based two-yearly recall is being trialled in certain parts of the UK. The DR screening classification system used in most of the UK is summarised in Table 10a.1, together with the recommended action based on fundoscopic findings. It is important to recognise signs of DR, as patients are often asymptomatic at the time of presentation, particularly in the absence of maculopathy. However, healthcare professionals outside eye-care specialties would not be expected to risk-stratify their patients accurately based on fundoscopic appearances. The screening programme has been an effective population-level intervention. Since its implementation around 20 years ago, there has been a reduction in the vision impairment due to diabetic eye disease [8]. Most patients (around 80%) receive retinal screening appropriately, but there is considerable variation in uptake, with factors such as younger age, duration of diabetes and social deprivation associated with poorer attendance. It is often helpful to signpost patients to their local eye clinic liaison officer, who may be able to direct them to relevant community groups that can provide appropriate support and discussion around helping to understand diabetic eye disease.

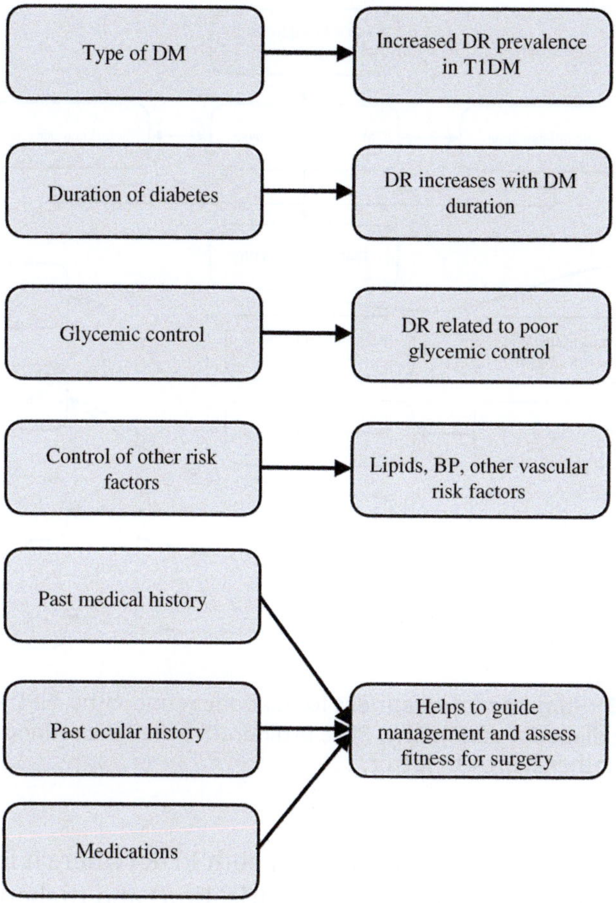

Figure 10a.2: Focused history to help guide ophthalmic investigation and management of suspected diabetic retinopathy (DR). BP, blood pressure; DM, diabetes mellitus; T1DM, type 1 diabetes mellitus.

Secondary Care

Treatments for sight-threatening DR are initiated by specialists, and include laser photocoagulation, intravitreal anti-VEGF, intraocular steroids and vitrectomy surgery [9]. These specialist treatments are summarised in Figure 10a.3 but are only covered briefly to help in advising patients of what may be offered to them after referral. Specialists will also usually perform further investigations such as optical coherence tomography to visualise the retinal layers and risk stratify existing disease more clearly.

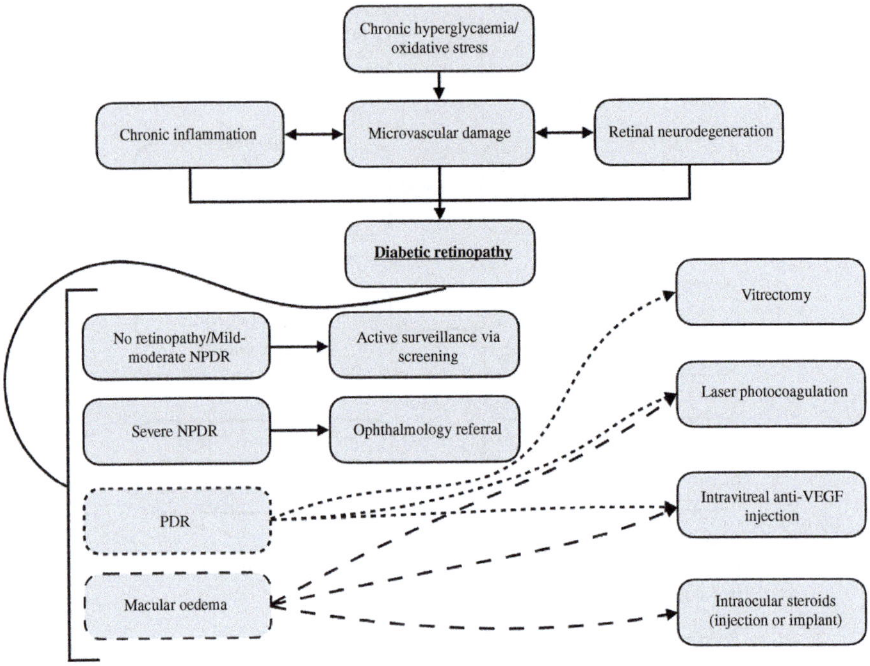

Figure 10a.3: Summary of treatment for diabetic retinopathy. NPDR, non-proliferative diabetic retinopathy; PDR, proliferative diabetic retinopathy; VEGF, vascular endothelial growth factor.

Laser photocoagulation is helpful in both PDR (where it is used pan-retinally to reduce further neovascularisation) and diabetic macular oedema (where it is used more focally, and has largely been superceded by anti-VEGF injections). Laser is used to create superficial thermal burns to the retina. Patients experience visual loss in the areas burnt by the laser, but this well-established treatment is known to be effective at protecting vision in most cases. Intravitreal anti-VEGF injections are a newer treatment option that has revolutionised the treatment of both macular oedema and, increasingly, PDR. This treatment has been shown to be superior to laser photocoagulation alone, and a number of anti-VEGF agents are licensed in the UK for this use [9]. Intravitreal anti-VEGF is not suitable for some patients, though, as it requires frequent follow-up and reinjection, particularly at the start of treatment (usually monthly).

Intraocular steroids are an alternative in such patients and are particularly effective in those with macular oedema. Steroids may be given via intravitreal injection (longer follow-up interval than anti-VEGF) or implant. However, the use of steroids is falling out of favour due to the higher rates of complications such as cataract and glaucoma. Vitrectomy surgery is rarely used as a first-line treatment, but is an option in patients with PDR if there are significant non-resolving retinal or vitreous haemorrhages or traction on the retina. Retinal surgery is also necessary in cases of tractional retinal detachment due to PDR.

Summary

Diabetic retinopathy is a gradually progressive but preventable cause of visual loss and blindness caused by chronic hyperglycaemia. While a number of specialist treatments exist for established disease, the best treatment is prevention by controlling diabetes and other vascular risk factors. Non-specialists play a crucial role in signposting patients to national retinal screening to ensure any disease is picked up in a timely manner to prevent devastating visual loss, and by referring appropriate cases to secondary care.

Clinical Practice Questions

Q1. A 75-year-old man with history of type 2 diabetes mellitus for 20 years presents to his general practitioner for review of routine blood results. His haemoglobin A1c, lipids and blood pressure are within the acceptable range. He has no visual symptoms, and fundoscopic examination is normal other than a few microaneurysms, but he has not attended any retinal screening appointments for the past five years. What is the most appropriate response?
Choose one option:

A. Urgent referral to ophthalmology service due to missing appointments.
B. Reschedule him in the regular screening programme.
C. It is unlikely that he has diabetic retinopathy in view of absent symptoms, so no action is necessary.
D. Microaneurysms alone are not diagnostic of diabetic retinopathy, so no action is necessary.
E. Controlled diabetes mellitus and risk factors put him at low risk of diabetic retinopathy so he does not need to be followed up.

Q2. A 65-year-old patient with type 1 diabetes presents to her general practitioner (GP) with gradually progressive visual loss in both eyes and new flashes/floaters, worse in the left eye since this morning. She has never attended retinal screening. Fundoscopic examination is challenging, but the GP wonders whether there is increased redness in both eyes, and a shadow at the back of the left eye. What is the most appropriate action?

Choose one option:

A. Urgent ophthalmology referral.
B. Optician assessment of her reduced visual acuity.
C. Refer her to routine retinal screening.
D. Prescribe antibiotic eye drops for her red eyes.
E. Check routine bloods to ensure tight glycaemic control.

References

1. Flaxman, S.R., RRA, B., Resnikoff, S. et al. (2017). Global causes of blindness and distance vision impairment 1990-2020: a systematic review and meta-analysis. *Lancet Glob. Health* 5: e1221–e1234.
2. National Institute of Diabetes and Digestive and Kidney Diseases (2017). Diabetic eye disease. https://www.niddk.nih.gov/health-information/diabetes/overview/preventing-problems/diabetic-eye-disease (accessed 26 October 2023).
3. Yau, J.W.Y., Rogers, S.L., Kawasaki, R. et al. (2012). Global prevalence and major risk factors of diabetic retinopathy. *Diabetes Care* 35: 556–564.
4. Cai, J. and Boulton, M. (2002). The pathogenesis of diabetic retinopathy: old concepts and new questions. *Eye* 16: 242–260.
5. Scanlon, P.H. (2017). The English National Screening Programme for diabetic retinopathy 2003–2016. *Acta Diabetol.* 54: 515–525.
6. Wang, W. and Lo, A.C.Y. (2018). Diabetic retinopathy: pathophysiology and treatments. *Int. J. Mol. Sci.* 19: 1816.
7. Dowler, J. Diabetic retinopathy. BMJ Best Practice 2024. https://bestpractice.bmj.com/topics/en-gb/532 (accessed 26 October 2023).
8. Lawrenson, J.G., Bourmpaki, E., Bunce, C. et al. (2021). Trends in diabetic retinopathy screening attendance and associations with vision impairment attributable to diabetes in a large nationwide cohort. *Diabetic Med.* 38: e14425.
9. Duh, E.J., Sun, J.K., and Stitt, A.W. Diabetic retinopathy: current understanding, mechanisms, and treatment strategies. *JCI Insight* 2: e93751.

10b Microvascular Complications: Diabetic Kidney Disease

Mohsen El Kossi
Nephrology Department, Doncaster Royal Infirmary, Doncaster, UK

Key Points

- Management of diabetic kidney disease in elderly patients is challenging.
- Careful interpretation of estimated glomerular filtration rate is required in this population, because of physiological decline with ageing.
- Prognosis of diabetic kidney disease is dependent on aggressive treatment of cardiovascular risk factors.
- Management of diabetic kidney disease complications will help improve uraemic symptoms and patients' quality of life.
- Timely referral of appropriate patients to nephrologist is important before irreversible decline in kidney function occurs.

Introduction

The prevalence of diabetes mellitus is progressively increasing worldwide, with an anticipated rise in diabetic kidney disease (DKD). This is likely to affect the elderly more, as they are the fastest growing group of patients with diabetes. Management of DKD in older people is challenging for several reasons. First, most of the available clinically useful

Care of Older People with Diabetes: A Manual for Healthcare Practice, First Edition.
Edited by Alan J. Sinclair and Ahmed H. Abdelhafiz.

Companion website: www.wiley.com/go/sinclair/1e

kidney function assessments rely on serum creatinine, which varies according to nutritional status, mobility and comorbidities. Second, the definition of chronic kidney disease (CKD) based on estimated glomerular filtration rate (eGFR) < 60 ml/minute/1.73 m^2 in the absence of albuminuria may be misleading in this age group. It does not discriminate between pathological kidney disease and physiological decline of kidney function with ageing [1]. Third, high prevalence of comorbidities in this age group would make appropriate management of DKD a real difficulty. Fourth, most of the available guidelines and evidence-based medicine may not be applicable to this group of patients, as many of the clinical trials excluded older people or those with advanced stages of CKD. This chapter reviews diagnostic challenges, assessment and management of older people with DKD.

Diabetic Kidney Disease

Kidney disease is a long-term complication of diabetes. Worldwide, DKD is the most common cause of CKD and end-stage renal disease (ESRD). Ageing is associated with a gradual decline in kidney function. Physiologically, eGFR drops by an average of 0.75 ml/minute/1.73 m^2/year in healthy individuals [2]. The number of nephrons is reduced from around one million per kidney in the age 18–29 years to around half a million in the age 70–75 years without compensatory hypertrophy in the remaining nephrons [3]. Prevalence of diabetes and its complications, including DKD, increase with ageing. This leads to a substantial increase in morbidity and mortality. This will also add more financial pressure on healthcare systems. Thus, early diagnosis and intervention may help improve outcomes.

Definitions and Diagnoses

Diabetic kidney disease is defined as a progressive worsening of urinary albumin excretion rate with eGFR decline. It is usually diagnosed in the context of long diabetes duration in the presence of diabetic neuropathy or retinopathy especially in type 1 diabetes, where correlation is good. On the other hand, DKD may exist at the time of type 2 diabetes diagnosis, as patients may remain asymptomatic for a considerable period of time. CKD is defined as abnormalities of kidney structure or function for more than three months [1]. An eGFR of 60 ml/minute/1.73 m^2

Prognosis of CKD by GFR and Albuminuria				Persistent albuminuria categories Description and range		
				A1	A2	A3
				Normal to mildly increased	Moderately increased	Severely increased
				< 30 mg/g < 3 mg/mmol	30–300 mg/g 3–30 mg/mmol	> 300 mg/g > 30 mg/mmol
GFR Categories (ml/min/1.73 m^2) Description and range	G1	Normal or high	≥ 90		Treat	Refer
	G2	Mildly decreased	60–89			
	G3a	Mildly to moderately decreased	45–59	Treat	Treat	Refer
	G3b	Moderately to severely decreased	30–44	Treat	Treat	Refer
	G4	Severely decreased	15–29	Refer	Refer	Refer
	G5	Kidney failure	<15	Refer	Refer	Refer

Figure 10b.1: Prognosis of chronic kidney disease (CKD) by glomerular filtration rate (GFR) and albuminuria category. Green, low risk (no markers of kidney disease, no CKD); yellow, moderately increased risk; orange, high risk; red, very high risk. Source: Adapted from KDIGO [1].

with albuminuria level higher than 3 mg/mmol is the basis of CKD diagnosis. Reduced eGFR alone, without albuminuria, would be debatable with increasing age because of physiological drop of eGFR. Two separate values of urine albumin–creatinine ratio (ACR) and/or eGFR in a three-month interval are required for CKD diagnosis. An early morning first-void urine sample is ideal for urine ACR measurement. CKD prognosis and referrals threshold are based on eGFR and urine ACR levels, as adopted by KDIGO (Kidney Disease Improving Global Outcome), are shown in Figure 10b.1.

Management

Lifestyle

Weight loss in individuals with obesity may help to reduce albuminuria and worsening kidney function. A low-protein diet can slow the progression of DKD to ESRD and improve quality of life; however, a strict low-protein diet should be avoided in frail anorexic patients. Low salt (< 2.3 g/day) intake is associated with reduced rate of serum creatinine doubling and progression to ESRD and is especially beneficial in patients with fluid retention. Exercise training, smoking cessation and reduced alcohol intake are all of cardiovascular and renal benefits in patients with DKD.

Glycaemic Control

Glycaemic control is important to delay the development and the progression of DKD in older people with new diagnosis of diabetes and those with low level of morbidities. However, the value of tight control in older people with long duration of diabetes and multiple morbidities is uncertain. Haemoglobin A1c (HbA1c) remains the gold standard for monitoring glycaemic control but should be carefully interpreted because its level is affected by factors common in CKD, such as shortened red blood cell lifespan, interference in assay by carbamylated haemoglobin, iron deficiency anaemia, erythropoietin use, iron treatment and repeated blood transfusions [4]. HbA1c range between 53 and 58 mmol/mol (7–7.5%) is suitable in healthy individuals with good physical and cognitive function. A more relaxed target of HbA1c 58–64 mmol/mol (7.5–8%) is suitable for patients with multiple morbidities including those with CKD of stage three or four. In patients with ESRD or on dialysis, less stringent levels of HbA1c 64–69 mmol/mol (8–8.5%) is appropriate due to high risk of hypoglycaemia.

In addition to glycaemic control, the newly introduced antihyperglycaemic agents of sodium glucose cotransporter-2 (SGLT-2) inhibitors and glucagon-like peptide receptor agonists (GLP-1) have added the benefits of cardiorenal protection beyond glycaemic control and can be used in patients with CKD up to an eGFR of 20 ml/minute/1.73 m^2. Furthermore, the benefits of these agents occur within few months of therapy and their risk of hypoglycaemia is minimal.

Blood Pressure Control

Hypertension is one of the common findings in DKD, and blood pressure control will slow down DKD progression and reduce cardiovascular risk. Renin–angiotensin–aldosterone system (RAAS) activation plays a central role in the pathogenesis of DKD. RAAS inhibition by angiotensin-converting enzyme inhibitors or angiotensin receptor blockers slows down DKD progression into ESRD and should be considered as a first-line therapy [5]. There is no eGFR cut-off point for the initiation of RAAS blockade but it would be advisable to avoid initiating these agents when eGFR < 20 ml/minute/1.73 m^2. Marginal increase of around 30% of serum creatinine is expected after initiation of RAAS blockade, otherwise investigations for the possibility of bilateral renal artery stenosis will be required if there is a significant worsening in renal function. Hyperkalaemia is another recognised adverse effect of RAAS blockade and should be monitored and treated to allow maximum tolerated dose of RAAS blockade before considering stopping these medications. Treatment of hyperkalaemia comprises dietary advice, the use of potassium-lowering agents such as patiromer or sodium zirconium and correction of metabolic acidosis by sodium bicarbonate to maintain serum bicarbonate level ≥ 22 mmol/l. Finerenone is a non-steroidal mineralocorticoid receptor antagonist, which slows down the progression of DKD in patients with eGFR >25 ml/minute/1.73 m^2 and albuminuria. The recommended dose is 10 mg/day for an eGFR between 25 and 59 ml/minute/1.73 m^2 and 20 mg/day for eGFR > 60 ml/minute/1.73 m^2 with careful monitoring of potassium levels.

Lipid Control

Guidelines recommend regular use of statins or combination of statins and ezetimibe in patients with DKD stages 3–5 not on dialysis. The recommended low-density lipoprotein level is < 70 mg/dl (< 1.8 mmol/l) [6, 7]. It is advisable to monitor serum lipid levels on annual basis with routine diabetes checks and probably once after 12 weeks from initiation of statins therapy. It is not advisable to combine statins with fibrates in advanced stages of DKD (G3b-5) because of risk of worsening renal function. In cases of intolerance of statins or hypertriglyceridaemia, fenofibrates may be an alternative option but the dose should be adjusted according to renal function. Several important considerations should be undertaken in older people. For instance, statins may increase the risk of muscle-related problems. These include muscle aches or weakness, which both can negatively impact patient quality of life. More importantly, these adverse effects may increase the risk of falls, which could be an avoidable disability in this group of patients in particular [8]. Statins with polypharmacy in these patients and potential drug interactions may increase rhabdomyolysis risk. This risk is also potentiated by the use of higher statin doses in frail patients with DKD who are over 80 years of age [9]. For this reason, careful attention should be paid to reducing the dose of statins, especially in very old or frail patients, to mitigate their potential adverse effects. This will also improve compliance. Lower doses of statin are also advisable in patients with polypharmacy, which may interfere with the clearance of statins and increasing their potential adverse effects.

Diabetic Kidney Disease-related Complications

With the progression of DKD and renal function decline, a number of recognised complications can occur, such as anaemia, mineral bone disorder, metabolic acidosis and fluid retention. These are of particular interest in older people and should be addressed.

Anaemia

Screening for anaemia is required at least biannually. DKD should be considered as a possible cause of anaemia when eGFR is <45 ml/minute/1.73 m^2. Iron deficiency anaemia is common in DKD and indications for oral or parenteral iron therapy include hypochromic red blood cells greater than 6%, serum ferritin less than 100 µg/l or transferrin saturation less than 20%. In anaemia not responding to iron therapy, erythropoiesis stimulating agent (ESA) injections or oral hypoxia inducible factor (HIF) stabilisers, such as roxadustat, will be required. Initiation and monitoring of these treatments under the care of renal physicians is advisable. Recommended haemoglobin levels for patients with DKD on ESA or HIF stabilisers range between 100 and 120 g/l.

Mineral Bone Disorder

Diabetic kidney disease carries the highest risk of fracture, with a hazard ratio of 1.45 compared with other causes of ESRD [10]. Abnormalities in phosphorus, calcium, vitamin D and parathyroid hormone levels associated with DKD result in impaired bone volume, turnover and mineralisation, which increase the risk of fracture. These abnormalities become evident more at eGFR <30 ml/minute/1.73 m^2 and severity is worse with CKD progression. Vitamin D supplements, together with bisphosphonates, can be used to reduce the risk of osteoporotic fractures. These medications should be used with caution in advanced stages of CKD (stage 3–5) to reduce the risk of adynamic bone disease. The latter is associated with a high risk of soft-tissue calcification, fracture and mortality. It is advisable to reserve active vitamin D preparations, such as calcitriol and alfacalcidol, for CKD stages 4–5 with severe and progressive secondary hyperparathyroidism.

Metabolic Acidosis and Fluid Retention

Correcting metabolic acidosis with oral sodium bicarbonate helps to maintain bone health, reduce hyperkalaemia, diminish protein degradation and increase muscle mass, and may slow down the progression of kidney disease. Before prescribing sodium bicarbonate, a risk–benefit assessment should be made in patients with fluid retention and heart failure, because of the elemental sodium content in these preparations, with the potential of worsening fluid retention. High dietary vegetable and fruit intake may help to reduce acidosis. Fluid retention can be managed by a low-salt diet, daily weight monitoring and maintenance of fluid balance, although diuretics can be used with close monitoring of renal function.

Nephrology Referral

It is important that patients with DKD are referred to nephrology service before they completely lose their kidney function. The aim of the referral is to address the following:

- To treat complications of advanced stages of DKD such as renal anaemia and CKD mineral bone disorder.
- To prepare patients for renal replacement therapy in suitable cases and to provide principles of conservative approach for those not receiving renal replacement therapy.
- To diagnose non-diabetic causes of CKD and offer specific treatments to avoid further decline in renal function.

Criteria for referral to nephrology service are summarised in Box 10b.1.

Box 10b.1: Criteria for Referral of Patients with Diabetic Kidney Disease to Nephrology

- Advanced stages of diabetic kidney disease: estimated glomerular filtration (eGFR) rate < 30 ml/minute.
- A change in eGFR stage within 12 months. Kidney failure risk equation is helpful online tool to estimate the two- and five-year risk of end-stage renal disease.
- Persistent microscopic haematuria with proteinuria on urine dipstick examination.
- Rapid worsening of kidney function or proteinuria in a short interval (days/weeks).
- Presence of systemic features of inflammation, such as haemoptysis, epistaxis, inflammatory arthritis with active urinary sediment (microscopic haematuria and proteinuria).
- Gross proteinuria with low serum albumin developing over the course of a short interval (weeks/months).
- Unexplained anaemia (haemoglobin < 110 g/l), abnormal potassium, calcium or phosphate.
- Acute kidney injury with no obvious cause.
- Resistant hypertension when four antihypertensives used with therapeutic doses failing to achieve the recommended blood pressure target.

Summary

Diabetic kidney disease is common in older people with diabetes; however, mortality is mostly related to cardiovascular disease, so management of cardiovascular risk factors will improve renal outcomes. Regular monitoring and management of DKD complications may help to relieve symptoms, improve outcomes, reduce deterioration in renal function and enhance overall quality of life of older people with diabetes. Patients who are taking many of the new medications that improve cardiovascular and renal outcomes, such as RAAS blockade or SGLT2 inhibitors, are advised to suspend these medications temporarily and follow the sick day rules with any intercurrent illness to minimise the risk of acute deterioration of kidney function.

Clinical Practice Question

Q1. An 88-year-old man who is normally fit and well was found on the floor. He has a background history of type 2 diabetes mellitus and hypertension. His diabetes control was previously poor, with a haemoglobin A1c of 85 mmol/mol one month ago. His diabetes nurse advised him to increase his bedtime insulin by four units. He also takes metformin 1 g twice a day and gliclazide SR 30 mg once a day. He is on aspirin 75 mg/day, atorvastatin 40 mg/day, ramipril 10 mg/day and bisoprolol 5 mg/day. He recently took over-the-counter painkillers for back pain. His baseline urea and electrolyte levels, taken one month ago, revealed serum creatinine 145 μmol/l and eGFR 40 ml/minute/1.73 m^2. The ambulance crew assessed his Glasgow Coma Scale score as 8/15, finger-prick blood glucose 1.5 mmol/l and blood pressure 70/40 mmHg, with a pulse rate of 82 beats per minute. Glucagon was give intramuscularly and intravenous glucose was administered. On arrival at hospital, his potassium level was 7.8 mmol/l, creatinine 201 μmol/l, and eGFR 27 ml/minute/1.73 m^2. His bicarbonate level was 10 mmol/l, lactate 8.2 mmol/l, and his blood pressure remained low at 85/50 mmHg. What should the next steps be?

Choose all the options that apply:

A. Hold metformin and ramipril.
B. Fluid resuscitation and correction of hyperkalaemia.
C. Stop gliclazide.
D. Medications education.
E. Increase his insulin dose in view of high haemoglobin A1c.

References

1. KDIGO (2013). KDIGO 2012 clinical practice guideline for the evaluation and management of chronic kidney disease. *Kidney Int. Suppl.* 3 (1): v, 1–xiii, 150.
2. Lindeman, R.D., Tobin, J., and Shock, N.W. (1985). Longitudinal studies on the rate of decline in renal function with age. *J. Am. Geriatr. Soc.* 33: 27885.
3. Denic, A., Lieske, J.C., Chakkera, H.A. et al. (2017). The substantial loss of nephrons in healthy human kidneys with aging. *J. Am. Soc. Nephrol.* 28: 313–320.

4. NGSP. Factors that interfere with HbA1c test results. `http://www.ngsp.org/factors.asp`. (accessed 23 November 2023).
5. Catalá-López, F., Macías Saint-Gerons, D., González-Bermejo, D. et al. (2016). Cardiovascular and renal outcomes of renin-angiotensin system blockade in adult patients with diabetes mellitus: a systematic review with network meta-analyses. *PLoS Med.* 13: e1001971.
6. Marx, N., Federici, M., Schütt, K. et al. (2023). 2023 ESC guidelines for the management of cardiovascular disease in patients with diabetes. *Eur. Heart J.* 44: 4043–4140.
7. ElSayed, N.A., Aleppo, G., Aroda, V.R. et al. (2023). Summary of revisions: standards of care in diabetes-2023. *Diabetes Care* 46 (Suppl 1): S5–S9.
8. Venegas Sanabria, L.C., Babosa Balaquera, S., Suarez Acosta, A.M. et al. (2017). Statin and risk of falls in the elderly: a sytematic review of the literature. *Rev. Esp. Geriatr. Gerontol.* 52: 317–321.
9. Chatzizisis, Y., Koskinas, K., Misirli, G. et al. (2010). Risk factors and drug interactions predisposing to statin-induced myopathy. Implications for risk assessment, prevention and treatment. *Drug Saf.* 33: 171–187.
10. Ziolkowski, S., Liu, S., Montez-Rath, M.E. et al. (2022). Association between cause of kidney failure and fracture incidence in a national US dialysis population cohort study. *Clin. Kidney J.* 15: 2245–2257.

10c Microvascular Complications: Peripheral Neuropathy

Mitra Tavakoli

Exeter Centre of Excellence for Diabetes Research, National Institute for Health and Care Research, University of Exeter Medical School, Exeter, UK

Key Points

- Diabetic neuropathy, the most common complication of diabetes, remains underdiagnosed and undertreated.
- Neuropathic complications can affect individuals of various age groups, not exclusively older diabetic patients. However, older patients often contend with additional health issues.
- Older patients may experience various types of neuropathies, such as peripheral sensorimotor polyneuropathy, small-fibre neuropathy, focal mononeuropathies, radiculoplexus neuropathies and autonomic neuropathy.
- Regular screening plays a crucial role in detecting subclinical neuropathy, identifying those at risk and minimising the risk of complications.
- Effectively managing diabetes-related neuropathic complications involves a dual focus on improving glycaemic control and implementing strategies for pain and symptom management.

Care of Older People with Diabetes: A Manual for Healthcare Practice, First Edition.
Edited by Alan J. Sinclair and Ahmed H. Abdelhafiz.

Companion website: www.wiley.com/go/sinclair/1e

Introduction

Globally, we are witnessing a surge in diabetes mellitus, with one person being diagnosed every 18 seconds [1]. This trend is evolving into an epidemic and endemic issue, imposing significant social and economic burdens across all age groups. However, the prevalence of diabetes, together with its associated comorbidities and mortality, is notably higher among middle-aged and ageing populations.

In the United States, diabetes mellitus affects approximately 10.9 million adults aged 65 years and older. Projections indicate that, by 2050, this number will escalate to 26.7 million, representing 55% of all diabetes cases [2]. These data underscore the increasing impact of diabetes within the ageing population and its anticipated future burden on healthcare systems.

Diabetic neuropathy, which is one of the most prevalent and costly complications of diabetes affects patients by increasing falls, causing pain, and reducing quality of life. This complication specifically affects peripheral nerves, leading to sensory loss, painful sensations and impaired motor function in the extremities. Additionally, diabetic neuropathy can potentially result in foot ulcers and, in severe cases, may necessitate amputations [3].

While diabetic neuropathy is a recognised complication across various age groups, its significance in older individuals is particularly noteworthy due to age-related vulnerabilities and potential coexisting health conditions. The mortality rate among older adults with diabetes surpasses that of their non-diabetic counterparts [4]. The interplay between diabetes and disability is amplified, particularly in older individuals with diabetes who are grappling with associated neuropathy. Therefore, it is imperative for healthcare providers overseeing the care of older individuals with diabetes to be vigilant about the hazards linked to medication polypharmacy, the assessment of functional capacity and the availability of home support when devising their care strategies [5].

Prevalence and Risk Factors

The true prevalence of diabetic neuropathy is underestimated as its assessment is challenging. However, it is recognised as the most common complication of diabetes and affects approximately 50% of people with diabetes. The occurrence of peripheral neuropathy in older individuals with diabetes is notably greater than in their younger counterparts. Advanced age stands out as one of the primary risk factors contributing to diabetic neuropathy. Longitudinal studies conducted in type 1 diabetes mellitus (T1DM), such as the Diabetes Control and Complications Trial and the Epidemiology of Diabetes Interventions and Complications study, have revealed a progressive rise in the prevalence of neuropathic symptoms and signs over time [6]. As individuals with T1DM age, the likelihood of neuropathy continues to increase, and this significantly impacts their physical function [7]. The prevalence of diabetic neuropathy is somewhat higher in patients with type 2 diabetes mellitus (T2DM) when compared with those with T1DM [8]. Longitudinal studies in T2DM indicate a higher risk of neuropathy development over time compared with those with T1DM [9]. Consequently, older individuals with either T1DM or T2DM face elevated risks of neuropathy as they age.

Additional risk factors for diabetic neuropathy encompass poorly managed blood sugar levels, uncontrolled blood pressure, elevated cholesterol levels, prolonged duration of diabetes, obesity, smoking, genetic predisposition, peripheral arterial disease, kidney disease, autoimmune factors and alcohol abuse [10].

The precise pathophysiology of diabetic neuropathy remains elusive [10]; however, it emerges from multifactorial aetiologies. Prolonged hyperglycaemia, suboptimal glycaemic control, microvascular complications and age-related neurophysiological alterations contribute intricately to heightened nerve susceptibility [11]. Addressing these determinants is pivotal in mitigating the impact of diabetic neuropathy in ageing individuals with diabetes mellitus.

Clinical Manifestations and Complications

In older individuals with diabetes, peripheral neuropathy manifests through a spectrum of clinical presentations, encompassing an array of sensory, motor and autonomic neuropathies. Sensory manifestations often manifest as numbness, tingling sensations and varying degrees of pain. Concurrently, motor impairments may include muscle weakness or loss of coordination. Additionally, autonomic dysfunction may surface, leading to disruptions in bodily functions regulated by the autonomic nervous system, such as digestion or blood pressure regulation.

This neuropathy significantly heightens the risk of falls among the senior diabetic population because of compromised sensation and motor function, contributing to an increased susceptibility to balance-related issues and falls. Concurrently, individuals with diabetic neuropathy are prone to foot complications, including ulcers and injuries, primarily due to reduced sensation in the lower extremities. These complications necessitate vigilant foot care to prevent the development of ulcers and other foot-related issues, which can lead to severe complications, including infections and amputations. Overall, the multifaceted clinical manifestations of diabetic neuropathy in older individuals with diabetes pose a heightened risk of falls and foot complications, emphasising the critical need for comprehensive management and preventive strategies.

Diagnosis and Assessment

Diabetic neuropathies encompass a varied spectrum of disorders exhibiting diverse clinical presentations. Remarkably, a significant proportion of individuals, up to 50%, may experience diabetic neuropathy without manifesting any discernible symptoms. Therefore, early and precise diagnosis, together with comprehensive assessment, holds paramount importance for effectively managing peripheral neuropathy in ageing patients with diabetes.

The American Diabetes Association and the International Working Group on the Diabetic Foot recommend regular examination of people with diabetes for the diagnosis of neuropathy and loss of protective sensation using simple standard tests for the identification of those at risk for diabetic foot ulcers. This includes a meticulous review of medical history and examination of small and large-fibre function, which is typically assessed through temperature or pinprick sensation, a 128-Hz tuning fork and 10-g monofilament testing to identify those at risks. In alignment with these recommendations, individuals diagnosed with diabetes should undergo assessment for peripheral neuropathy promptly upon diagnosis in T2DM and five years post diagnosis in T1DM. Subsequently, regular evaluations, at least annually thereafter, are crucial [12]. Table 10c.1 summarises the current tests that are available for the diagnosis of diabetic neuropathy.

The current clinical approach frequently misses the early stages of neuropathy, emphasising the urgency for timely intervention to halt its

Table 10c.1: Some available diagnostic tests for assessing diabetic neuropathy.

	Nerve Fibres	Advantages	Limitations	Assessed
Symptoms and signs	Questionnaires	Large (Aβ) and small (Aδ and C) fibres	Easy to administer. Used for monitoring symptoms [13]	Lack of sensitivity, accuracy and reproducibility, subjective [14]
	NDS	Large (Aβ) and small (Aδ and C) fibres	Does not require specialist equipment. Assesses large- and small-fibre function [15]	Not sensitive or reproducible, low correlation with small-fibre quantitative tests [16]
	10-g monofilament	Large (Aβ) fibres	Simple, quick and inexpensive [17]	No standardisation of methods. Cannot detect early neuropathy [17]
	Ipswich touch test	Large (Aβ) fibres	Simple. Requires no specialist equipment [18]. Can test at home	Can only detect advanced neuropathy [17]
	QST (thermal and vibration thresholds)	Large (Aβ) and small (Aδ and C) fibres	Measures small- and large-fibre function [13]. Good repeatability [19]	Unable to differentiate between peripheral and central abnormalities [20]. High interoperator variability [21]
Large-fibre tests	**DPNCheck**	Large, sural nerve (Aβ) fibres	Quick, easy to perform. Good sensitivity (92–95%) compared with NCS [22, 23]	Relies on the accessibility of sural nerve [24]. Validation studies had small patient numbers [22, 23]
	NCS	Large (Aβ) fibres	A sensitive measure of large nerve function [25]. Reproducible [26]	Does not assess small fibres. Uncomfortable [27]. Does not assess early neuropathic changes

(*Continued*)

Table 10c.1: Continued

	Nerve Fibres	Advantages	Limitations	Assessed
Small-fibre tests	**Skin biopsy (IENFD)**	Small (C) fibres	Gold standard for SNF. Quantitative. Good sensitivity. Detects early nerve changes [28, 29]	Invasive, risk of infection. Repeatability. Requires trained personnel and special laboratories [13]
	CCM	Small (Aδ and C) fibres	Non-invasive. Good reproducibility [30]. Rapid and objective [31, 32]	Relatively expensive. Requires specialist equipment and personnel. Manual analysis is time consuming [13]
Autonomic tests	**Neuropad**	Small (C) fibres	Can be self-administered, suitable for screening. Non-invasive. Good sensitivity [23, 33–38]	Varied interpretation of the results [23, 33–36]
	Sudoscan	Small (C) fibres	Non-invasive. Easy to perform	Unclear if measuring sudomotor function. Variable specificity (53–92%) [39–43]
	QSART	Small (C) fibres	Sensitive for SFN (82%) [44] Gold standard for measuring sudomotor function	Time-consuming. Requires specialist equipment and trained personnel [45]. Uncomfortable

IENFD, intra-epidermal nerve fibre density; NCS, nerve conduction studies; QSART, quantitative sudomotor axon reflex test; CCM, corneal confocal microscopy; NDS, neuropathy disability score; QST, quantitative sensory testing; SFN, small-fibre neuropathy.

advancement. Addressing this gap is crucial, emphasising the necessity for a clear, precise test or a series of tests capable of identifying and diagnosing diabetic neuropathy in its nascent phases [46]. This approach will enable mitigation of the risk of foot ulcers and diminish the probability of amputations – a vital necessity for the expanding ageing diabetic population, especially given the heightened prevalence rates within this demographic.

Management of Diabetic Neuropathy

Diabetic neuropathy lacks a targeted pharmaceutical intervention, underscoring the pivotal role of stringent glycaemic control as a primary management strategy. This emphasis aims to curtail nerve damage progression and mitigate its impact. However, addressing the distressing pain associated with this condition requires a comprehensive and nuanced approach.

At present, there are only four US Food and Drug Administration-approved treatments for painful peripheral neuropathy: pregabalin, duloxetine, tapentadol and the 8% capsaicin patch. Each of these treatments employs distinct mechanisms to address pain [47].

Managing pain and neuropathy in ageing patients with diabetes necessitates a comprehensive approach involving diverse interventions. These encompass pharmacological treatments, lifestyle adjustments, foot care practices and rehabilitation programmes. Central to this approach is the emphasis on patient-centred care and the development of tailored treatment plans to suit individual needs.

In the management of neuropathic pain, pharmacotherapy assumes a prominent role. This may involve anticonvulsants, tricyclic antidepressants, serotonin–norepinephrine reuptake inhibitors or, in some cases, opioid medications [48]. Figure 10c.1 presents an algorithm for approaching pain management [49].

Concurrently, lifestyle modifications play a crucial role in pain management. Regular physical activity serves as an indispensable facet, contributing to improved nerve function and diminished discomfort. Maintaining an optimal body weight, adhering to a well-balanced diet and abstaining from alcohol and smoking significantly impact the alleviation of neuropathic pain.

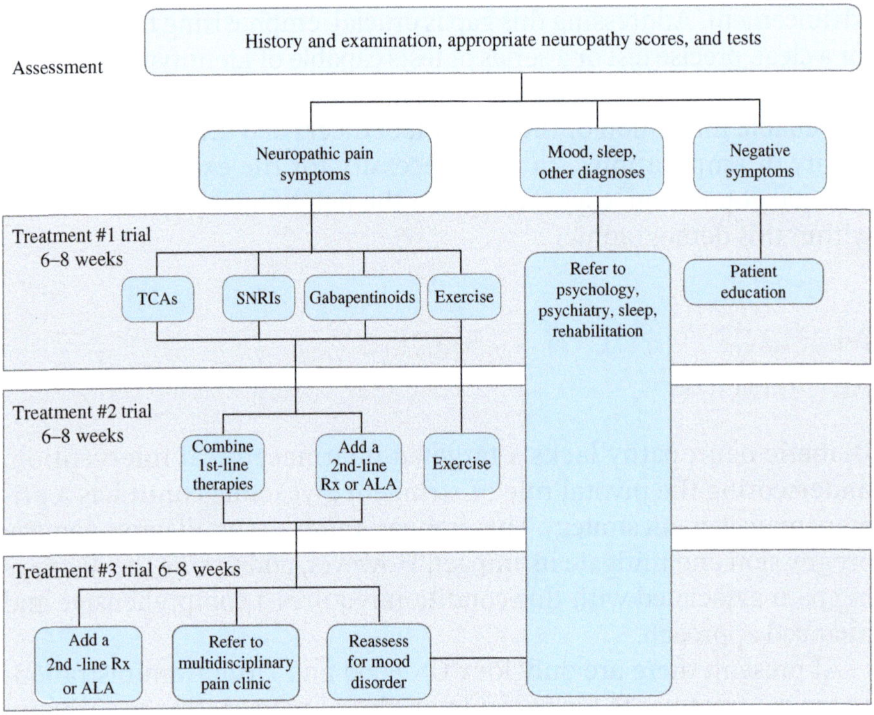

Figure 10c.1: Algorithm for approaching pain management [49]. ALA, alpha-lipoic acid; SNRIs, serotonin and norepinephrine reuptake inhibitors; TCAs, tricyclic antidepressants; Rx, medical prescription.

In conjunction with pharmaceutical and lifestyle interventions, complementary and alternative therapies, such as acupuncture, transcutaneous electrical nerve stimulation and biofeedback, stand as promising adjuncts in alleviating neuropathic pain. These modalities complement conventional medical approaches, offering supplementary avenues for pain management. This holistic approach may help to enhance the overall well-being and quality of life for individuals affected by diabetic neuropathy.

Diabetes Foot Care in Care Homes

By 2050, the UK is expected to have over 8 million people aged 85 years and above. The ageing population will lead to a significant rise in older individuals living with diabetes, creating a growing demand for care in their later years. Notably, one in four residents in care homes has diabetes. This highlights the urgent need for targeted strategies in diabetes management within care-home settings to address the unique needs of this demographic and ensure their wellbeing [50].

Diabetes UK figures highlight a troubling reality: individuals living with diabetes in care homes are currently hospitalised every 25 minutes, with this rate expected to sharply increase to one person every 10 minutes. These statistics emphasise the urgent need for improved diabetes care strategies within care-home settings to address the growing frequency of hospital admissions and prioritise the wellbeing of residents with diabetes [51]. Recognising and addressing neuropathic pain is essential, given its tendency to be underestimated among the elderly, leading to various health issues. Strict guidelines for regular neuropathy screenings and meticulous foot care should be followed and implemented [52].

In care homes, managing diabetes poses specific challenges for residents, particularly concerning lower extremities. A comprehensive evaluation upon entry, considering appearance, circulatory health and sensory status of lower limbs is crucial. Inquiries into balance, activity limitations, pain and prior foot issues should be conducted and, if available, screening tests can aid in assessing neuropathy and identifying risks [53, 54]. Upon identifying risk levels, residents benefit from personalised footcare plans, involving regular examinations and sensory testing according to National Institute for Health and Care Excellence guidelines [55]. Documenting findings, such as redness or calluses, helps monitor progress and address concerns like oedema, skin issues, foot deformities and toenail conditions. Ensuring continuity of care is vital, especially during transitions between care settings, as environmental changes may impact blood glucose levels. Trained staff need to conduct routine assessments, ensuring adherence to personalised footcare routines, emphasising proper footwear choices, implementing tailored exercise plans and making necessary environmental adjustments.

Continuous collaboration with healthcare professionals is integral for prompt intervention in emerging foot-related concerns. This unwavering commitment to proactive neuropathy and foot care measures stands as a cornerstone, reinforcing the overarching goal of maintaining the health and comfort of residents in the care homes setting.

Summary

Diabetic neuropathy remains a pressing concern among older people coping with diabetes, significantly influencing their daily lives and overall wellbeing and quality of life, and the clinical complications can be profoundly severe.

A comprehensive understanding of its prevalence, risk factors and effective management approaches is vital to provide optimal care for this demographic. Implementing early detection, meticulous assessment and personalised interventions empowers healthcare professionals to adeptly address diabetic neuropathy, thereby enhancing the lives of older diabetic patients.

While diabetic neuropathy affects individuals across various age groups, its impact on older adults is particularly profound due to age-related vulnerabilities and potential comorbidities. Recognising and addressing the specific challenges faced by older individuals contending with diabetes-related peripheral neuropathy are critical for optimising their care.

As healthcare providers, delving into these unique challenges underscores the necessity for tailored management strategies that navigate the complexities of diabetic peripheral neuropathy in older populations. By adopting and implementing these refined approaches, healthcare providers can substantially augment the quality of life for older people navigating the intricate landscape of diabetes-related neuropathies. There is unmet need for further research aimed at developing effective curative treatments for diabetic neuropathy to better serve this vulnerable population.

Clinical Practice Question

Q1. In an 82-year-old care-home resident with diabetes, which of the following are true statements:

- **A.** Signs and symptoms of peripheral neuropathy are often difficult to detect by care staff working in the care home.
- **B.** Peripheral neuropathy in care home residents with diabetes is usually easily managed once detected and does not affect future quality of life.
- **C.** Acupuncture can be used as an adjunct to drug therapy in the treatment of peripheral neuropathy.
- **D.** A 256-Hz tuning fork can be used to identify residents at risk of peripheral neuropathy.
- **E.** Peripheral vascular disease is a recognised risk factor for the development of peripheral neuropathy.

References

Key references only are listed here. For a full list of references visit: https://www.wiley.com/go/sinclair/1e.

3. Pop-Busui, R., Boulton, A.J., Feldman, E.L. et al. (2017). Diabetic neuropathy: a position statement by the American Diabetes Association. *Diabetes Care* 40 (1): 136–154.
5. LeRoith, D., Biessels, G.J., Braithwaite, S.S. et al. (2019). Treatment of diabetes in older adults: an Endocrine Society clinical practice guideline. *J. Clin. Endocrinol. Metab.* 104 (5): 1520–1574.
7. Martin, C.L., Trapani, V.R., Backlund, J.C. et al. (2022). Physical function in middle-aged and older adults with type 1 diabetes: long-term follow-up of the diabetes control and complications trial/epidemiology of diabetes interventions and complications study. *Diabetes Care* 45 (9): 2037–2045.
10. Tesfaye, S., Chaturvedi, N., Eaton, S.E. et al. (2005). Vascular risk factors and diabetic neuropathy. *N. Engl. J. Med.* 352 (4): 341–350.
12. ElSayed, N.A., Aleppo, G., Aroda, V.R. et al. (2023). Retinopathy, neuropathy, and foot care: standards of care in diabetes-2023. *Diabetes Care* 46 (Suppl 1): S203–S215.
20. Themistocleous, A.C., Ramirez, J.D., Serra, J., and Bennett, D.L. (2014). The clinical approach to small fibre neuropathy and painful channelopathy. *Pract. Neurol.* 14 (6): 368–379.
46. Carmichael, J., Fadavi, H., Ishibashi, F. et al. (2021). Advances in screening, early diagnosis and accurate staging of diabetic neuropathy. *Front. Endocrinol.* 12: 671257.
47. Ziegler, D., Papanas, N., Schnell, O. et al. (2021). Current concepts in the management of diabetic polyneuropathy. *J. Diabetes Investig.* 12 (4): 464–475.
50. Sinclair, A.J. and Abdelhafiz, A.H. (2022). Multimorbidity, frailty and diabetes in older people-identifying interrelationships and outcomes. *J. Pers. Med.* 12 (11): 1911.
52. Sinclair, A., Morley, J.E., Rodriguez-Manas, L. et al. (2012). Diabetes mellitus in older people: position statement on behalf of the International Association of Gerontology and Geriatrics (IAGG), the European Diabetes Working Party for Older People (EDWPOP), and the International Task Force of Experts in Diabetes. *J. Am. Med. Dir. Assoc.* 13 (6): 497–502.

11a Vascular Risk Factors: Hypertension

Pann Ei Hnynn Si[1] *and Ahmed H. Abdelhafiz*[2]

[1] *Sheffield Kidney Institute, Sheffield Teaching Hospitals, Sheffield, UK*

[2] *Department of Geriatric Medicine, Rotherham General Hospital, Rotherham, S60 2 UD, UK*

Key Points

- Ageing is associated with vascular changes that promote the development of hypertension.
- Hypertension often correlates with diabetes and stands as a significant cardiovascular risk element.
- Fit older individuals with diabetes are advised to maintain strict blood pressure regulation.
- Patients with concurrent conditions, particularly dementia or frailty, might benefit from more lenient blood pressure targets.
- Older individuals with diabetes warrant specific considerations due to factors such as orthostatic hypotension, polypharmacy and an elevated risk of falls.

Introduction

Hypertension is the most prevalent cardiovascular risk factor that increases the risk of major adverse cardiovascular events (MACE). Globally intertwined with type 2 diabetes mellitus, hypertension affects approximately 1 billion individuals and contributes to around

Care of Older People with Diabetes: A Manual for Healthcare Practice, First Edition.
Edited by Alan J. Sinclair and Ahmed H. Abdelhafiz.

Companion website: www.wiley.com/go/sinclair/1e

7–8 million cardiovascular deaths annually [1]. The prevalence of hypertension increases proportionally with increasing age due to age related cardiovascular changes, which predispose to the development hypertension. Consequently, with the continued ageing of the population, the prevalence of hypertension is anticipated to rise persistently. Hypertension is a systemic disease associated with the increased risk of other morbidities such as chronic kidney disease (CKD) and cognitive impairment. In addition, in older people with diabetes, the presence of hypertension, alongside other morbidities, increases the risk of frailty [2]. This chapter reviews the challenges of management of hypertension in this complex and diverse group of patients.

Age-related Blood Pressure Changes

Both systolic blood pressure (SBP) and diastolic blood pressure (DBP) increase with age until around 60 years old. After this point, SBP continues to rise, while DBP either stabilises or declines, resulting in an elevation of pulse pressure. This shift stems primarily from increased stiffness in the arterial walls as individuals age. Arterial wall stiffness occurs as a result of increased arterial-wall thickening, calcification, atheroma formation, increased collagen deposition and fragmentation of elastin network. Impaired vascular endothelial function and modification of smooth-muscle cell reactivity also contribute to the arterial wall stiffness [3]. As a consequence, arterial-wall stiffness intensifies variations in blood pressure on changes in posture, leading to orthostatic hypotension. Orthostatic hypotension will be exaggerated in the presence of other morbidities that cause autonomic neuropathy such as diabetes mellitus. These age-related blood pressure changes including orthostatic variability are associated with increased risk of MACE (Figure 11a.1).

Definition

Despite the progressive changes in blood pressure with increasing age, the definition of hypertension remains the same across all age groups as ≥140/90 mmHg based on three or more measurements at two or more visits to a medical practitioner as reported by European Society of Cardiology. However, the American Diabetes Association defined hypertension at a lower level of blood pressure ≥130/80 mmHg (Table 11a.1).

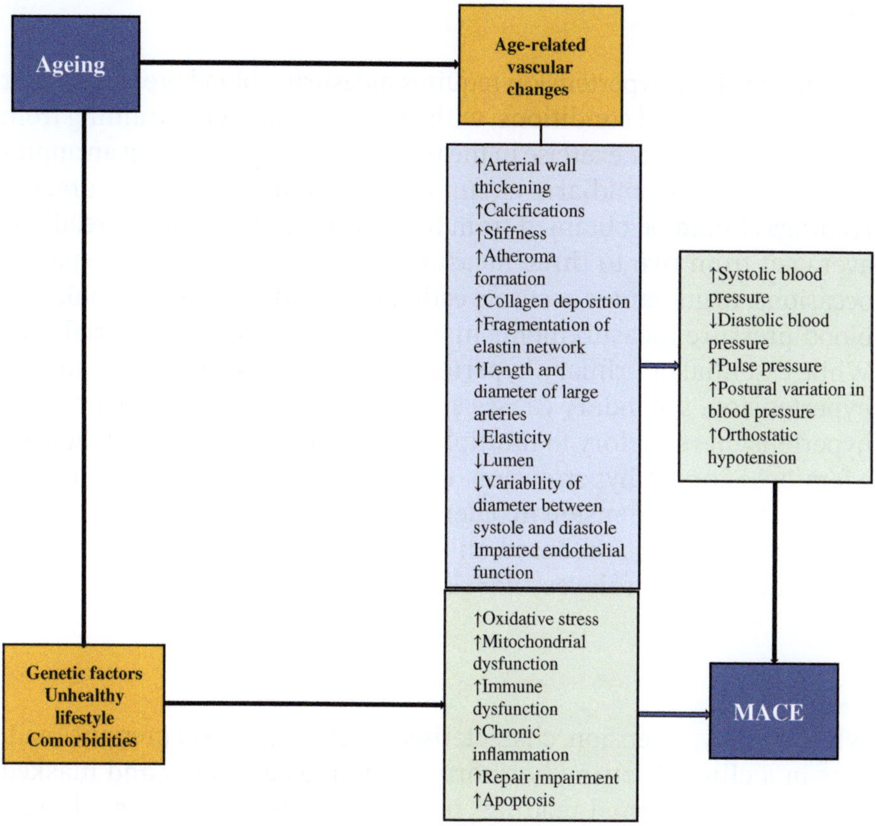

Figure 11a.1: Age-related vascular changes predispose to the development of hypertension and increased risk of cardiovascular disease and cardiovascular events. MACE, major adverse cardiovascular events.

Table 11a.1: Main guidelines for blood pressure targets in diabetes.

European Society of Cardiology	American Diabetes Association
Treat blood pressure in individualised manner; start treatment when blood pressure ≥ 140/90 mmHg; target SBP for older people (> 65 years) 130–139 mmHg, SBP target of <130 mmHg in people at high risk of stroke	Blood pressure ≥ 130/80 mmHg qualifies for treatment; target < 130/80 mmHg; individualised target through shared decision making

Diagnosis

The diagnosis of hypertension requires measuring blood pressure under resting and relaxed conditions, with an empty bladder, refraining from smoking, caffeine or exercise in the past 30 minutes, and using an appropriate cuff size for mid-arm circumference. To minimise inaccuracies, readings should be obtained from both arms, and the higher readings averaged from two to three measurements on two to three separate occasions, to guarantee accurate estimate. In older people, ambulatory blood pressure measurements may be required to reduce variability. While essential or primary hypertension is the most common cause of hypertension, secondary causes should be screened for patients with hypertension refractory to multiple drug therapy or in those who lack a family history of hypertension. Owing to the high prevalence of isolated systolic hypertension in older people, it is appropriate to diagnose and treat hypertension based on systolic readings alone due to their correlation with cardiovascular risk.

Types

White-coat hypertension, characterised by elevated blood pressure readings in a clinical setting but normal readings at home, and masked hypertension (normal readings in clinical setting but elevated readings at home) represent distinct forms of hypertension best diagnosed through ambulatory blood pressure monitoring. Resistant hypertension is uncontrollable blood pressure despite the use of three or more antihypertensives, including a diuretic. Isolated systolic hypertension (blood pressure $\geq 140/<90$ mmHg) is the most common type, accounting for 60–80% of cases, which increases proportionally with age.

Orthostatic hypotension, identified by a blood pressure drop of more than 20/10 mmHg within three minutes of standing, probably stems from autonomic dysfunction, diminished baroreceptor sensitivity or a reduced compensatory heart rate response to postural changes [4]. Pseudohypertension, characterised by high blood pressure due to non-collapsing sclerotic arteries, should be considered in patients with resistant hypertension but lacking evidence of end organ damage. Nocturnal hypertension occurs when blood pressure fails to drop physiologically (non-dipper patients) by 10–20% at night and is associated with end-organ damage. Nocturnal hypotension occurs when blood pressure

Table 11a.2: Common types of hypertension in older people.

Type of hypertension	Definition
White-coat	High office but normal home blood pressure
Masked	Normal in clinic but high home blood pressure
Resistant	Uncontrollable blood pressure despite treatment with ≥3 agents including a diuretic
Isolated systolic	≥140/<90 mmHg.
Orthostatic	A drop of >20/10 mmHg after standing for at least 1 minute
Pseudo	Falsely elevated SBP due to atherosclerotic arteries
Nocturnal (non-dippers)	Blood pressure does not drop physiologically by 10–20% at night
Nocturnal (dippers)	Blood pressure drops ≥20% at night

drops by ≥20% at night, increasing the risk of cerebral hypoperfusion (Table 11a.2) [5].

Management

Control of the blood pressure is crucial to reduce MACE, CKD, cognitive decline, frailty and mortality. The first line of therapy is lifestyle modification, such as regular exercise, achieving ideal body weight and maintaining a healthy low-salt diet. In mild cases, these lifestyle modifications might suffice as the sole intervention, with pharmacological therapy introduced only when necessary.

Recommended Targets

Older people with diabetes will benefit more from blood pressure reduction compared with those without diabetes, because of their higher baseline risk. For example, in the Systolic Hypertension in Europe trial, for a comparable 22 mmHg reduction in SBP, the reduction in the risk of mortality was 76% for participants with diabetes compared with only 13% in those without diabetes [6]. A SBP target of 140 mmHg is associated with a reduction in cardiovascular risk compared with SBP > 140 mmHg. In the International Verapamil SR-Trandolapril Study, SBP < 130 mmHg was not associated with better cardiovascular outcomes compared with a blood pressure of 140–130 mmHg. In addition, SBP < 130 mmHg was associated with slightly increased risk of mortality (11.0% vs. 10.2%) [7]. Further lowering of SBP (< 120 mmHg) compared with standard treatment (SBP < 140 mmHg) was not associated with statistically significant reductions in cardiovascular events, as demonstrated in the ACCORD-Blood Pressure study, but was associated with modest reduction in stroke at the expense of increased rates of serious adverse events [8]. For most older people with diabetes, the current evidence suggests a target SBP of 140 mmHg. A lower SBP of 130 mmHg may be considered in patients with high risk of stroke or those with CKD and albuminuria [9]. This lower target should considered only after taking into account the balance between benefits and risks. Although evidence for the benefit of blood pressure reduction was only seen in individuals up to the age of 80 years, the Hypertension in the Very Elderly Trial provides evidence that antihypertensive treatment was associated with reduced risks of heart failure, all-cause mortality and fatal stroke in individuals 80 years and over, although only around 7% of participants had diabetes [10]. Suggested targets based on three different categories of older people are illustrated in Figure 11a.2.

Medications

All major antihypertensive drug classes such as thiazides, beta-blockers, calcium channel blockers (CCBs), angiotensin converting

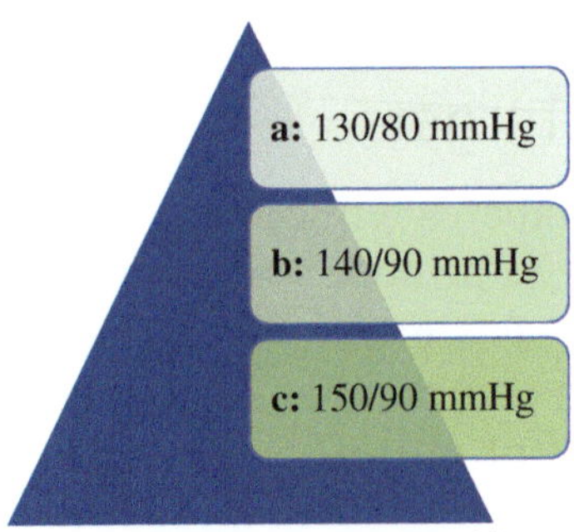

Figure 11a.2: Escalation of blood pressure control based on category. (a) Fit older people with high stroke risk. (b) Fit older people. (c) Frail older people.

enzyme (ACE) inhibitors and angiotensin receptor blockers (ARBs) can be used in older people with diabetes. A meta-analysis has shown no difference between antihypertensive classes in reducing all-cause or cardiovascular mortality [11]. This suggests that lowering blood pressure to improve outcomes is more important than using a particular class of antihypertensive agents. Usually, more than one antihypertensive agent is required to achieve target blood pressure. Data from five clinical trials demonstrated that the average number of antihypertensive agents required to achieve a target blood pressure of 130/85 mmHg is 2.6–4.3 in people with diabetes [12]. Blocking the renin–angiotensin–aldosterone system by ACE inhibitors or ARBs reduced the risk of diabetic kidney disease; however, the combination of ACE inhibitors with ARBs should be avoided in older people because of the increased risk of adverse effects. Certain antihypertensive agents such as older generation beta-blockers are less effective in reducing blood pressure and may worsen blood glucose control, especially if combined with thiazide diuretics. In a meta-analysis of 12 studies including 94 492 patients, beta-blocker therapy resulted in 22% increased risk of new-onset diabetes (relative risk 1.22, 95% confidence interval 1.12–1.33) compared with non-diuretic antihypertensive agents. On the other hand, CCBs and ACE inhibitors or ARBs resulted in 21% and 23% reductions, respectively, in the risk of new-onset diabetes, and their antihypertensive efficacy was superior compared with beta-blockers [13]. Another meta-analysis demonstrated that the effect of the antihypertensive class of drugs on new-onset diabetes was lowest for ARBs and ACE inhibitors, followed by CCBs then beta-blockers and diuretics, in that order [14]. The newer generation of beta-blockers, such as bisoprolol, carvedilol and nebivolol, are more effective antihypertensives, have less effect on blood glucose levels and can be used as a first-line therapy, especially in older people with diabetes and associated coronary artery disease or heart failure.

Considerations in Older People

Orthostatic Hypotension

Antihypertensive medications effectively lower both supine and standing blood pressure. Older people have a higher incidence of insomnia, which can be exacerbated by conditions such as overactive bladder. While the practice of administering antihypertensive medications at night is typically recommended for younger patients to manage nighttime hypertension and prevent morning orthostatic hypotension, in older individuals this approach warrants caution as it may increase the risk of nocturnal orthostatic hypotension and falls. Adequate control of supine hypertension may improve orthostatic hypotension, although patients should be closely observed for adverse effects such as presyncope and falls.

Falls

Treatment with antihypertensive medications can lead to an increased risk of injurious falls, especially in people with previous history of falls. Risk of falls also increases with the use of higher doses of medications. Therefore, when starting or intensifying antihypertensive therapy, the risk of falls should be discussed with the patients from the outset and preventive strategies should be in place.

Systolic Hypertension

Systolic hypertension, common in older people, is caused by arterial stiffness. Antihypertensive medications work mainly by reducing peripheral resistance, making it difficult to control SBP. Increasing intensity of antihypertensive medications to reduce SBP may unduly reduce DBP, compromising coronary artery perfusion and increasing the risk of cardiac events. Therefore, in patients with systolic hypertension, DBP should not be reduced to levels <60 mmHg or <65 mmHg in those with known coronary artery disease or <70 mmHg in patients over 80 years of age.

Frailty

Frailty may modify or attenuate the association between blood pressure and outcomes. The relationship is U-shaped and a higher blood pressure (above 140 mmHg) may be more appropriate in frail older people. Low blood pressure in frail older people could be an expression of malnutrition, heart failure and other comorbidities that are associated with poor prognosis rather than being a direct consequence of antihypertensive therapy.

Dementia

Patients with dementia are likely to be frail with multiple comorbidities. Intensive blood pressure lowering in these patients with limited life expectancy is likely to be associated with an increased risk of adverse events that may outweigh any benefits in cardiovascular risk reduction. Lower blood pressure levels may contribute to a more decline in cognitive function and worsening of dementia; thus, a higher blood pressure above 140 mmHg is more appropriate in this population.

Comorbidity

The burden of comorbidities increases with increasing age and may shorten life expectancy and reduce the benefits of antihypertensive medications. Even in absence of clinical disease, subclinical pathology may be prevalent and affect health outcomes. Comorbidities should therefore be considered as part of a holistic assessment of the complex older patient.

Polypharmacy

Polypharmacy increases with increasing age and older people may be taking regular medications that increase blood pressure, such as non-steroidal anti-inflammatory drugs, decongestants or glucocorticoids, which may make blood pressure control more challenging and may result in a vicious circle of increased polypharmacy. Regular medications review and rationalisation, and reducing medications that have hypertensive effects may help to reduce polypharmacy and improve adherence to blood pressure treatment (Box 11a.1).

Summary

High blood pressure is very common among older individuals with diabetes, and managing blood pressure effectively contributes to better cardiovascular outcomes. While tighter blood pressure control is advised for healthier individuals, higher targets are more suitable

Box 11a.1: Considerations When Treating Hypertension in Older People with Diabetes

- Intensity of blood pressure lowering increases the risk of falls, especially in patients with a prior history of falling.
- Intensive blood pressure lowering may be a contributing factor to a decline in cognitive function.
- Higher SBP (130–145 mmHg) may be more protective for cognitive function in older people with cognitive impairment.
- Presence of frailty may modify the relationship between blood pressure control and outcomes.
- A SBP >140 mmHg may be more appropriate in frail individuals.
- Isolated systolic hypertension in people with diabetes is associated with adverse outcomes.
- Treatment of isolated systolic hypertension with multiple antihypertensives may unduly reduce DBP to a critically low level compromising coronary artery perfusion and increasing the risk of cardiac events.
- In treating isolated systolic hypertension, DBP should be maintained at or above 60 mmHg.
- Postural hypotension, common in older people with diabetes, is associated with an increased risk of falls, syncope and cardiac events.
- Better control of hypertension may reduce the incidence of postural hypotension.
- Clinical practice should focus on achieving blood pressure targets with careful monitoring of postural symptoms.
- Hypertensive medications should be temporally withheld in an acute illness, which cause volume loss such as vomiting and diarrhoea to avoid severe hypotension.
- Regular review and rationalisation of medications may help reduce polypharmacy and improve adherence to antihypertensive therapy.

SBP, systolic blood pressure; DBP, diastolic blood pressure.

for those with compromised function, particularly for individuals with cognitive impairments or frailty. In managing hypertension in older individuals, it is crucial to consider specific factors such as orthostatic hypotension and the increased risk of falls.

Clinical Practice Question

Q1. An 88-year-old woman with type 2 diabetes mellitus and hypertension for > 30 years. She lives in a care home and takes amlodipine 10 mg od, bendroflumethiazide 2.5 mg once a day and ramipril 2.5 mg once a day for hypertension, together with metformin 1 g twice a day, linagliptin 5 mg and insulin glargine 28 units daily for diabetes. She was admitted to hospital with a fall and was found to have sustained a fracture of the surgical neck of her left humerus. Her blood pressure was 112/78 mmHg with no postural drop. She had no history of hypoglycaemia, haemoglobin A1c 62 mmol/mol and estimated glomerular filtration rate 39 ml/minute/1.73 m^2. She scored 18/30 on the Montreal Cognitive Assessment (MoCA) and 6/9 on the clinical frailty scale. She should have the following antihypertensive medications adjustment.

Choose one option:

- **A.** Stop ramipril in view of reduced renal function.
- **B.** No change, as there is no postural drop in blood pressure.
- **C.** Stop both ramipril and bendroflumethiazide to reduce risk of dehydration and acute kidney injury.
- **D.** Stop both ramipril and bendroflumethiazide to reduce amlodipine to 5 mg once daily.
- **E.** Consider withdrawing all antihypertensive medications.

References

Key references only are listed here. For a full list of references visit: `https://www.wiley.com/go/sinclair/1e`.

1. Danaei, G., Finucane, M.M., Lin, J.K. et al. (2011). National, regional and global trends in systolic blood pressure since 1980: systematic analysis of health examination surveys and epidemiological studies with 786 country-years and 5.4 million participants. *Lancet* 377: 568–577.

2. Castrejón-Pérez, R.C., Gutiérrez-Robledo, L.M., Cesari, M. et al. (2017). Diabetes mellitus, hypertension and frailty: a population-based, cross-sectional study of Mexican older adults. *Geriatr. Gerontol. Int.* 17: 925–930.
3. Xu, X., Wang, B., Ren, C. et al. (2017). Age-related impairment of vascular structure and functions. *Aging Dis.* 8: 590–610.
4. Applegate, W.B., Davis, B.R., Black, H.R. et al. (1991). Prevalence of postural hypotension at baseline in the systolic hypertension in the elderly program (SHEP) cohort. *J. Am. Geriatr. Soc.* 39: 1057–1064.
5. Holt-Lunstad, J., Jones, B.Q., and Birmingham, W. (2009). The influence of close relationships on nocturnal blood pressure dipping. *Int. J. Psychophysiol.* 71: 211–217.
6. Tuomilehto, J., Rastenyte, D., Birkenhäger, W.H. et al. (1999). Effects of calcium-channel blockade in older patients with diabetes and systolic hypertension. *N. Engl. J. Med.* 340: 677–684.
7. Cooper-DeHoff, R.M., Gong, Y., Handberg, E.M. et al. (2010). Tight blood pressure control and cardiovascular outcomes among hypertensive patients with diabetes and coronary artery disease. *JAMA* 304: 61–68.
8. ACCORD Study Group, Cushman, W.C., Evans, G.W. et al. (2010). Effects of intensive blood-pressure control in type 2 diabetes mellitus. *N. Engl. J. Med.* 362: 1575–1585.
9. Brunström, M. and Carlberg, B. (2016). Effect of antihypertensive treatment at different blood pressure levels in patients with diabetes mellitus: systematic review and meta-analyses. *BMJ* 352: i717.
10. Beckett, N.S., Peters, R., Fletcher, A.E. et al. (2008). Treatment of hypertension in patients 80 years of age or older. *N. Engl. J. Med.* 358: 1887–1898.

11b Vascular Risk Factors: Dyslipidaemia

Pann Ei Hnynn, Si[1] *and Ahmed H. Abdelhafiz*[2]

[1]*Sheffield Kidney Institute, Sheffield Teaching Hospitals, Sheffield, UK*

[2]*Department of Geriatric Medicine, Rotherham General Hospital, Rotherham, UK*

Key Points

- Ageing and diabetes synergistically increase the risk of dyslipidaemia, especially the most atherogenic small low-density lipoprotein particles.
- Atherosclerotic cardiovascular disease is the most common cause of death in older people with diabetes.
- Older people with diabetes stand to benefit most from lipid-lowering therapy due to their high baseline risk.
- Aggressive lipid lowering therapy is required in fit older people with diabetes who have established atherosclerotic cardiovascular disease.
- Clinical discretion about the intensity of lipid-lowering therapy should be considered in frail older people with diabetes.

Introduction

Diabetes is associated with high risk of micro- and macrovascular disease, which increases with age and duration of diabetes. Macrovascular disease is caused by diabetes-related atherosclerosis and manifests as coronary artery disease, cerebrovascular disease and peripheral

Care of Older People with Diabetes: A Manual for Healthcare Practice, First Edition.
Edited by Alan J. Sinclair and Ahmed H. Abdelhafiz.

Companion website: www.wiley.com/go/sinclair/1e

vascular disease. Dyslipidaemia, in diabetes, is one of the major risk factors that causes the development of atherosclerotic cardiovascular disease (ASCVD), which is the leading cause of diabetes-related mortality. Diabetes-associated dyslipidaemia is a cluster of lipoprotein abnormalities characterised by an increase in triglyceride levels, decrease in high-density lipoprotein (HDL) levels and an increase in the atherogenic small low-density lipoprotein (LDL) particles. The cardiovascular benefit of treating dyslipidaemia with lipid-lowering drugs is well established. Although older people stand to benefit most from dyslipidaemia treatment, many older people with high baseline cardiovascular risk are excluded from clinical trials and results are extrapolated from clinical trials conducted on younger populations. This chapter reviews the effect of ageing on lipid profile, investigates the characteristics of dyslipidaemia in older people with diabetes and explores the safety consideration of lipid-lowering agents in this group of patients.

Ageing and Lipid Profile

With increasing age, total cholesterol, triglyceride and LDL levels increase but HDL remains unchanged. In addition, postprandial lipid clearance diminishes, especially in people with a sedentary lifestyle. Therefore, ageing is associated with increased postprandial atherogenic lipid particles leading to increased arterial atherosclerosis and prevalence of cardiovascular disease. Ageing-related atherosclerosis is associated with arterial stiffness, fibrosis and calcification of the atherosclerotic plaques. With increasing age, atherosclerotic plaques tend to be more stable and the occurrence cardiovascular events is more likely to be caused by arterial stiffness rather than by rupture of unstable plaques. Cholesterol-lowering medications usually work by stabilisation of unstable atherosclerotic plaques and, as a result, they may be less effective with increasing age.

Diabetes and Lipid Profile

Dyslipidaemia is very common in type 2 diabetes mellitus (T2DM), affecting up to 85% of patients, and is likely caused by insulin resistance rather than hyperglycaemia [1]. People with T2DM often have an increase in serum triglyceride levels, increased very-low-density lipoprotein and their remnants and decreased HDL. There is also an increase in small, dense LDL, a lipoprotein particle that may be particularly pro-atherogenic. However, LDL remains normal or slightly increases with a predominance of the most atherogenic small dense particles. Increased glycation and oxidation of these small particles increases its permeability into arterial intima, leading to an increased risk of atherosclerosis and cardiovascular disease. These small particles cannot normally be detected in routine blood testing. As LDL may remain normal, the routine testing of the lipid profile may not reflect the serious nature of diabetes-associated dyslipidaemia. Therefore, the measurement of non-HDL cholesterol levels may be a better reflection of lipid profile in patients with diabetes (Figure 11b.1).

Diabetes and Risk of Atherosclerotic Cardiovascular Disease

Diabetes is associated with a fourfold increased risk of ASCVD and 75% increased risk of mortality compared with people without diabetes [2]. Because of the high ASCVD risk associated with diabetes, patients with T2DM who have no other additional cardiovascular risk factors are classified as moderate cardiovascular risk. Many older people with diabetes have multiple morbidities and diabetes-related clinical or subclinical end-organ damage, so the ASCVD risk in this group of patients is likely to be high. In addition, ASCVD may develop before the diagnosis of diabetes is made. For example, prediabetes has been shown to be associated with an increased risk of all-cause mortality (relative risk [RR] 1.13, 95% confidence interval [CI] 1.10–1.17), cardiovascular disease (RR 1.15, CI 1.11–1.18), coronary heart disease (RR 1.16, CI 1.11–1.21) and stroke (RR 1.14, CI 1.08–1.20) after a median follow-up of 9.8 years [3]. Cardiorenal end-organ damage have also been demonstrated in a large proportion of patients before the clinical diagnosis of T2DM [4]. Older patients with diabetes are thus likely have high cardiovascular risk and the earlier the start of lipid-lowering drugs the better.

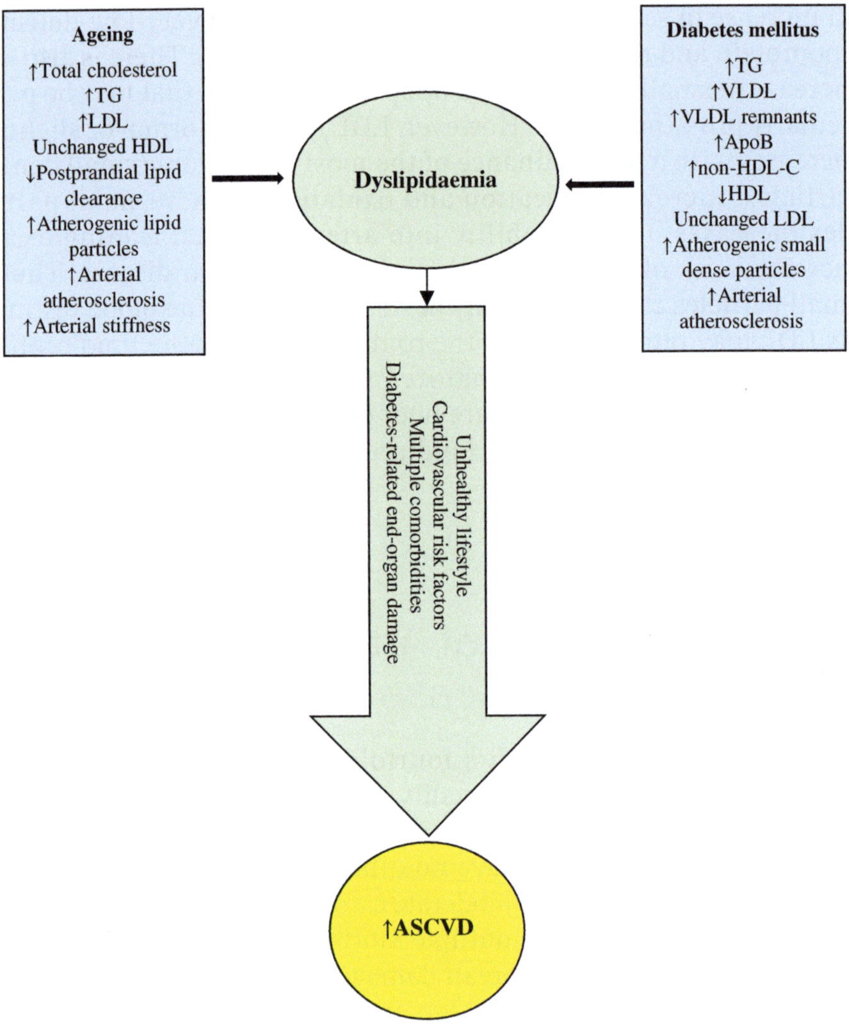

Figure 11b.1: Synergistic effects of ageing and diabetes on dyslipidaemia, increasing the risk of atherosclerotic cardiovascular disease (ASCVD). HDL, high-density lipoprotein; LDL, low-density lipoprotein; TG, triglyceride; VLDL very-low-density lipoprotein.

Atherosclerotic Cardiovascular Disease Risk Reduction

The aim of lipid-lowering therapy in older people with diabetes is to reduce the risk of ASCVD, defined as vascular disease of atherosclerotic origin, such as stable angina, unstable angina, myocardial infarction, ischaemic stroke, transient ischaemic attack, peripheral arterial disease, aortic aneurysm or the need for revascularisation procedures. Most of lipid-lowering studies to date have been conducted on younger participants. The Prospective Study of Pravastatin in the Elderly at Risk (PROSPER) was designed for older people aged 70–82 years (10.5% had diabetes) and included people with either pre-existing vascular disease (secondary prevention) or with increased cardiovascular risk due to smoking or presence of hypertension or diabetes (primary prevention) [5]. The study showed a 15% reduction in cardiovascular endpoints in the cholesterol-lowering group [5]. Similar results were shown in the heart protection study (primary prevention), which included a total of 20 536 patients between the ages of 40–80 years (28% were > 70 years and 28% had diabetes) [6]. The magnitude of risk reduction in older people appears to be similar to younger patients but the absolute benefit of cholesterol-lowering therapy is likely to be higher in older people due to their higher baseline risk. This was demonstrated in the post hoc analysis of the Collaborative Atorvastatin Diabetes Study, which included 1129 patients aged 65–75 years and 1709 younger patients. Relative risk reduction of cardiovascular events was similar in both groups (38% in older vs 37% in younger group) but the absolute risk reductions were 3.9% vs 2.7% and the numbers needed to treat were 21 and 33, respectively [7].

Lipid-lowering Agents

Lifestyle modification of regular physical exercise, achieving ideal body weight, smoking cessation, reduced alcohol intake and adherence to healthy diet is the first line of lipid-lowering therapy. In addition to lifestyle modifications, pharmacological intervention will be required to treat dyslipidaemia. There are several classes of lipid-lowering agents (Table 11b.1) The hydroxymethylglutaryl coenzyme A reductase inhibitors or statins are the first line of therapy and their efficacy in reducing ASCVD risk is established (Table 11b.2) [5–7]. Ezetimibe, cholesterol absorption inhibitor, can be used in cases of intolerance to statins or when statins are not sufficient to treat dyslipidaemia. The combination of statins with ezetimibe is associated with greater efficacy, than statins alone, in reducing the incidence of cardiovascular disease and stroke in patients with diabetes (RR 0.69, 95% CI 0.67–0.73 and 0.74, 0.56–0.98, respectively) [8]. Fibrates reduces triglyceride, increases HDL and decreases small, dense LDL. Fibrates are mainly used to lower triglyceride levels and to reduce the risk of pancreatitis, but they have

Table 11b.1: Lipid-lowering agents.

Agent	Actions	Cautions
Statins	HMG-CoA reductase inhibitors, highly effective, first line therapy. ↓LDL, ↓TG, ↑HDL	Nausea, diarrhoea, constipation, stomach pain, muscle pain, myositis, rhabdomyolysis, elevated liver enzymes, new-onset diabetes. Caution in patients with pre-existing muscle or liver disease. Drugs that inhibit cytochrome P450 3A4 (CYP3A4) such as macrolide antibiotics can increase the risk of statin-induced myopathy
Ezetimibe	Inhibits intestinal absorption of cholesterol, moderate efficacy, can be used in combination with statins to enhance efficacy and in FH. ↓LDL, ↓TG, ↑HDL	Upper respiratory tract infection, diarrhoea, abdominal pain, fatigue, muscle pain. Caution in patients with elevated transaminase levels, especially those on statins therapy
Fibrates	Mainly used to reduce triglyceride levels and risk of pancreatitis. No clear effects on cardiovascular outcomes. ↓LDL, ↓TG, ↑HDL	Nausea, abdominal and muscle pain. Not used in patients with active liver disease such as primary biliary cirrhosis, persistent liver function abnormality or gall bladder disease. Severe renal impairment or ESRD, including dialysis
Nicotinic acid	Increases HDL, can help reduce LDL in FH. No clear effects on cardiovascular outcomes. ↓LDL, ↓TG, ↑HDL	Flushing, dyspepsia, itching and increased blood glucose. Not used in patients with active liver disease, elevated transaminases, active peptic ulcers, hypotension or arterial haemorrhage
BAS	In combination with other lipid lowering agents, can be used in FH. Safe in patients with liver problems. ↓LDL, ↑HDL	GI adverse effects such as bloating, constipation, nausea and abdominal pain. Not used in biliary obstruction or severe hypertriglyceridaemia. Malabsorption of other drugs like fat-soluble vitamins such as vitamin K leading to impaired clotting

Table 11b.1: Continued

Agent	Actions	Cautions
PCSK9 inhibitors	Very effective new class, used in FH requiring further reduction of LDL despite statin therapy. Do not cause muscle or liver damage. ↓↓LDL	Reaction on injection site such as erythema, swelling, pain and itching. Parenteral route of administration and cost implications are issues
Omega-3 fatty acids	Adjuvant treatment to statins. ↓TG, ↑HDL	Indigestion, belching, fishy taste, may increase risk of bleeding
ACL inhibitors	Adjuvant treatment to statins. ↓LDL	Muscle spasms, joint pain and acute gout

ACL, adenosine triphosphate-citrate lyase; BAS, bile acid sequestrants; ESRD, end-stage renal disease; FH, familial hypercholesterolemia; GI, gastrointestinal; HMG-CoA, hydroxymethylglutaryl coenzyme A; PCSK9, proprotein convertase subtilisin/kexin type 9.

Table 11b.2: Statins strengths.

Statin	Intensity		
	Low (<30% ↓ LDL) (mg)	Moderate (30–50% ↓ LDL) (mg)	High (>50% ↓ LDL) (mg)
Simvastatin	10	20–40	–
Pravastatin	10–20	40–80	–
Fluvastatin	20–40	80	–
Pitavastatin	1	2–4	–
Lovastatin	20	40	
Atorvastatin	–	10–20	40–80
Rosuvastatin	–	5–10	20–40

no effects on ASCVD when added to statins. Nicotinic acid increases HDL, reduces triglyceride and LDL levels and can be combined with statins to increase efficiency in patients with familial hypercholesterolaemia. However, the combination of nicotinic acid and statins do not have additional benefits on ASCVD reduction compared with statins monotherapy. Bile acid sequestrants can be used in combination with other lipid-lowering agents to reduce total cholesterol and LDL but have no effects on ASCVD risk reduction. Proprotein convertase subtilisin/kexin type 9 (PCSK9) inhibitors comprise a new class of effective lipid-lowering agents, which can be used in combination with other lipid-lowering classes in patients with familial hypercholesterolaemia or in patients who require further reduction of LDL despite statins therapy. The addition of PCSK9 inhibitors to statins therapy further reduces the risk of ASCVD [9]. Omega-3 fatty acids and adenosine triphosphate–citrate lyase inhibitors are adjuvant to statins therapy, which can further reduce LDL.

Goals of Therapy in Old Age

Moderate intensity statins can be used in older people with diabetes who have no other cardiovascular risk factors without a need for risk assessment. A meta-analysis of clinical trials found that moderate-intensity statins therapy to be associated with ASCVD risk reduction by 25%. In older people with diabetes and other cardiovascular risk factors, high-intensity statins should be used with the aim to reduce LDL by 50% or more [10]. The evidence for cholesterol-lowering therapy is established for older people with diabetes up to the age of 80 years, whether for primary or secondary prevention. Observational studies showed some extra evidence, although not significant, of the benefit of cholesterol-lowering for people older than 80 years [11]. There was also a trend towards mortality benefit in those aged 80–85 years compared with those above the age of 85 years [11]; however, there are no clear data for benefits for patients above the age of 85 years.

Recommendations from Guidelines

The European Society of Cardiology and the European Association for the Study of Diabetes recommend a target LDL of <2.6 mmol/l in patients with diabetes and moderate risk of ASCVD. In patients at high risk, a target LDL of <1.8 mmol/l and $\geq 50\%$ reduction of LDL is recommended. In patients with very high risk, a target LDL of <1.4 mmol/l and $\geq 50\%$ reduction of LDL is recommended. A secondary goal of non-HDL target of <2.2 mmol/l in patients at very high risk and

< 2.6 mmol/l in those at high-risk is recommended [12]. The American Diabetes Association recommends the use of high-intensity statins in individuals with diabetes and established ASCVD to reduce LDL by ≥ 50% from the baseline and target LDL < 1.4 mmol/l. High-intensity statins are recommended in individuals aged 40–75 years with diabetes and having one or more ASCVD risk factors, to reduce the LDL by ≥ 50% of the baseline and to target LDL < 1.8 mmol/l. In patients aged > 75 years, moderate-intensity statin can be initiated, or the original statins regimen continued if they were already receiving therapy. If the goal is not achieved on maximum tolerated statins therapy, the addition of ezetimibe or a PCSK9 inhibitor is recommended (Table 11b.3) [13].

Table 11b.3: Guidelines for dyslipidaemia treatment in older people with diabetes.

European Society of Cardiology/European Association for the Study of Diabetes	
ASCVD risk	**Low-density lipoprotein**
Moderate[a]	< 2.6 mmol/l
High	< 1.8 mmol/l, aim for ≥ 50% reduction
Very high	< 1.4 mmol/l, aim for ≥ 50% reduction
A secondary goal of non-HDL target of <2.2 mmol/l in very high risk and <2.6 mmol/l in high risk patients is recommended.	
American Diabetes Association	
Diabetes and established ASCVD	High-intensity statins, LDL < 1.4 mmol/l and reduce by ≥ 50% of baseline
Age 40–75 years with diabetes and ≥ 1 ASCVD risk factors.	High-intensity statins, LDL < 1.8 mmol/l and reduce by ≥ 50% of baseline
Aged > 75 years	Continue statins if already on therapy or initiate at moderate intensity statin if newly starting
If the goal is not achieved on maximum tolerated statins therapy, the addition of ezetimibe followed by PCSK9 inhibitor is recommended.	

[a] Moderate ASCVD risk = young patients (type 1 diabetes mellitus aged < 35 years or type 2 aged < 50 years), diabetes duration < 10 years and without other risk factors. High ASCVD risk = patients with diabetes duration > 10 years without target organ damage plus any other additional cardiovascular risk factor. Very high ASCVD risk = patients with diabetes and established cardiovascular disease or target organ damage or ≥ 3 major cardiovascular risk factors or type 1 diabetes of > 20 years.

Goals in Frailty

There are no clinical trials on the benefits of cholesterol-lowering therapy in frail older people with diabetes. Frailty is a wasting disease characterised by significant weight loss and malnutrition. In some frail patients, the weight loss is so severe to the extent of normalisation of haemoglobin A1c, which requires the withdrawal of hypoglycaemic therapy. These patients are likely to have low cholesterol and low albumin levels as markers of malnutrition. Review of statins therapy will be required for these patients. For example, the effects of high- or moderate-intensity statins therapy in care-home residents may not have positive effects on avoiding hospital admissions or reducing mortality [14]. In this group of fully dependent frail people, clinical discretion is required for the reduction of the intensity or the complete withdrawal of cholesterol-lowering therapy, with the aim of focusing on quality of life and reduction of unnecessary polypharmacy (Figure 11b.2).

Summary

Dyslipidaemia is common in older people with diabetes and is one of the major risk factors for ASCVD. Aggressive lipid-lowering therapy is required in fit older people with diabetes, while clinical discretion should be considered in frail individuals.

Clinical Practice Question

Q1. An 81-year-old man with diabetes mellitus for 27 years. He is an ex-smoker and has a past medical history of hypertension, ischaemic heart disease and transient ischaemic attack. His body mass index is 31 kg/m^2. He walks with a stick and needs some assistance in activities of daily living. His medications include metformin 1 g twice a day, empagliflozin 10 mg once a day, dulaglutide 1.5 mg/week, ramipril 10 mg once a day and atorvastatin 10 mg once a day. His haemoglobin A1c is 60.7 mmol/mol (7.6%), total cholesterol 3.9 mmol/l, low-density lipoprotein 2.1, high-density lipoprotein 0.93 and triglyceride 2.7 mmol/l. What is the most appropriate treatment?

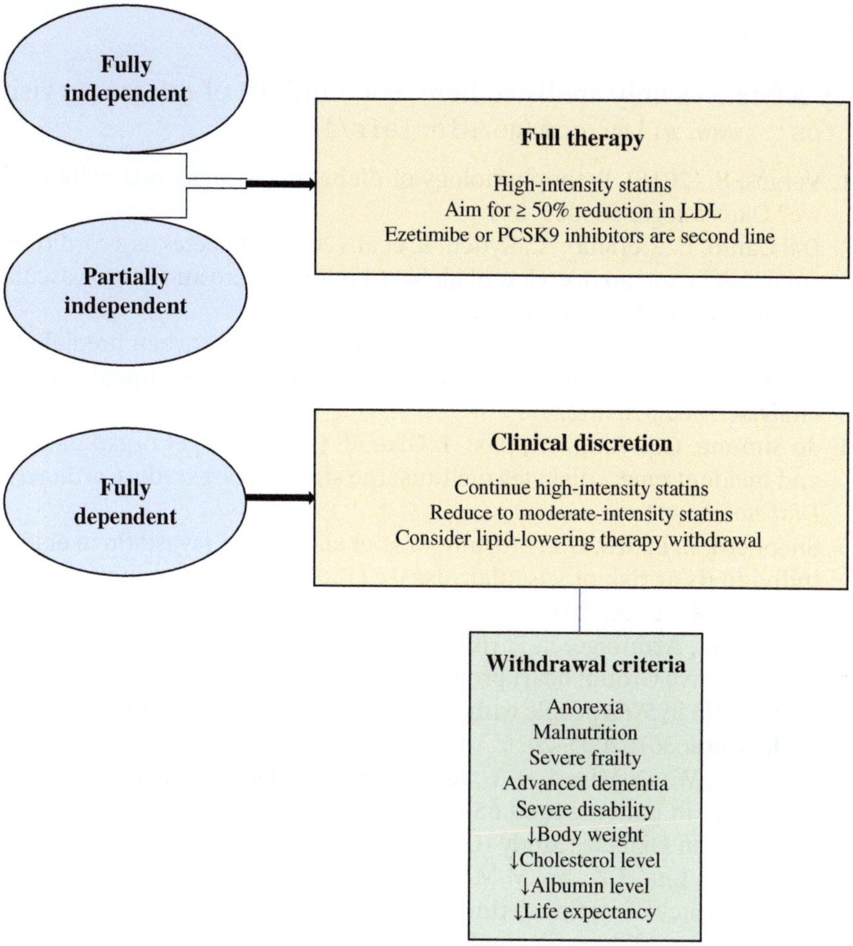

Figure 11b.2: Suggested lipid-lowering therapy in older people with diabetes based on function. Fully independent, no physical or cognitive impairment and no assistance in activities of daily living (ADL); partially independent, mild cognitive/physical impairment needing some assistance in ADL; dependent, moderate-severe cognitive/physical impairment needing full assistance in ADL. LDL, low-density lipoprotein; PCSK9, proprotein convertase subtilisin/kexin type 9.

Choos one option:

A. Add another hypoglycaemic agent for better control of diabetes.
B. Encourage lifestyle changes to reduce body weight.
C. Increase atorvastatin to 20 mg once a day.
D. Increase atorvastatin to reach at least 40 mg once a day.
E. Add fibrates to reduce triglycerides.

References

Key references only are listed here. For a full list of references visit: https://www.wiley.com/go/sinclair/1e.

1. Vergès, B. (2015). Pathophysiology of diabetic dyslipidaemia: where are we? *Diabetologia* 58: 886–899.
2. Dal Canto, E., Ceriello, A., Rydén, L. et al. (2019). Diabetes as a cardiovascular risk factor: an overview of global trends of macro and micro vascular complications. *Eur. J. Prev. Cardiol.* 26: 25–32.
3. Cai, X., Zhang, Y., Li, M. et al. (2020). Association between prediabetes and risk of all cause mortality and cardiovascular disease: updated meta-analysis. *BMJ* 370: m2297.
4. de Simone, G., Wang, W., Best, L.G. et al. (2017). Target organ damage and incident type 2 diabetes mellitus: the strong heart study. *Cardiovasc. Diabetol.* 16: 64.
5. Shepherd, J., Blauw, G.J., Murphy, M.B. et al. (2002). Pravastatin in elderly individuals at risk of vascular disease (PROSPER): a randomised controlled trial. *Lancet* 360: 1623–1630.
6. Collins, R., Armitage, J., Parish, S. et al. (2003). Heart Protection Study Collaborative Group: heart protection study of cholesterol lowering with simvastatin in 5963 people with diabetes: a randomised placebo-controlled trial. *Lancet* 361: 2005–2016.
7. Neil, H.A.W., DeMicco, D.A., Luo, D. et al. (2006). Analysis of efficacy and safety in patients aged 65–75 years at randomisation. Collaborative Atorvastatin Diabetes Study (CARDS). *Diabetes Care* 29: 2378–2384.
8. Miao, X.Y., Liu, H.Z., Jin, M.M. et al. (2019). A comparative meta-analysis of the efficacy of statin-ezetimibe co-therapy versus statin monotherapy in reducing cardiovascular and cerebrovascular adverse events in patients with type 2 diabetes mellitus. *Eur. Rev. Med. Pharmacol. Sci.* 23: 2302–2310.
9. Sabatine, M.S., Leiter, L.A., Wiviott, S.D. et al. (2017). Cardiovascular safety and efficacy of the PCSK9 inhibitor evolocumab in patients with and without diabetes and the effect of evolocumab on glycaemia and risk of new-onset diabetes: a prespecified analysis of the FOURIER randomised controlled trial. *Lancet Diabetes Endocrinol.* 5: 941–950.
10. de Vries, F.M., Denig, P., Pouwels, K.B. et al. (2012). Primary prevention of major cardiovascular and cerebrovascular events with statins in diabetic patients: a meta-analysis. *Drugs* 72: 2365–2373.

12a Metabolic Decompensation: Hyperglycaemic Crisis

Puja Merwaha and Ahmed H. Abdelhafiz

Department of Geriatric Medicine, Rotherham General Hospital, Rotherham, United Kingdom

Key Points

- Older people with diabetes are most vulnerable to hyperglycaemic crisis because of their risk of acute stressful events, comorbidities and reduced immunity.
- Hyperglycaemic crisis may be the first presentation of diabetes in this age group.
- Atypical neurological symptoms can be the dominant manifestation of a hyperglycaemic crisis in older people.
- In old age, a hyperglycaemic crisis is associated with worse morbidity and mortality than younger people.
- Close follow-up after recovery from a hyperglycaemic crisis is required as there is a high risk of recurrence.

Introduction

Diabetic ketoacidosis (DKA) and hyperosmolar hyperglycaemic state (HHS) are the two main hyperglycaemic crises in older people with diabetes. DKA is characterised by a triad of hyperglycaemia, metabolic acidosis and ketosis. DKA is common in type 1 diabetes mellitus (T1DM), due to insulin insufficiency, but it occasionally occurs in type 2 diabetes mellitus (T2DM). DKA in older people is associated with more adverse outcomes and healthcare- related costs compared with the

Care of Older People with Diabetes: A Manual for Healthcare Practice, First Edition.
Edited by Alan J. Sinclair and Ahmed H. Abdelhafiz.

Companion website: www.wiley.com/go/sinclair/1e

same condition in younger people [1]. HHS is characterised by a triad of severe hyperglycaemia, hyperosmolarity and severe dehydration. HHS is not usually associated with acidosis. However, DKA and HHS may overlap and present simultaneously in up to one third of cases [2]. This chapter reviews the epidemiology, clinical presentation and management of hyperglycaemic crises in old age.

Epidemiology

In a retrospective study, DKA represented 2% of acute hospitalisations of older people with diabetes [3]. The incidence of HHS is estimated to be about 1% of all acute diabetes-related hospital admissions and tends to occur later in life than DKA [4]. Hyperglycaemic crises affect slightly more women than men and the incidence is also higher in populations with a high prevalence of diabetes [3, 5]. Increasing age and duration of diabetes are associated with increased risk of hospitalisation due to hyperglycaemic crisis [6]. Diabetes may present for the first time with DKA, which is referred to as DKA-onset diabetes. Patients with T2DM prone to ketosis are susceptible to DKA due to significant impairment of β-cell function leading to insulin insufficiency.

Precipitating Factors

Older patients' characteristics predispose them to risk of hyperglycaemic crisis, including comorbidities, cardiovascular events, polypharmacy, risk of infection, non-compliance with glucose lowering medication and dehydration (Box 12a.1). Polypharmacy, especially atypical antipsychotics increase the risk of metabolic syndrome and persistent hyperglycaemia [7]. Morbidities with reduced oral intake increases risk of dehydration, which is the leading factor in precipitation of HHS. Hospital-acquired DKA is another form of DKA common in older people and is caused largely by errors in insulin administration during hospital admissions, such as reducing the dose, holding or interruption of insulin, as well as hospital- acquired infections [8]. Parenteral solutions rich in dextrose or fat content increase blood glucose levels and, in patients with insulin resistance, may precipitate HHS.

Box 12a.1: Precipitating Factors of Hyperglycaemic Crisis in Older People with Diabetes

- Increasing age
- Long duration of diabetes
- Impaired thirst perception
- Acute febrile illness
- Acute fluid loss
- Dehydration
- Hypothermia
- Burns
- Acute vascular event
- Acute pancreatitis
- Multiple morbidities:
  - Congestive cardiac failure
  - Chronic kidney disease
  - Peritoneal dialysis
  - Dementia
  - Debility
  - Institutionalisation
  - Immobility
  - Endocrine disorders (e.g. Cushing's, acromegaly and thyrotoxicosis)
- Medications:
  - Glucocorticoids
  - Anti-psychotics
  - Anti-epileptics
  - Thiazide diuretics
  - Alcohol
  - Immunosuppressants
  - Sodium glucose transporter-2 inhibitors
  - Statins
  - Beta-blockers
- Non-compliance with hypoglycaemic therapy
- Trauma
- Emergency surgery
- Neglect or abuse

Pathogenesis

Older people have reduced number and function of the pancreatic β-cells. Acute illness leads to increased secretion of stress hormones, such as cortisol and catecholamine, and growth-hormone potentiating hyperglycaemia. The relative insulin deficiency prevents peripheral uptake of glucose; this intracellular starvation leads to increased hepatic gluconeogenesis, which further increases hyperglycaemia.

In DKA, due to a lack of available glucose, lipolysis occurs leading to the formation of ketone bodies and metabolic acidosis. In HHS, insulin levels are sufficient to prevent lipolysis and ketone bodies formation but is insufficient to keep blood glucose at normal levels. Hyperglycaemia leads to osmotic diuresis and a reduction of total body water. The continuous osmotic diuresis leads to hypovolaemia and hypotension.

Acute kidney injury and oliguria may occur due to severe dehydration. Reduction of level of consciousness and coma are the final steps in this process (Figure 12a.1).

Clinical Presentation

Hyperglycaemic crisis in older people may present with general non-specific symptoms such as general decline, reduced oral intake, lethargy, confusion, falls and, in some cases, it may be the first presentation of diabetes [9, 10]. A high index of suspicion for hyperglycaemic crisis is needed as it can be masked by the presenting complaint or the triggering factor.

DKA classically presents with acute gastrointestinal symptoms such as nausea, vomiting and acute abdominal pain. The severity and acuteness of symptoms correlate with the severity of acidosis. Ketosis may lead to a fruity smell to the breath. However, in older people with reduced reserve, reduced stress response and comorbidities, the gastrointestinal symptoms may be subtle or absent. Tachypnoea and Kussmaul breathing, due to acidosis, may be misinterpreted as a respiratory or a cardiac cause. In addition, in older people, an altered mental state such as delirium may mask the diagnosis and the precipitant [11].

The onset of HHS occurs more gradually over few days or weeks and is slower than that of DKA. Dehydration over a period is a key trigger of HHS, especially in patients with a premorbid condition, which causes reduced oral intake. In advanced cases, focal neurological symptoms such as seizures or coma may occur. Symptoms and signs of the primary

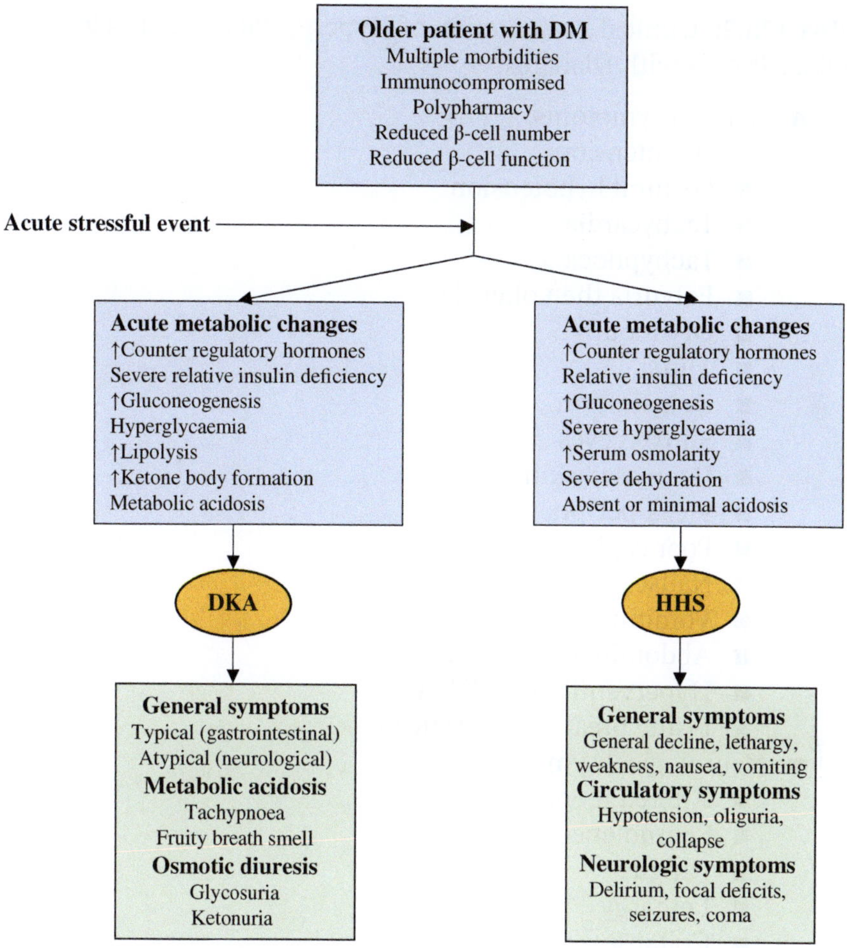

Figure 12a.1: Pathogenesis of hyperglycaemic crisis in older people with diabetes. DM, diabetes mellitus; DKA, diabetic ketoacidosis; HHS, hyperosmolar hyperglycaemic state.

triggering event may coexist in addition to those in hyperglycaemic crisis (Box 12a.2).

Diagnosis

Hyperglycaemic crises should be suspected in all older people presenting with diabetes or acute hyperglycaemia even if they do not present with the classic symptoms. The classic laboratory findings of DKA are high blood glucose, high blood ketones, metabolic acidosis or low bicarbonate, glycosuria and ketonuria. In patients taking sodium glucose transporter-2

Box 12a.2: Clinical Presentation of Hyperglycaemic Crisis in Older People with Diabetes

- General symptoms:
  - Hypotension
  - Postural hypotension
  - Tachycardia
  - Tachypnoea
  - Polyuria then oliguria
  - Dry mouth
  - Thirst
  - Dehydration
  - Sunken eyes
  - Decreased skin turgor
  - Weak peripheral pulses
  - Poor capillary refill
  - Nausea
  - Vomiting
  - Abdominal pain (DKA)
  - Hyperventilation (DKA)
  - Fruity breath smell (DKA)
- Neurological symptoms:
  - Altered mental state
  - Somnolence
  - Fatigue
  - Lethargy
  - Collapse
  - Falls
  - Delirium
  - Lack of concentration
  - Disturbed visual acuity
  - Seizures (HHS)
  - Focal neurological deficits (HHS)
  - Coma (HHS)

DKA, diabetic ketoacidosis; HHS, hyperglycaemic hyperosmolar state.

Table 12a.1: Diagnostic criteria of hyperglycaemic crisis in older people with diabetes.

Diabetic ketoacidosis	Hyperglycaemic hyperosmolar state
Typical or atypical symptoms plus:	General or neurological symptoms plus:
Ketonaemia ≥3 mmol/l or ketonuria >2+ on urine dipsticks	Severe hyperglycaemia (blood glucose >30 mmol/l)
Hyperglycaemia >11 mmol/l or history of diabetes mellitus	Hyperosmolarity (>320 mOsm/kg)
Metabolic acidosis (serum HCO_3 <15 mmol/l or pH <7.3)	No or minimal acidosis (HCO_3 >15 mmol/l or pH >7.3)
	No significant ketonaemia (ketone bodies <3 mmol/l)

inhibitors and those with alcohol excess or liver cirrhosis, DKA may present with normal blood glucose levels termed euglycaemic DKA.

In HHS, history taking of consumption of high sugary items or starting of new medications such as diuretics may be a trigger for HHS. Patients with HHS presenting with neurological symptoms may need neurological investigation to rule out intracerebral infection or an acute cerebrovascular event. The underlying cause of hyperglycaemic crisis such as infection may present with fever and symptoms of the corresponding site of infection, such as productive cough or burning micturition. All patients with hyperglycaemic crises should have blood glucose level, serum electrolytes, renal function, blood ketones, arterial blood gases, serum osmolarity and urine ketones checked. Acidosis is not common in HHS but it can occur due to renal failure or lactic acidosis associated with sepsis and severe dehydration (Table 12a.1).

Management

Management of hyperglycaemic crisis includes general assessment of the patient, identifying and treating the precipitating factor, volume repletion, treatment of hyperglycaemia and correction of acidosis and

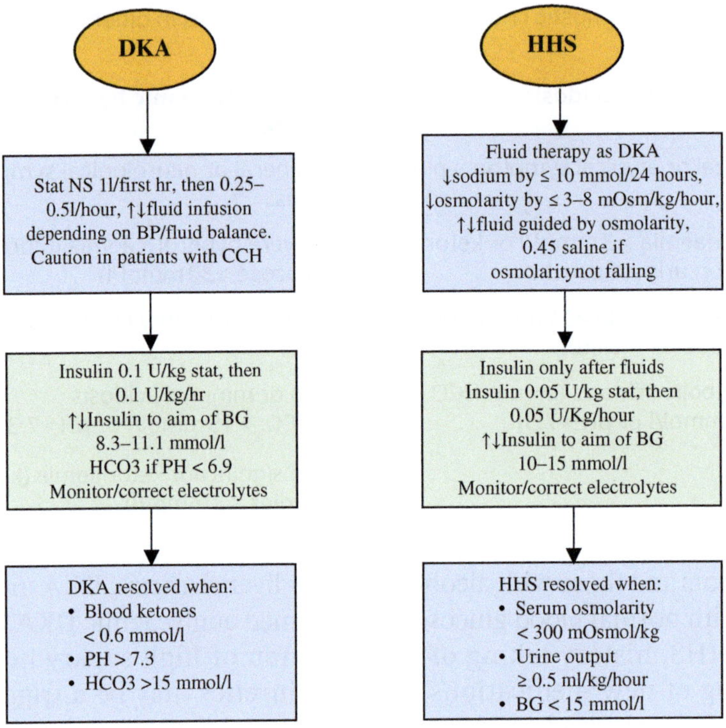

Figure 12a.2: Management of hyperglycaemic crisis in older people with diabetes. NS, physiological saline; BP, blood pressure; CCF, congestive cardiac failure; BG, blood glucose; DKA, diabetic ketoacidosis; HHS, hyperosmolar hyperglycaemic state.

electrolyte imbalances. Initial management can be in an acute ward, which provides close monitoring, but intensive care admission may be required in severe cases (Figure 12a.2; Table 12a.2).

Correction of Hypovolaemia

Intravascular volume should be corrected to maintain blood pressure and urine output. Initially, intravenous administration of 0.9% saline at 1.0 l in the first hour then followed by a slower correction with a reduced rate of 0.25–0.5 l 0.9% saline/hour is appropriate. The rate is guided by the maintenance of blood pressure, clinical fluid status and urine output with regular reviews and fluid input–output charts. Caution with fluid therapy should be considered to avoid fluid overload in frail elderly patients and those with renal or cardiovascular morbidities. The aim is to correct half of the patient's fluid deficit in the first 24 hours.

Table 12a.2: Criteria for intensive care admission of older people with hyperglycaemic crisis.

Diabetic ketoacidosis	Hyperglycaemic hyperosmolar state
Severe acidosis: serum ketones >6 mmol/l or serum HCO_3 <5 mmol/l or pH<7.1 or anion gap >16	Sodium >160 mmol/l
Hypokalaemia (K<3.5 mmol/l)	Osmolality >350 mOsm/kg
Altered conscious level (GCS score <12)	pH<7.1
Organ failure[a]	Admission potassium <3.5 or >6.0 mmol/l
Hypokalaemia (K<3.5 mmol/l)	Oxygen saturation<92%
	Altered conscious level (GCS score <12)
	Systolic blood pressure <90 mmHg
	Heart rate <60 or >100 bpm
	Organ failure[a]
	Hypothermia
	Oliguria (urine output <0.5 ml/kg/hour)
	Acute vascular events

GCS, Glasgow Coma Scale.
[a]Renal, cardiac, circulatory, respiratory or liver.

Choice of fluids should take into account the electrolyte imbalances. Correction of serum sodium should not be greater than 10 mmol/24 hours to avoid hyponatraemia and fluid shifts. In HHS, the reduction of plasma osmolarity should be by ≤3–8 mOsm/kg/hour to avoid neurological complications. If osmolality is falling at rate >8.0 mOsm/kg/hour consider reducing the infusion rate. Half-normal (0.45%) physiological saline may be required when osmolarity is not declining despite adequate fluid repletion.

Correction of Hyperglycaemia

In DKA, insulin should be given at a fixed rate of 0.1 U/kg/hour. An initial bolus dose could be considered of 0.1 U/kg followed by infusion of 0.1 U/kg/hour. The expected reduction of blood glucose is 2.8–4.2 mmol/l in the first hour; otherwise, insulin doses may need to be adjusted. The aim is to maintain blood glucose within 8.3–11.1 mmol/l.

In HHS, insulin therapy should start only after initial fluid resuscitation as rapid correction of hyperglycaemia may cause fluid shifts leading to further hypotension and vascular collapse. Initial fluid resuscitation will reduce the production of counter regulatory hormones therefore, reducing the intensity of hyperglycaemia. Insulin therapy should start intravenously at a fixed rate of 0.05 U/kg/hour. The aim is to reduce blood glucose by a rate of ≤5.0 mmol/l/hour. Insulin rate can be increased to 0.1 units/kg/hour if glucose levels are not falling and fluid balance is adequate. The aim is to keep blood glucose at 10-15 mmol/l in the first 24 hours.

In both conditions, patients normally on long-acting insulin should continue alongside regular insulin infusion. When blood glucose falls to less than 14 mmol/l, continue 0.9% saline and commence glucose 5% or 10% as well, to avoid hypoglycaemia. Recent guidelines recommend 10% glucose and also a reduced rate of insulin. When biochemical parameters are corrected and the patient is able to eat and drink with no vomiting, their usual insulin regimen can be started. Intravenous insulin infusion can then be stopped after one to four hours of starting usual regimen. If not tolerating adequate oral intake commence a variable rate insulin infusion with close monitoring of blood glucose levels.

Correction of Acidosis

In DKA, acidosis starts to improve with the correction of hypovolaemia and hyperglycaemia. Ketone body testing, which measures acetoacetic acid, may remain positive as it takes some time for the conversion of β-hydroxybutyric acid to acetoacetic acid. Serum pH and bicarbonate improve with insulin/saline therapy although serum bicarbonate may take up to 24 hours to normalise. Intravenous bicarbonate should be administered if pH drops to less than 6.9, with the aim of slow pH correction. A bicarbonate dose of 50–100 mmol should be given over two hours with repeated measurement of serum pH. Continuous intravenous insulin/saline solution should be continued until urine is consistently negative for ketone bodies and serum pH is normal. Bicarbonate should be undertaken only on specialist advice and in intensive care settings.

Correction of Electrolytes

Hyperglycaemia causes osmotic diuresis, which leads to dehydration and urinary loss of electrolytes, especially sodium and potassium. Hyponatraemia or hypernatraemia may occur depending on body fluid status. This will be corrected during insulin/saline infusion. In DKA, acidosis is associated with potassium shifting out of cells. Therefore, the initial serum potassium level is likely to be high, but normal serum potassium indicates potassium depletion and should be corrected by adding potassium to the crystalloid solution. Hypokalaemia should be avoided as it can lead to serious cardiac arrhythmias. The aim is to keep serum potassium level between 4 and 5 mmol/l. Hypophosphataemia may occur during treatment but does not require routine phosphate repletion unless it is associated with neurological symptoms, haemolysis or rhabdomyolysis. Correction of hypophosphataemia may be associated with hypocalcaemia, therefore calcium levels need to be monitored. Severe electrolyte abnormalities requiring intensive care admission may occur (Table 12a.2).

Complications

Diabetic ketoacidosis is associated with more complications in older compared with younger people, such as longer length of hospital stays (five vs three days, $p < 0.001$) and increased mortality (16.7% vs 1.6%, $p < 0.001$) [1]. In addition, in old age, recurrent DKA is associated with acute neuronal dysfunction, which does not return to baseline leading to progressive neurological decline [12]. The most common complications of HHS are hypokalaemia and hypoglycaemia. Mortality in HHS is about 5–20% and most likely related to the underlying clinical conditions [13]. Overlap cases of DKA–HHS have higher mortality (8%) than isolated DKA (3%) or HHS (5%) [2].

Rapid fluid correction may lead to non-cardiogenic pulmonary oedema. This should be avoided with cautious rehydration especially, in those at risk. Cerebral oedema is less common but the risk increases in HHS, with acute drop in serum osmolality. Mannitol infusion and mechanical ventilation are used to treat cerebral oedema.

Other key complications include arrhythmias secondary to electrolyte imbalances. Thrombotic complications or disseminated intravascular coagulation may occur; therefore, prophylactic anticoagulation is part of management. Foot care must be taken to avoid pressure ulcers.

Prevention

Patient and carer education on medication compliance, adequate hydration, regular nutrition and sick day rules is important. Carer's detection of early symptoms of dehydration or mental decline may help prevent hyperglycaemic crises. Regular review of medications and maintenance of good glycaemic control is required. The differences between DKA and HHS are summarised in Table 12a.3.

Clinical Practice Question

Q1. 82 year old woman with known dementia and type 2 diabetes mellitus presented with worsening confusion, shortness of breath and productive cough. Medications included metformin 1 g twice a day, linagliptin 5 mg once a day and memantine 20 mg once a day. Her haemoglobin A1c was 63 mmol/mol. On examination, her Glasgow Coma Scale score was 11/15, respiratory rate 36/minute, heart rate 110/minute. Chest auscultation revealed bibasal chest crackles. Investigations: Ph 7.17, HCO_3 11.1 mmol/l, glucose 43.9 mmol/l, blood ketones 5.1 mmol/l, urea 21.7 mmol/l,

Table 12a.3: Comparison of diabetic ketoacidosis and hyperglycaemic hyperosmolar state in older people with diabetes.

Diabetic ketoacidosis	Hyperglycaemic hyperosmolar state
Common in type 1 diabetes mellitus	Common in type 2 diabetes mellitus
Lower mortality (up to 2%)	Higher mortality (up to 20%)
Acute onset within hours or days	Less acute onset within days or weeks
Severe relative insulin deficiency	Relative insulin deficiency
Hyperglycaemia	Sever hyperglycaemia
Ketoacidosis common	Ketoacidosis less common
Tachypnoea with acidotic breathing	Tachypnoea
General neurologic features	General or focal neurologic features
Immediate insulin therapy required	Insulin only after fluid therapy.
Anion gap monitoring required	Serum osmolarity monitoring required

creatinine 187 µmol/l, sodium 163 mmol/l, serum osmolality 391.6 mOsm/kg.
What is the most appropriate treatment?
Choose one option:
A. Admit to the acute medical ward with close monitoring.
B. Start fluid therapy first to bring osmolarity down, then add an insulin infusion.
C. Start fluid combined with insulin at a rate of 0.05 U/kg/hour.
D. Start fluid and insulin infusion at a rate of 0.1 U/kg/hour.

References

Key references only are listed here. For a full list of references visit: https://www.wiley.com/go/sinclair/1e.

1. Schwarzfuchs, D., Rabaev, E., Sagy, I. et al. (2020). Clinical and epidemiological characteristics of diabetic ketoacidosis in older adults. *J. Am. Geriatr. Soc.* 68: 1256–1261.
2. Pasquel, F.J., Tsegka, K., Wang, H. et al. (2020). Clinical outcomes in patients with isolated or combined diabetic ketoacidosis and hyperosmolar hyperglycemic state: a retrospective hospital-based cohort study. *Diabetes Care* 43: 349–357.
3. Lin, W., Chen, C., Guan, H. et al. (2016). Hospitalization of elderly diabetic patients: characteristics, reasons for admission, and gender differences. *BMC Geriatr.* 16: 160.
4. Bradford, A.L., Crider, C.C., Xu, X., and Naqvi, S.H. (2017). Predictors of recurrent hospital admission for patients presenting with diabetic ketoacidosis and hyperglycemic hyperosmolar state. *J. Clin. Med. Res.* 9: 35–39.
5. Nugent, B.W. (2005). Hyperosmolar hyperglycemic state. *Emerg. Med. Clin. North Am.* 23: 629–648.
6. Huang, E.S., Laiteerapong, N., Liu, J.Y. et al. (2014). Rates of complications and mortality in older patients with diabetes mellitus: the diabetes and aging study. *JAMA Intern. Med.* 174: 251–258.
7. Guenette, M.D., Hahn, M., Cohn, T.A. et al. (2013). Atypical antipsychotics and diabetic ketoacidosis: a review. *Psychopharmacology (Berl.)* 226: 1–12.
8. Williams, D.M., Taverner, S., Watson, R. et al. (2022). A series of patients with hospital-acquired diabetic ketoacidosis (HADKA): a descriptive analysis. *Clin. Med. (Lond.)* 22: 549–552.
9. Shekaraiah, T. and Evans, P.J. (2019). Never too late for diabetic ketoacidosis (DKA). *Age Ageing* 48: i20.
10. Kitabchi, A.E., Umpierrez, G.E., Miles, J.M. et al. (2009). Hyperglycemic crises in adult patients with diabetes. *Diabetes Care* 32: 1335–1343.

12b Metabolic Decompensation: Hypoglycaemia

Srikanth Bellary[1,2], *Ahmed H. Abdelhafiz*[3] *and Alan J. Sinclair*[4]

[1] *Diabetes and Endocrinology, University Hospitals NHS Trust Birmingham, Birmingham, UK*
[2] *Metabolic Medicine, School of Biological Sciences, Aston University, Birmingham, UK*
[3] *Department of Geriatric Medicine, Rotherham General Hospital, Rotherham, UK*
[4] *Foundation for Diabetes Research in Older People, Diabetes Frail Ltd, UK*

Key Points

- Hypoglycaemia in older people with diabetes is less recognised and under reported.
- Hypoglycaemia in older people with diabetes is associated with significant morbidities of reduced physical and cognitive function, leading to frailty and disability.
- Hypoglycaemia occurs in frail undernourished older people regardless of diabetes status.
- Tighter glycaemic control is reasonable in fit older adults but a relaxed approach is more appropriate in frail older adults at risk of hypoglycaemia.
- Targets in frail older people with diabetes should focus on short-term day-to-day blood glucose levels to avoid hypoglycaemia, rather than basing on diabetes care around a long term haemoglobin A1c strategy.

Care of Older People with Diabetes: A Manual for Healthcare Practice, First Edition.
Edited by Alan J. Sinclair and Ahmed H. Abdelhafiz.

Companion website: www.wiley.com/go/sinclair/1e

Introduction

Achieving tight blood glucose control over sustained periods is a fundamental aspect of diabetes management and hypoglycaemia is a significant barrier towards achieving this aim. Non-iatrogenic hypoglycaemia in the setting of diabetes is extremely rare and is invariably associated with the treatment most commonly with sulfonylureas or insulin. Frequent episodes of hypoglycaemia have significant impact on individual health and is a predictor of future hypoglycaemia. It is also associated with significant morbidity and substantial direct and indirect healthcare costs. This chapter reviews the epidemiology, pathophysiology, clinical impacts and management of hypoglycaemia in older people with diabetes.

Definition

Opinions vary as to the optimal threshold used to define hypoglycaemia, but it is widely accepted that a glucose value of less than 3.9 mmol/l (70.2 mg/dl) [1] would be consistent with hypoglycaemia while a value of less than 3.5 mmol/l (63 mg/dl) as accepted by most as clinically significant. Based on the severity, hypoglycaemia is classified as mild (usually self-treated on appearance of symptoms) or severe (often requiring third-party assistance). Hypoglycaemia can also be classified as symptomatic and asymptomatic. The latter when associated with poor recognition of symptoms despite falling glucose values is also known as hypoglycaemia unawareness.

Recognition

The recognition of hypoglycaemia may be difficult due to the predominance of neurological rather than autonomic symptoms resulting in misdiagnosis [2]. Another diagnostic challenge is the similarities in the clinical presentation of hypoglycaemia with that of dementia, where patients present with agitation, increased confusion or behavioural changes. Symptoms can also be generally non-specific such as fatigue or weakness, leading to under-recognition and under-reporting by patients and physicians, subsequently leading to underestimated frequency (Box 12b.1) [3].

Box 12b.1: Difficulties in Recognising Hypoglycaemia in Older People

- Symptoms are non-specific
- Easily misdiagnosed (e.g. stroke, vertigo or visual disturbance)
- Misinterpreted as dementia-related symptoms (e.g. agitation or behaviour change)
- Atypical presentation (e.g. confusion or passive delirium)
- Little warning or unawareness of autonomic symptoms
- Patients with dementia are unable to communicate their feelings or symptoms

Epidemiology

The real incidence of hypoglycaemia in older people with diabetes may be underestimated. Hypoglycaemia incidence is likely to be higher in older age due to associated comorbidities and polypharmacy and tends to be less recognised due to altered adaptive physiologic responses to low glucose levels, as we get older. There is scarce literature on the incidence of hypoglycaemia specific to older people because of the heterogeneity of this age group, particularly in those living in care homes. The incidence of serious hypoglycaemia (defined as an episode leading to fatal outcome or hospital admission) was 1.23% for patients treated with sulfonylureas and 2.76% for those treated with insulin in a US retrospective population-based study of 19932 Medicaid patients, aged ≥65 years [4]. The incidence of hypoglycaemia of any severity was 14.1% over a 12-month period in a more recent prospective study of DiaRegis (multicentre registry of patients with diabetes) in Germany which included 3347 patients (median age 66.1 years) [5]. Older age seems to be associated with increased incidence of hypoglycaemia (12.8% for those ≥75 vs 9.0%, for those <60 years, $p < 0.01$) in a prospective observational study of 3810 patients in primary care [6]. In care homes, the incidence of hypoglycaemic episodes is higher occurring in 41.9% of patients in one study over a one-year period (median 2, range 1–10 episodes per patient per year) due to older age and higher level of comorbidities in this population [7].

Pathophysiology

The pathophysiology of hypoglycaemia involves attenuated counter regulatory response in the presence of relative or absolute insulin excess and falling glucose levels. Under physiological conditions, a drop in

Box 12b.2: Risk Factors for Hypoglycaemia in Older People

- Old age, malnutrition, multiple comorbidities
- Acute illness, insulin or sulfonylurea therapy
- History of hypoglycaemia, care-home residency, recent hospitalisation
- Hypoglycaemia unawareness, blunted counter-regulatory responses
- Chronic hepatic or renal dysfunction, stroke or transient ischaemic attack
- Multiple medications (≥ 5), dementia, depression, heart failure and social isolation

glucose levels to less than 3.9 mmol (< 70.2 mg/dl) triggers counter-regulatory response with the release of glucagon and adrenaline. This counter-regulatory response manifests as autonomic symptoms such as palpitations, hunger, sweating and tremors prompting patients to take corrective action. Neuroglycopaenic symptoms develop when glucose levels drop further often to less than 2 mmol/l (36 mg/dl) and present as impaired cognition, seizures and coma. If untreated, severe hypoglycaemia can therefore be fatal. The ability to recognise symptoms of hypoglycaemia, particularly during early stages and the onset of counter-regulatory response is modified by several factors, particularly longer duration of diabetes and advancing age. Studies comparing older adults with younger individuals have shown that older adults are prone to more severe cognitive impairment during hypoglycaemia than their younger counterparts, less likely to experience warning symptoms and have delayed recovery following an episode of hypoglycaemia. These responses are attributed to physiological changes associated ageing and is further accentuated in the presence of other comorbidities such as declining renal function [8]. Multiple risk factors can be present in older people with diabetes and add to the risk of unwanted hypoglycaemia as summarised in Box 12b.2 [9].

Clinical Consequences

Older people with diabetes are likely to be at a higher risk of the adverse consequences of hypoglycaemia due to the increased prevalence of multiple comorbidities, undernutrition and polypharmacy compared with younger people. Severe hypoglycaemia may lead to serious acute vascular events such as stroke, myocardial infarction, acute cardiac failure and ventricular arrhythmias. On the other hand, the morbidity due to recurrent episodes of hypoglycaemia is associated with silent and chronic complications, which could lead to significant physical and cognitive dysfunction and eventually to frailty, disability and increased mortality. In addition, severe hypoglycaemia in older adults is also associated with increased risk of falls and injuries [9].

Impact on Cognition

The dose–response relationship between the frequency of severe hypoglycaemic episodes and the incidence of dementia has also been shown in a large Taiwanese national population database study of 15404 patients with type 2 diabetes mellitus (T2DM) and no history of dementia. The incidence rate of dementia was about 3% in those with history of hypoglycaemia compared with 1% in those without after seven years of follow-up. The increased number of hypoglycaemic episodes enhanced the risk of developing dementia ($p < 0.001$) [10]. In the Edinburgh Type 2 Diabetes Study in 831 patients with T2DM aged 60–75 years, there was a correlation between cognitive function and self-reported history of severe hypoglycaemia. A history of severe hypoglycaemia was associated with poorer initial cognitive ability and a more rapid rate of cognitive decline after four years of follow up [11]. A negative association between hypoglycaemia and dementia has been shown in the ACCORD-MIND and ADVANCE trials, in which patients in the intensive therapy arm, with more frequent hypoglycaemic episodes, had a similar decline in cognitive function compared to those in the usual care arm with less hypoglycaemia. However, these studies were not designed to directly investigate the relationship between hypoglycaemia and cognitive decline as a primary end point. It is also plausible that better glycaemic control in the intervention arm may have improved cognitive function diluting any deleterious effect of hypoglycaemia on cognition [12, 13].

Impact on Frailty

Frailty is a condition characterised by a reduction in physiological reserve and in the ability to resist physical or psychological stressors. Its definition is based on the presence of three or more of the following phenotypes: weight loss, weakness, decreased physical activity, exhaustion or slow gait speed. Frailty is likely to be a result of multi-system physiological dysregulation including cardiovascular, neuroendocrine, metabolic, immune and nervous systems. Sarcopenia or muscle mass loss is a component of frailty, which seems to be accelerated when diabetes is present. The relationship between frailty and hypoglycaemia seems to be bidirectional. It has been previously shown in a population-based study of 19932 patients with diabetes aged ≥65 years that frail older people (defined as oldest old, those on multiple medications and those with frequent hospitalisations) are at a higher risk of hypoglycaemia [4]. On the other hand, hypoglycaemia may lead to significant morbidity, disability and frailty as well as exerting a negative impact on quality of life in older people with diabetes [14].

Recurrent episodes of hypoglycaemia may occur unnoticed due to the impaired autonomic response in old age, which may result in frequent falls and progressive physical frailty. In addition, frequent hospital admissions due to severe hypoglycaemia are likely to lead to more deterioration in patients' physical function and eventually lead to frailty. Hypoglycaemic events seem to be common in older people with diabetes, especially in those who are frail and suffered significant weight loss. This group of patients currently appear to be over treated and seem to be inappropriately using medications that likely increase the risk of hypoglycaemia. Therefore, as patients with diabetes get older or develop dementia, overtreatment should be avoided, targets need to be reset and the effect of frailty and weight loss should be considered with a view of reducing or even completely withdrawing hypoglycaemic medications. New guidelines are needed to clarify when to deintensify hypoglycaemic medications and to balance the performance measures that incentivise both appropriate intensification as well as appropriate deintensification of hypoglycaemic therapy [15]. Characteristics of hypoglycaemia in older people with diabetes is illustrated in Figure 12b.1.

Management

General management on avoidance of hypoglycaemia and enhancing patient safety can be summarised as (Figure 12b.2):

- All health professionals involved in the care of older patients with T2DM should assess the risk of hypoglycaemia and adjust glycaemic targets to levels appropriate to the functional capacity, comorbid load, frailty level and life expectancy of the individual.

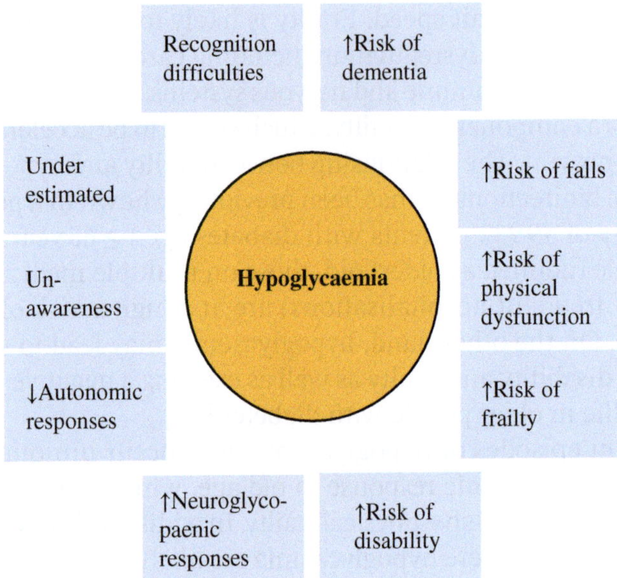

Figure 12b.1: Characteristics of hypoglycaemia in older people with diabetes mellitus.

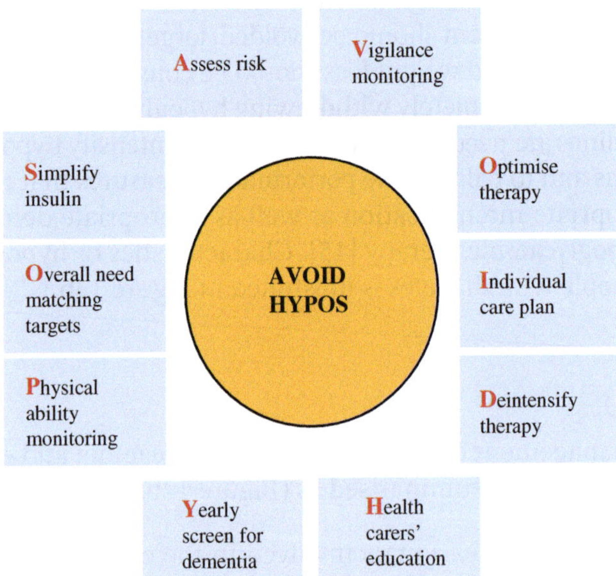

Figure 12b.2: AVOID-HYPOS acronym in older people with diabetes mellitus.

- All older people should have regular medicines review to assess potential hypoglycaemic risks. This should include minimising exposure to sulfonylureas, particularly long-acting agents, using low-risk insulin regimens such as once daily neutral protamine Hagedorn or long-acting analogue and reducing polypharmacy.
- All insulin treated patients should be assessed for capacity to self-administer, where this is not possible, third-party administration should be considered. It is important to ensure good education support for both patients and carers in respect of injection timing and blood glucose monitoring.
- Patients at high risk (low glycated haemoglobin or frailty) or those that experience either frequent or severe hypoglycaemia should be subject to a multidisciplinary review to reduce exposure to hypoglycaemic agents and to assess cognitive capacity in respect of medicines safety.
- Extravagance of hypoglycaemia is required in patients with type 1 diabetes of older age, as they may become hypoglycaemia unaware and their physiological response is blunted. This may require changes in glucose targets, correction factors, insulin dose and mode of delivery. In severe cases, glucose sensors may be indicated.

Summary

Hypoglycaemia continues to be a common feature of living with diabetes in many older people. Hypoglycaemia in any adult with diabetes must not only be viewed as a serious adverse drug event, but also as a failure of system process and clinical review by healthcare organisations. However, prevention of hypoglycaemia in older patients with diabetes remains a major challenge. Providing education and advice on avoiding hypoglycaemia should be a priority in their individualised care plan.

Clinical Practice Question

Q1. A 78-year-old man with type 2 diabetes for 10 years presents to his general practitioner (GP) with a history of non-injurious falling for the past three months. His current diabetes therapy is metformin 2 g daily and modified release gliclazide 60 mg once daily.

His haemoglobin A1c (HbA1c), recorded one month previously, was 48 mmol/mol (6.5%) and recent estimated glomerular filtration rate was 70 ml/minute/1.73 [2]. He has complained of fatigue for six months and he has lost more than 10% of his body weight during the past year. He is self-managing his diabetes. His GP noted his HbA1c result and suspects episodes of hypoglycaemia. What factors below may be operating?

A. Poor renal function
B. Dementia
C. Frailty
D. Over-tight glycaemic control
E. Undiagnosed malignancy

References

Key references only are listed here. For a full list of references visit: `https://www.wiley.com/go/sinclair/1e`.

1. NHS England. Low blood sugar (hypoglycaemia). https://www.nhs.uk/conditions/low-blood-sugar-hypoglycaemia (accessed 6 May 2024).
2. Jaap, A., Jones, G., McCrimmon, R. et al. (1998). Perceived symptoms of hypoglycemia in elderly type 2 diabetic patients treated with insulin. *Diabet. Med.* 15: 398–401.
3. Bonds, D.E., Miller, M.E., Dudl, J. et al. (2012). Severe hypoglycemia symptoms, antecedent behaviors, immediate consequences and association with glycemia medication usage: secondary analysis of the ACCORD clinical trial data. *BMC Endocrine Disorders* 12: 5.
4. Shorr, R.I., Ray, W.A., Daugherty, J.R. et al. (1997). Incidence and risk factors for serious hypoglycaemia in older persons using insulin or sulfonylureas. *Arch. Intern. Med.* 157: 1681–1686.
5. Tschöpe, D., Bramlage, P., Binz, C. et al. (2012). Incidence and predictors of hypoglycaemia in type 2 diabetes: an analysis of the prospective DiaRegis registry. *BMC Endocr. Disord.* 12: 23.
6. Bramlage, P., Gitt, A.K., Binz, C. et al. (2012). Oral antidiabetic treatment in type-2 diabetes in the elderly: balancing the need for glucose control and the risk of hypoglycaemia. *Cardiovasc. Diabetol.* 11: 122.
7. Chen, L.K., Lin, M.H., Lai, H.Y. et al. (2008). Care of patients with diabetes mellitus in long-term care facilities in Taiwan: diagnosis, glycemic control, hypoglycemia, and functional status. *J. Am. Geriatr. Soc.* 56: 1975–1976.

8. Munshi, M. (2017). Hypoglycemia. In: *Diabetes in Old Age*, 4e (ed. A.J. Sinclair, T. Dunning, L. Rodroguez Manas, and M. Munshi), 350–359. Chichester: Wiley.
9. Abdelhafiz, A.H., Rodríguez-Mañas, L., Morley, J.E., and Sinclair, A.J. (2015). Hypoglycemia in older people – a less well recognized risk factor for frailty. *Aging Dis.* 6: 156–167.
10. Lin, C.H. and Sheu, W.H.H. (2013). Hypoglycaemic episodes and risk of dementia in diabetes mellitus: 7-year follow-up study. *J. Intern. Med.* 273: 102–110.

13a Management of Diabetes in Hospital

Julie Lewis[1] *and Chris Cottrell*[2]

[1] *Lead Nurse for Diabetes in Wales, Clinical Lead for Diabetes North Wales, Betsi Cadwaladr University Health Board, Bangor, Wales, UK*

[2] *Lead for Diabetes Nurse Education, Swansea Bay University Health Board, Port Talbot, Wales, UK*

Key Points

- Individualised care planning that is co-created to attend to the unique requirements for the older person with diabetes will reduce the likelihood of unscheduled hospital attendance.
- Effective care planning incorporates fundamental processes that, when followed properly and communicated effectively, will yield less harm and promote safety and quality of life for the older person with diabetes.

Introduction

This chapter considers the key aspects of caring for the older person with diabetes as an inpatient, and the influencing factors that, when adjusted to account for the person's unique circumstances, can reduce the need for hospital admission and improve their quality of life.

Care of Older People with Diabetes: A Manual for Healthcare Practice, First Edition.
Edited by Alan J. Sinclair and Ahmed H. Abdelhafiz.

Companion website: www.wiley.com/go/sinclair/1e

Fundamentals of Care

Adhering to the fundamentals of care described in Table 13a.1 will ensure an accurate and safe individualised approach and avoid unnecessary harm in the inpatient setting.

Advancing age in itself is a risk for developing diabetes. In the UK, it is estimated that 33% of adults over the age of 65 years have a diagnosis of diabetes [1]. In many cases this is combined with other chronic conditions and higher cardiovascular risk. The degree of functional independence will vary widely in and problems such as sarcopenia, dexterity difficulties, eyesight degeneration and decline in cognitive

Table 13a.1: Fundamentals of care.

Care	Description
Type of diabetes	Confirm the 'type' of diabetes. There are an increasing number of people with type 1 diabetes living well into older age
Functional independence	Assess at defined intervals and more regularly during acute episodes of intercurrent illness. Degree of independence can vary widely and change quickly for the older person
Nutrition and hydration	Can often be compromised, especially in acute illness. Poor nutrition and dehydration will increase the degree of frailty. Avoid long periods of fasting. Provide detailed nutritional assessment and review
Sick day rules	Acute illness such as sepsis and acute kidney injury often require a change in diabetes management and medication reviews. These may not be intended as permanent changes. Communicate clearly with the person with diabetes and relevant primary and community teams
Glucose targets 6–12 mmol/l	Individualised glucose targets, accounting for all of the above that seek to maintain safe glucose levels to prevent complications of hypoglycaemia, and hyperglycaemia
Continuity and communication	Avoid unnecessary disruptions: moving between departments, unfamiliar surroundings and discontinuity in care can increase vulnerability to adverse outcomes. Keep communication channels open with those who assist with care in the person's usual place of residence

function will affect the ability to effectively self-manage diabetes in the midst of competing health challenges [1].

Where the person lives and who they rely on for support will impact on how well diabetes is managed. Interruptions in diabetes management, which can be a common factor in cared-for situations, including missed or mistimed medications, poorly managed hypo- or hyperglycaemia, pose a high risk for unnecessary unscheduled hospital care. The collective burden of other significant comorbidities, disability, frailty and deteriorating cognition heightens the susceptibility for acute admission and readmissions to hospital. Education and training gaps, low staff to resident ratios and high workforce turnover contribute to the sub-optimal management of people with diabetes.

In the hospital setting, US inpatient diabetes data observed that the older person with diabetes inpatient statistics were 20% for adults aged 65–75 years, doubling to 40% for inpatients with diabetes over 80 years of age [2]. Compared similarly with those without diabetes, they observed a higher rate of hospital related complications, greater mortality and increased length of stay [2].

English data on inpatient clinical episodes across all age bands during 2021–22 coded for diabetes (type 1 diabetes [T1DM] = E10, type 2 diabetes [T2DM] = E11) [3] revealed that 44 704 finished consultant episodes (FCEs) in T1DM, of which 5630 (12.6%) were aged from 65 years to over 90 years. The mean age and length of hospital stay were 37 years and 4 days, respectively [4]. In T2DM during the same period, there were 55 440 FCEs, of which 30 316 (54.7%) were aged from 65 years to over 90 years. The mean age and length of stay were 66 years and 8 days, respectively [4].

These data demonstrate a considerable amount of inpatient activity for older people who have diabetes. While diabetes-specific admissions may not be the principal cause of admission, mismanagement of diabetes will have either contributed to the admission risk in the first place or hindered recovery while an inpatient, leading to excess length of stay, avoidable diabetes-related inpatient harm requiring additional discharge care support.

The total figures across all age groups in T1DM do not reflect the split in prevalence (estimated 90% of total diabetes will be T2DM) but there is a significant proportion of older people aged over 65 years with T1DM generating inpatient hospital activity. This is likely to be underestimated by many healthcare professionals and may lead to inaccurate clinical management plans (e.g. stopping insulin due to hypoglycaemia). This information serves us well enough to highlight how important it is to be clear about the type of diabetes to produce an individualised, robust plan of care to support discharge and avoid readmission.

An increasing number of hospital diabetes services are undertaking the processes of evaluation matched to high standards of inpatient care through the Diabetes Care Accreditation programme (inpatient) [4]. This helps to ensure that standards of evidence-based care are being promoted and audited against. If the value of education for care providers is not prioritised or supported, it is unlikely that a change in unscheduled admissions for older people with diabetes will be possible.

Key Considerations for Effective Inpatient Care for Older People with Diabetes

The Inpatient Setting

The admission of older people to hospital is often a challenge. The environment and impact of moving the person to different units or wards and the unfamiliarity of staff, lighting, noise, sensory overload and language barriers can increase their anxiety and confusion. Clinical teams need to think about how these disruptions will affect the person's routine diabetes self-care.

Stress, infection, steroids (and other medications), dietary changes, inactivity, delayed or mistiming of medication can lead to both hypoglycaemia and hyperglycaemia. If the person has been admitted with an infection this may require increased medication (e.g. insulin to help manage hyperglycaemia temporarily). Admission for an acute event such as diabetic ketoacidosis or hyperosmolar hyperglycaemic state is more likely to warrant admission and tend to have a greater mortality risk and increased length of stay. Acute kidney injury is a more common reason for admission for the older person. Treatment often requires a change to usual medications, including glucose lowering therapies that can destabilise glycaemia.

Timing of meals and snacks, with long periods of fasting, especially in the evening and overnight, can cause unwarranted diabetes inpatient harm [5]. Many older people with diabetes are already malnourished and dehydrated on admission, this may worsen or develop as a new problem while in hospital.

Prolonged admission may result in hospital acquired infections further delaying discharge. This may impact on their functional status, enhancing frailty. The person may have been independent prior to admission but very quickly becomes dependent requiring care services on discharge to support their diabetes care.

Pressure Damage and Footcare Assessment

There may be a risk to skin integrity and development of thrombosis and diabetes-related foot disease [6] in this vulnerable group. National guidelines promotes that routine monitoring and surveillance should be observed [7–9]. All measures should be in place to prevent pressure damage or prevent deterioration to avoid complications of infection or sepsis, which will promote patient flow and timely discharge. Foot checks should be conducted within the first 24 hours of admission with continuing regular assessments throughout their stay. High-risk feet should be referred in timely fashion to the podiatry team to prevent further deterioration [7]. All active foot disease should be referred within 24 hours to the podiatry team. Communication is vital on discharge to ensure that community and primary care colleagues are informed to promote continuation of care and timely management.

Planning Care

It is clear to see how easily the person becomes disorientated, confused and clinically vulnerable to avoidable harm without a clearly communicated individualised care plan. The hospital environment is pressured and clinical demands compete minute by minute, so time to plan care can easily be compromised. Key themes to help good care planning for the older person with diabetes in hospital are shown in Box 13a.1.

Key Considerations to Reduce Unscheduled Admission to Hospital

Avoidable admissions associated with diabetes can be minimised with individualised care planning, taking account of the type of diabetes, promoting safe management, ensuring that quality of life is at the forefront of care that is supported with consistent education and training for health professionals and carers.

Box 13a.1: Inpatient Care: What Needs to be Included

- Establish the degree to which the person is generally (preadmission) able to self-manage their diabetes, including monitoring and medications.
- Clarify support structures at home. Individuals may have relied on support that is no longer available.
- Assess nutrition, hydration on admission and again at intervals pertinent to individual need. Avoid long periods of fasting, especially where hypoglycaemia is a risk.
- Minimise the risks of immobility and frailty through assessment and frequent reassessment of pressure areas, including foot assessments as standard.
- Identify the key contributors to the admission and provide a clear discharge plan that will minimise the risk for readmission and enhance continuity of safe care. Specify the diabetes support needs in discharge planning.
- Prescribed treatments often change in hospital. Ensure that there is clear discharge guidance for monitoring requirements, prescription changes (temporary measures, acute or repeat prescriptions).
- Avoid a discharge out of daytime hours. Ensure the receiving venue (usual place of residence or new) is appropriately prepared to meet the required care needs.
- Ensure re-enablement and care providers are fully prepared to assure safe continuity of care.
- Document the discharge follow-up plan.

Functional independence can deteriorate suddenly in the presence of acute illness and in advancing age, the likelihood of regaining pre-illness levels of independence cannot be assured and care needs may be temporarily or permanently increased as a result. It is therefore important to review the care plan at regular intervals, and additionally where there is a disruption in care due to acute illness.

The Independent Diabetes Federation working group (2013) has proposed three categories to influence care planning for elderly people who have diabetes [8]:

- Category 1 – those who are functionally independent

- Category 2 – those who are functionally dependent, owing to either frailty or dementia
- Category 3 – those in end-of-life care, defined as a life expectancy of less than one year.

The key aspects that contribute to more effective care planning with the older person are shown in Box 13a.2. These considerations will influence effective care planning within the context of promoting safety and quality of life for the older person with diabetes [9].

It is essential that the older person with diabetes has the opportunity to participate to their best potential in decisions about how

Box 13a.2: Considerations for Care Planning for the Older Person With Diabetes

- The known wishes and decisions of the person. Involve all who are supporting care for the older person with diabetes, such as relatives, carers, primary and community support teams.
- Type of diabetes with usual treatment regimen and method of glucose surveillance.
- Admission and readmission avoidance: a care plan that incorporates agreed modifications to treatments that can restore glucose levels to the agreed range. Realistic target/goal setting to minimise acute ill health. Incorporate triggers (where agreed glucose levels are breeched) to provide timely adjustments to treatment.
- Safety – quality over quantity of life expectancy where complex comorbidities are high and life expectancy is short (e.g. medication reviews and adjustment to achieve a safe balance between clinical effectiveness and quality of life).
- Incorporate regular nutrition and hydration assessments to avoid malnourishment and dehydration where the preferred food choices of the individual are included.
- Timely reviews with regular functional and frailty assessments. Improved management and care may help to improve risks factors and frailty scores from moderate to low risk. Deterioration in function and frailty can be avoided and improved.
- Encourage activity that is suited to the individual's needs with a focus on muscle strengthening, resistance and balance.

their diabetes should be managed, and that the regimen is assessed at agreed intervals to maintain stability of diabetes management and avoid unnecessary harm [2].

Monitoring Requirements

An assessment should be undertaken within an acceptable time frame determined by the complexity of treatment changes made and degree of monitoring required. Local guidance should be adapted from national evidence-based guidance to direct correct and timely management. Maintenance glucose targets and action ranges for prevention of both hypo- and hyperglycaemia should be agreed because the environment has changed [10]. Setting maintenance targets of 6.0–12.0 mmol/l can support patient flow in reducing length of stay and earlier discharges, which could be continued or individualised in this vulnerable group in any setting [10–12]. Many changes to medication made in hospital are not intended to be permanent. Indeed, some medication may have been discontinued to minimise harm and regulate diabetes management which also provide clinical benefit for other conditions. It is therefore important to review the reintroduction of these medications in the context of the individual's presenting needs and contributory benefit to clinical safety and quality of life.

Often, when insulin is commenced in hospital for a person who is not able to self-monitor glucose or administer their own insulin, such tasks can fall to family members or community nursing teams. The role of the community diabetes specialist nurse is a growing resource for communities and primary care services to provide education and enhance the clinical assessment of the person. This may include de-escalation of treatments that pose a high risk of adverse effects, reviewing of insulin regimens to offer flexibility for timing visits, and supporting the use of diabetes technology such as continuous glucose monitoring.

Education and Training

Mismanagement and errors are commonly reported in all care settings. Reports of adverse events via the Datix system should be accessible to diabetes teams to evaluate, prioritise and target education to improve learning and outcomes. Protocols and guidance are useful to guide management but the turnover of staff, employing agency and

Box 13a.3: Educational Resources

- Diabetes courses for healthcare professionals: Diabetes UK (www.diabetes.org.uk)
- Diabetes self-management education: Diabetes UK
- Diabetes Education and Information Resource, aimed at carers: Diabetes Multidisciplinary Working Group (http://www.diabetes-care.wales)
- Diabetes films: PocketMedic film library (http://PocketMedic.org)
- Eden Training: Leicester Diabetes Centre, University Hospitals of Leicester NHS Trust (https://www.edendiabetes.com/training)
- Trend Diabetes (https://trenddiabetes.online)
- Trend Diabetes Learning Platform, specialising in diabetes training for healthcare professionals: (https://trenddiabeteslearning.co.uk)

recruitment of overseas staff presents a huge challenge. The National Diabetes Inpatient Audit reports that 18% of inpatients have diabetes yet, diabetes education is not mandatory in all care settings [5]. Education and training will be instrumental in implementing improvements to ensure standardised diabetes care. Box 13a.3 lists some useful educational resources.

Summary

This chapter has reviewed the key themes that need careful consideration to design safe, quality care to the older person with diabetes. The intention is to minimise unnecessary variability in diabetes management that reduces the risk for unscheduled hospital attendance.

Effective care planning that accompanies the older person across settings can encourage continuity of safe care, which often unravels due to gaps in communication. Matching access to consistent education with investment in the contribution of care provided by many untrained staff and family members would place a value that will yield clinical and cost-effective savings in pressurised hospital settings, enabling the older person with increasing levels of support to be cared for comprehensively in their usual place of residence.

When the older person with diabetes is admitted to hospital, clinical and functional distress often manifests. We can strive in the midst of clinical demands to deliver the basic fundamentals of assessment generally and specifically to diabetes. Clear communication, engaging with relevant support teams engineered through considerate individualised care planning will help to reduce future hospital events.

Clinical Practice Questions

An 80-year-old woman with type 2 diabetes mellitus, Alzheimer's disease and chronic kidney disease was admitted from a care home where district nurses attend once daily to administer her insulin. She is on insulin glargine 42 units once a day, metformin 500 mg twice a day and oral semaglutide. The dose was increased to 14 mg maximum dose prior to previous admissions when her haemoglobin A1c was 101 mmol/mol (8 months prior to first admission).

She presents at this admission with a history of falls. Her weight was decreasing with poor oral intake and significant weight loss. She was cachexic on admission with significant sarcopenia in her lower limbs. Her blood glucose levels ranged between 3.5 and 5 mmol/l. The patient had not been reviewed since increasing the oral semaglutide to maximum dose several months ago.

Q1. What key factors have contributed to this patient's hypoglycaemia? Select all options that apply.

- A. Oral semaglutide
- B. Insulin
- C. Chronic kidney disease
- D. General deterioration and frailty
- E. No recent assessment

Q2. Any changes in management should be reviewed but this has not been done. This patient has clearly been missed to follow-up, resulting in hypoglycaemia and falls, all of which are contributing to her frailty and sarcopenic state. What key factors have contributed to the weight loss?

Select all options that apply:

- A. Increasing frailty and weakness
- B. Hypoglycaemia
- C. Recall not arranged to review response to treatment change
- D. Patient not taking their glucose-lowering medication

Q3. How will a readmission of this type be prevented and what continuing management plan will support her safer care?
Select all options that apply:
A. Ensure regular monitoring and agree safe glucose targets in view of her age, frailty and chronic kidney disease.
B. Dietetic review with possible food supplementation to restore nutritional status using an individualised management plan to build her back up
C. Re-enablement team involvement for strength and resistance activities.
D. Communication with all involved in her care to support and agree a plan going forward.
E. Arrange timely recalls.
F. Provide education regarding sick day rules if taking a sodium glucose transporter-2 inhibitor.
G. Discharge with no treatment change
H. No need for recall or review.
I. Discharge without a plan of care.
J. Treat every person on this treatment the same way.

Q4. What medication changes might be considered?
Select all options that apply:
A. Stop Oral semaglutide.
B. Review insulin dose.
C. Review safety of the metformin dose aligned to current renal function.
D. Continue oral semaglutide.
E. Continue the same dose of insulin.
F. Increase her insulin dose by 20%.
G. Increase the dose of metformin.

References

Key references only are listed here. For a full list of references visit: `https://www.wiley.com/go/sinclair/1e`.

1. LeRoith, D., Biessels, G.J., Braithwaite, S.S. et al. (2019). Treatment of diabetes in older adults: an endocrine society clinical practice guide. *J. Clin. Endocrinol. Metab.* 104 (5): 1520–1574.
2. Umpierrez, G.E. and Pasquel, F.J. (2017). Management of inpatient hyperglycemia and diabetes in older adults. *Diabetes Care* 40: 509–517.

3. McKay, A.J., Gunn, L.H., and Vamos, E.P. (2021). et al, Associations between attainment of incentivised primary care indicators and emergency hospital admissions among type 2 diabetes patients: a population-based historical cohort study. *J. R. Soc. Med.* 114 (6): 299–312.
4. Royal College of Physicians Diabetes Care Accreditation Programme (2023). Accreditation Standards. London: Royal College of Physicians.
5. NHS Digital (2021). *National Diabetes Inpatient Audit (NaDIA) Harms,* 2020 England 8 Jul 2021 V1.0 Annual Report. London: Healthcare Quality Improvement Partnership. https://digital.nhs.uk/data-and-information/publications/statistical/national-diabetes-inpatient-audit---harms/national-diabetes-inpatient-audit---harms-2020 (accessed 2 August 2024).
6. Game, F.L., Chipchase, S.Y., and Hubbard, R. (2006). et al, Temporal association between the incidence of foot ulceration and the start of dialysis in diabetes mellitus. *Nephrol. Dial. Transplant* 21: 3207–3210.
7. National Institute for Health and Care Excellence (2019). Diabetic Foot Problems: Prevention and Management. NICE Guideline NG19. London: NICE. https://www.nice.org.uk/guidance/NG19 (accessed 2 August 2024).
8. International Diabetes Federation (2013). Managing Older People with Type 2 Diabetes: Global Guideline. Brussels: IDF.
11. Joint British Diabetes Societies for Inpatient Care (2022). Guidelines for the Management of Inpatient Diabetes. London: JBDS.
12. Dhatariya, K.K. and Umpierrez, G. (2023). Gaps in our knowledge of managing inpatient dysglycaemia and diabetes in non-critically ill adults: a call for further research. *Diabet. Med.* 40 (3): e14980.

13b Management of Diabetes in Care Homes

Lynne Reedman[1] *and Alan J. Sinclair*[2]

[1] *DUET Diabetes Ltd, Cambridge, UK*
[2] *Foundation for Diabetes Research in Older People and King's College, London, UK*

Key Points

- Identifying whether a new or existing resident has diabetes is important.
- The individual requirements of each resident living with diabetes should be understood, monitored, documented and acted upon. Responding to changes delivers a truly person-centred, safe and responsive service.
- Role-specific diabetes training has the potential to significantly increase the knowledge, confidence and skills of staff.
- A knowledgeable, skilled and empowered care-home team can subsequently improve the quality of life of residents.
- Effective communication and collaboration (internally and externally) is key to laying the foundations for comprehensive policies, aligned working practices and better outcomes for residents.

Introduction

Quality of life is paramount for people living with diabetes, regardless of their age or circumstances. There has been increased focus in recent years regarding diabetes care for older people and, in particular, those residing in care homes. Diabetes is an independent risk factor for

Care of Older People with Diabetes: A Manual for Healthcare Practice, First Edition.
Edited by Alan J. Sinclair and Ahmed H. Abdelhafiz.

Companion website: www.wiley.com/go/sinclair/1e

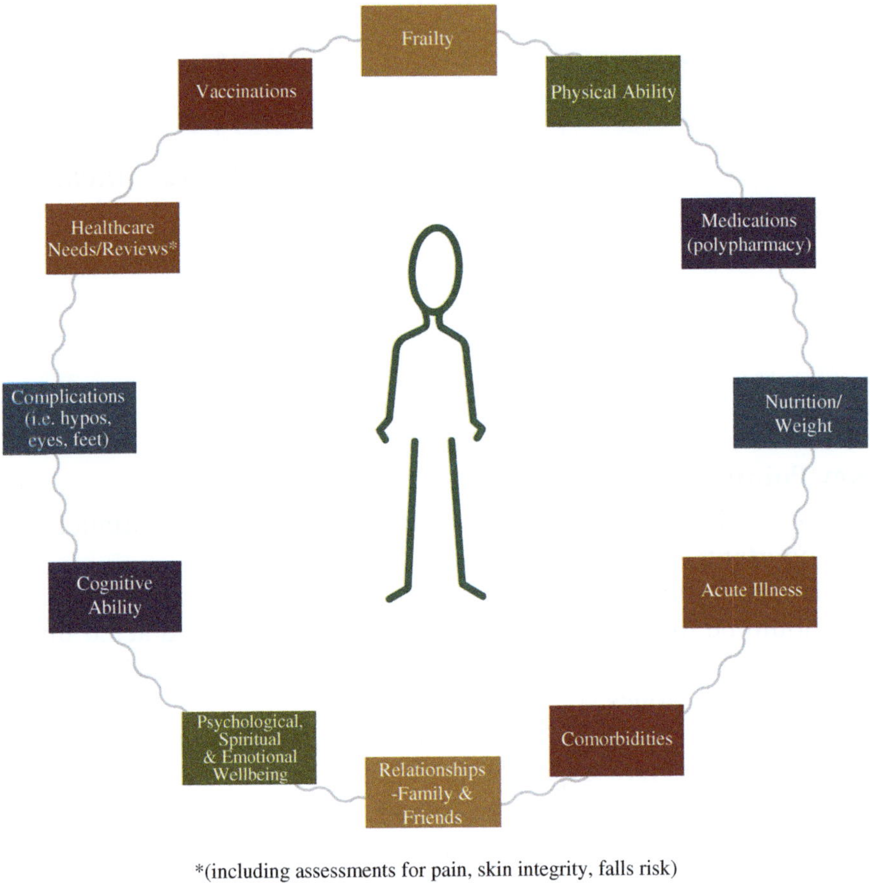

Figure 13b.1: Diabetes and the older person.

admission to a care home and up to 25% of residents live with diabetes. There are multiple considerations and areas of interest in older people with diabetes (Figure 13b.1).

The British Geriatrics Society has recognised that there are 'increasing levels of clinical acuity' in the care home sector [1]. The numbers of people aged over 65 years continue to increase and people living in care homes do so with increasingly complex and advanced healthcare conditions. The care home workforce, together with allied healthcare professionals, need to collaborate on how best to meet the clinical, health and wellbeing needs of residents.

Residents living with diabetes in care homes are at higher risk of infections, leg and foot ulceration and complications associated with hypo- and hyperglycaemia [2]. Specific training in the awareness and management of diabetes for care home staff is generally, at best, basic, which leads to a workforce with a lack of knowledge and understanding of this complex condition. This can then lead to poorer health and wellbeing outcomes for residents who are living with diabetes.

Another key aspect to be aware of is that frailty is emerging as a new complication of diabetes and may affect 32–48% of adults with diabetes over the age of 65 years [3]. It has a significant impact and is associated with poor outcomes, including reduced survival rate.

Relevant questions that care home staff and their allied healthcare team should ask include:

- Do we screen for diabetes when new residents move in?
- What is the person's frailty status?
- Are the treatment targets still appropriate, including the blood glucose range?
- How detailed are the care plans? Are they individualised (i.e. do they include details of type of diabetes, diabetes medication, hypoglycaemia risk, preferred hypoglycaemia treatment? Are there specific hypoglycaemia warning signs/symptoms)?
- What comorbidities exist (i.e. dementia, cardiovascular disease, kidney disease)?
- When was the last diabetic foot examination and what was the outcome?
- What diabetes training is provided to employees, in what format and how frequently?

Important Considerations for Diabetes Care

Every person living with diabetes will have differing health status, comorbidities and medications, all of which will alter over time. As someone ages, these aspects of care need to be regularly reviewed.

To maintain (or even improve upon) effective diabetes care, there are some key metrics that care homes should be incorporating into their policies, records, care environment, skills and capabilities of team members, summarised in Table 13b.1. In addition, key areas of management within a care-home setting are summarised in Table 13b.2.

Table 13b.1: Key metrics for use in care home diabetes management.

Metric	Considerations
Type of diabetes and treatment	Document within care record, plus current medication and an individualised care plan (including whether the resident can self-manage their diabetes)
Increased risk of hypoglycaemia episodes (hypo)	Document in care record: could their treatment cause hypos (such as sulfonylureas or insulin? Has the person experienced a hypo before? If yes, were any signs/symptoms evident?
Hypo kit availability	At the care home? 'Travel hypo kit' for when leaving the setting? Hypo treatment preference documented for each individual
Diabetic foot disease	When was the last diabetic foot screening examination performed? Is a 'risk calculation and assessment tool for diabetes foot disease' available? Document current risk and when next examination required plus any continuing treatment
Nutritional deficiency and weight loss	Is there a nutritional screening tool, such as MUST, in use?
Communication difficulties	Is cognitive impairment assessed? Is 'quality of life and wellbeing' being assessed?
Frailty	Has frailty been identified? What frailty assessment tool is used?
Training and education to ensure appropriate knowledge, skills and confidence	Is role relevant training and education provided, documented and kept up to date?
Communication and collaboration to ensure integrated and holistic treatment and care	Internally (care records, policies and procedures), audits to highlight successes and gaps to address Externally with allied services and healthcare professionals to ensure appropriate monitoring and medication to avoid over- or under-treatment

MUST, Malnutrition Universal Screening Tool.

There is an opportunity, prior to moving into a care home, for the individual's diabetes status and management to be reviewed. As someone ages, their health status may change due to increasing frailty or additional challenges, such as dementia [4]. These all contribute to the need

Table 13b.2: Key Metrics and Areas of Management in Care Homes.

Area of management	Details
Type of diabetes and treatment	Document within care record plus current medication and an individualised care plan (including whether the resident can self-manage their diabetes)
Increased risk of hypoglycaemia episodes (hypo)	Document in care record: could the treatment cause hypos (such as sulfonylureas or insulin?[a]). Has the person experienced a hypo before? If yes, were any signs/symptoms evident?
Hypo kit availability	At the care home? 'Travel hypo kit' for when leaving the setting? Hypo treatment preference documented for each individual
Diabetic foot disease	When was the last diabetic foot screening examination performed? Is a 'risk-calculation and assessment tool for diabetes foot disease' available? Document current risk and when next examination required plus any ongoing treatment
Nutritional deficiency and weight loss	Is there a nutritional screening tool, such as MUST[b], in use?
Communication difficulties	Is cognitive impairment assessed? Is 'quality of life and wellbeing' being assessed?
Frailty	Has frailty been identified? What frailty assessment tool is used?
Training and education to ensure appropriate knowledge, skills and confidence	Is role relevant training and education provided, documented and kept up to date?
Communication and collaboration to ensure integrated and holistic treatment and care	Internally (care records, policies and procedures), audits to highlight successes and gaps to address. Externally with allied services and healthcare professionals to ensure appropriate monitoring and medication to avoid over- or under-treatment

[a] Metformin is unlikely to cause hypoglycaemia as a monotherapy; however, there have been anecdotal reports of older frail individuals experiencing hypoglycaemia when taking metformin.
[b] MUST, Malnutrition Universal Screening Tool.

for a different approach and different 'targets' such as for blood glucose management, to prevent avoidable issues such as hypoglycaemia (and possible falls). It should be pointed out that people living with diabetes (types 1 and 2) have between 1.5 and fivefold increased risk of dementia [5].

Ineffective or lacking care plans can lead to miscommunication and missed opportunities to prevent future unwanted events or problems. For example, low blood glucose (hypoglycaemia), high blood glucose (hyperglycaemia) or foot ulcers can all lead to unnecessary hospital admissions. Robust and comprehensive care plans tailored to each person can make a tangible difference, made all the easier with the adoption of technology such as electronic care record systems, which are becoming more commonplace.

Effective communication channels, internally and externally, are crucial to maintain or even improve the quality of life for people living with diabetes, as is role-appropriate, engaging and inclusive training, accommodating differing learning styles and meeting the needs of the setting.

In the United Kingdom (UK), the National Institute for Health and Care Excellence does not have guidance for managing diabetes care in care homes. *A Strategic Document of Diabetes Care*, compiled by the National Advisory Panel on Care Home Diabetes, was published in April 2022 [6]. This is a UK-wide multidisciplinary initiative that was designed to enhance diabetes care within care homes and may have useful relevance to other geographies.

For older people living in care homes, high levels of frailty and comorbidities, together with the high frequency of acute illness and repeated infections, make monitoring an important activity to achieve effective diabetes care.

Haemoglogin A1c (HbA1c) is used to make decisions about treatment (to increase or reduce glucose lowering therapies); however, high levels of frailty and multimorbidity make this group of people more vulnerable to rapid change. Waiting to undertake a HbA1c every six months is far too long to detect important deviations in control and are likely to increase the risk of 'overtreatment'.

Nutritional and functional status can change from one HbA1c test to the next, increasing their vulnerability to acute illness and/or less effective control of their diabetes.

No one should act to change medication on the back of one individual capillary blood glucose reading. If it was out of range (high), increased monitoring would be advised, together with additional observations to ascertain whether or not the resident had eaten additional carbohydrates, of which the carers where unaware, or if an infection is 'brewing' and clinical input is required to potentially alter medication.

Importance of Monitoring Glucose Levels

Regular blood glucose monitoring is essential. An older person's blood glucose may indicate an issue prior to presenting with symptoms (of high or low blood glucose). Older people do not always display symptoms in the same way a younger person would (and/or may not be able to communicate them) and so to reduce the occurrence of 'surprises', twice-weekly blood glucose checks are proposed for residents on 'diet/tablet' (non sulfonylurea) medication. More regular monitoring would be indicated for those being treated with sulfonylurea medication or insulin.

The main focus should be on achieving the best control possible without producing (hyperglycaemic) symptoms and avoiding hypoglycaemia and metabolic decompensation. The COVID-19 pandemic has shown the importance of having in place policies for acute illness in residents and for those with diabetes. It is quite clear that improved monitoring is crucial and that failure to monitor sufficiently or only make changes at six monthly intervals would now be described as poor practice. Each resident should have their own range included in their care plan, together with actions to take if the result is out of range.

If weekly blood glucose levels begin to indicate that treatment may need to be altered, provided that the previous HbA1c was at least three-months ago, a test can be performed and acted upon accordingly. Having their medication altered may subsequently positively affect the resident's behaviour. They may become more alert and interactive (if, for example, their glycaemic control was below target). This then contributes to maintaining or improving the individual's quality of life.

Other Management Issues

The social care workforce are essentially the eyes, ears and hands of the wider healthcare team. They are in a great position to undertake a range of tasks and spot potential problems in a timely manner, thus contributing to a 'prevention/proactive approach' rather than a 'reactive environment'.

One of the stumbling blocks of optimal diabetes management in care homes can simply be the lack of understanding of the condition by the workforce. Improving knowledge and confidence of team members at all levels within the setting is key for not just everyday support of the person living with diabetes but also for identifying potential problems and 'raising the flag' to senior colleagues or allied clinical teams. This improvement in knowledge allows for prompt decisions as to whether or not an individual needs admitting to hospital, an urgent referral or continued management and support in their home.

People working within care homes are closest to the residents they support and spend more time with them than anyone else. They should be seen as part of the wider team responsible for an individual's diabetes care (whether it be the general practitioner, community nurse, secondary care diabetes team or other allied healthcare professionals). Role relevant education and training will empower care homes to deliver the best possible person-centred care for people living with diabetes; not just maintaining but in some cases even improving the quality of life for some individuals.

Hypoglycaemia

Hypoglycaemia (or a 'hypo') is an abnormally low blood-glucose level (below 4 mmol/l). It needs to be treated quickly and effectively to avoid further reduction in blood glucose. Hypoglycaemia is the most common adverse effect of insulin and sulfonylureas; however, there have been anecdotal reports of older people experiencing 'hypos' when being treated with other oral medications, such as metformin. It should therefore not be discounted, regardless of what medication the resident may be taking.

Communication is key, such as documenting particular signs or treatment preference (pointless encouraging Mrs Jones to eat some jelly babies if she does not like them, for example). Capturing relevant information in care plans and ensuring it is kept up to date is essential.

Care home teams should be informed if medication could cause hypoglycaemia. To minimise the possible detrimental impact of hypoglycaemia for an older person, a medication review may indicate the need to alter the type of medication (such as changing from a sulfonylurea to a class less likely to cause hypoglycaemia).

For all organisations, it is important to have a fully stocked, accessible hypoglycaemia kit to ensure that treatment is carried out in a calm and controlled manner. A useful tip is to paste a copy of a hypoglycaemia treatment algorithm to the top of their hypoglycaemia kit so that anyone treating a hypo can be confident that they have taken all the appropriate steps.

For any resident who is at risk of having a hypoglycaemic episode, when they leave the care home they (or whoever is accompanying them) should have the ability to test for and treat a hypo.

With the advance of technology, an increasing number of older people will be making use of continuous glucose monitoring (CGM). The use of CGM devices may help to overcome the increased risk of hypoglycaemia for older people, particularly the use of the alarm features (audible and vibrating options). The ability to share CGM data may help care givers and clinicians to identify triggers of hypoglycaemia and to help people maintain less glucose variability. Appropriate communication and monitoring needs to be agreed between the care provider and the healthcare team.

Diabetes Foot Disease

Feet should be inspected regularly (ideally daily). Any injury, wound or sign of infection, skin discolouration or swelling should be treated immediately and referred to the healthcare team. Care home staff should be trained on preventative footcare and how to carry out a diabetic foot screening examination (using a risk stratification assessment tool), document in care plans and take action in line with local guidelines [6–9].

The use of tools such as the Neuropad® (TRIGO International, Wiehl, Germany) allow for neuropathy to be identified; particularly useful in those individuals who are unable to take part in a 10-g monofilament test because of cognitive impairment, for example [10].

Nutritional Deficiency and Weight Loss

It is important that particular needs are catered for, such as food intolerances and preferences (i.e. vegetarian diets). Dietetic advice (and training) should be sought, as required, from local dieticians to ensure an appropriate approach for optimisation of health status and outcomes, to avoid unintentional weight loss, malnutrition and dehydration.

In the UK, as a result of a national survey, the prevalence of under nutrition in care homes was estimated to be 41%, with a range of 30–40% on admission [11].

Residents who are frail or have borderline malnourishment (using a tool such as the Malnutrition Universal Screening Tool) should have a documented personalised nutritional plan as the maintenance of weight is essential [12, 13].

Frailty

All residents should be regularly assessed for functional status, which will help to identify early signs of frailty and/or cognitive decline, if not previously identified or documented. Further decline in frailty can be potentially halted or slowed by easily implemented interventions to maintain muscle strength, mass and function. The aim is to improve mobility and balance and subsequently reduce the risk of falls, adverse health outcomes and increased dependency [14]. The Clinical Frailty Scale (Rockwood frailty scale) is a visual and easy tool to use in the care home setting [15].

Education

In the UK, there is currently no national programme (funded or otherwise) for diabetes in care homes. One of the challenges is that 'diabetes training' is not deemed a mandatory training requirement by the Care Quality Commission (the national body in England responsible for inspecting and assuring safety and quality of care delivered by care homes). In many cases, if training is offered within care settings, it is e-learning.

If people undertake e-learning in isolation, where does the learner go when they have questions? Is it tailored to their setting (i.e. does it discuss the older person)? If they are learning a new skill, such as how to perform a capillary blood glucose test or diabetic foot examination, how can that be embedded online without a practical session with an experienced educator overseeing the capabilities of the learner?

If possible, care providers should identify a team member as a 'diabetes champion'. Investing in face-to-face training for care homes to increase knowledge and confidence will elevate standards of care (updated policies and improved care plans) and enable team development through enhanced skills and better advocacy for residents when communicating and collaborating with allied healthcare providers [Rayner et al., personal communication; 6, 16].

Communication and Collaboration

The overall goal of health and social care providers is to make a difference for people living with diabetes, to help them maintain, or even improve, their health and wellbeing, and prevent (or at the very least minimise the chances of) complications associated with their condition. In summary, the goal is to ensure that people's quality of life is the best it can be, regardless of their age or circumstances.

Implementing joint and supportive working arrangements (between social care and healthcare providers) are crucial to ensure the best quality of life of people for living in care homes. To achieve this aim, education, communication and collaboration are key and need to be established. Doing so will help to avoid paramedic visits for avoidable hypoglycaemia, and avoid hospital admission for avoidable hyperglycaemia (DKA or HHS).

Early detection of elevated blood glucose with a swift response could lead to either effective management within the home or a more rapid admission to hospital prior to the individual deteriorating to such an extent that poorer outcomes prevail.

Use of Audit

Numerous articles and audits highlight that a number of problems exist in managing diabetes in care home residents [2, 6, 17]. The main issues highlighted, together with the under-reporting of diabetes within the care home setting, were:

- lack of or inadequate diabetes policies (including no written hypoglycaemia policy)
- lack of awareness of the existence of national guidelines for diabetes care in care homes

- the significant percentage of residents at moderate or high risk of developing a diabetic foot problem
- lack of access to diabetes education and training for their teams (at all levels).

Care home providers need to ensure that robust policies and audits are in place, and that diabetes management in line with best practice and guidelines are adopted alongside role-specific training. A focus on establishing relevant clinical skills and appropriate monitoring of diabetes within care homes, and effective communication channels with allied healthcare professionals will go a long way to helping residents living with diabetes to live the best life they can.

The same high-quality person-centred diabetes care (both clinical and holistic) that you would expect if the person living with diabetes was still living in their own home and able to visit the general practitioner and other appointments, must be strived for in the care home setting.

Measuring Outcomes

Outcome measures enable the quality of care being delivered to each resident living with diabetes to be assessed. Identifying the impact that diabetes has on an individual and, in turn, the affect that care home resources and implementation of monitoring, planning, educational initiatives have can positively elevate the provision of a person-centred, safe and responsive service. Potential outcome measures are shown in Box 13b.1.

Summary

It is to be hoped that adoption of national guidelines and sharing of best practice would drive a reduction of inequalities, promote staff development, increase joint and supportive working arrangements, improve efficiencies and, very importantly, maintain or even improve the quality of life for people living with diabetes in care homes. Improvement of knowledge, skills and confidence as a result of role relevant training, combined with a strong communication and collaborative approach, internally and externally, has the potential to reduce the risk of avoidable hospital admissions and enable high quality every day care [16, 18].

Box 13b.1: Potential Outcome Measures

- Percentage of residents achieving agreed haemoglobin A1c, blood pressure and weight during previous 12 months
- Frequency and severity of hypoglycaemic episodes in previous 12 months
- Complication rates of foot ulceration, visual loss, renal impairment, falls and angina
- Change in level of frailty during the previous 12 months
- Change in cognitive ability during the previous 12 months
- Frequency of diabetes related hospital admissions in the last 12 months
- Percentage of residents with individualised comprehensive care plans in the past 12 months
- Regular review of role relevant training needs of all team members
- Effective communication channels with allied healthcare services and clinicians
- Percentage of residents having regular comprehensive review of their medical needs, including vaccinations in the past 12 months

Clinical Practice Question

Q1. The general practitioner of an 89-year-old care-home resident with diabetes on a twice-daily insulin regimen is concerned about the patient's recent history of repeated episodes of hypoglycaemia and recent weight loss. She has just received the resident's estimated glomerular filtration rate, which is 30. Which of the following are potential risk factors or causes?

Choose all the options that are relevant:

A. Her known diagnosis of frailty
B. Polypharmacy – the resident is on six medications
C. Renal impairment
D. Insulin
E. Advanced age
F. Malnourishment

References

Key references only are listed here. For a full list of references visit: https://www.wiley.com/go/sinclair/1e.

2. Sinclair, A.J., Gadsby, R., Abdelhafiz, A.H., and Kennedy, M. (2018). Failing to meet the needs of generations of care home residents with diabetes: a review of the literature and a call for action. *Diabet. Med.* 35 (6): 1144–1156.
3. Morley, J.E. (2008). Diabetes, sarcopenia, and frailty. *Clin. Geriat. Med.* 24: 455–469.
6. National Advisory Panel on Care Home Diabetes (2022). A Strategic Document of Diabetes Care for Care Homes. London: Foundation for Diabetes Research in Older People. http://fdrop.net/napchd (accessed 2 August 2024).
7. Goodwin, J., Underwood, V., Housley, A., and Rajbhandari, S. (2008). High-risk foot care is necessary for people in residential care. *Diabetic Foot J.* 11 (2): 64.
9. International Working Group on the Diabetic Foot (2023). IWGDF Guidelines on the Prevention and Management of Diabetes-related Foot Disease. Maastricht, Netherlands.
10. Zografou, I., Iliadis, F., Sambanis, C., and Didangelos, T. (2020). Validation of neuropad in the assessment of peripheral diabetic neuropathy in patients with diabetes mellitus versus the Michigan neuropathy screening instrument, 10g monofilament application and biothesiometer measurement. *Curr. Vasc. Pharmacol.* 18 (5): 517–522.
14. Sinclair, A.J. and Gallagher, A. (2019). Managing frailty and associated comorbidities in older adults with diabetes: Position Statement on behalf of the Association of British Clinical Diabetologists (ABCD). London: Association of British Clinical Diabetologists. https://abcd.care/resource/managing-frailty-and-associated-comorbidities-older-adults-diabetes-position-statement (accessed 2 August 2024).
15. Rockwood, K., Song, X., MacKnight, C. et al. (2005). A global clinical measure of fitness and frailty in elderly people. *CMAJ* 173: 489–495.
17. Institute of Diabetes in Older People and Association of British Clinical Diabetologists (2014). *England-wide Care Home Diabetes Audit*. Luton: Institute of Diabetes in Older People.
18. Boyle, P.J., O'Neil, K.W., Berry, C.A. et al. (2013). Improving diabetes care and patient outcomes in skilled-care communities: successes and lessons from a quality improvement initiative. *J. Am. Med. Dir. Assoc.* 14 (5): 340–344.

14

Nutrition

Rihan Said[1] *and Grace Zaman*[2]

[1]*Department of Diabetes and Endocrinology, Rotherham General Hospital, Rotherham, UK*

[2]*Department of Nutrition and Dietetics, Rotherham General Hospital, Rotherham, UK*

Key Points

- Older people, including those with diabetes mellitus, are at increased risk of malnutrition.
- Nutritional screening is required to identify individuals at risk of malnutrition.
- Psychosocial factors, neurocognitive disorders, dysphagia and adverse effects of medication are primary contributors to decreased dietary intake.
- Interventions to improve dietary intake include meal-time assistance, texture-modified diet, shared meals and deprescribing of medications.
- Dietary restriction should be avoided in the elderly, as management of malnutrition is prioritised over glycaemic control.
- Patients on enteral or parenteral nutrition will require regular monitoring and liaison with the diabetes team to achieve reasonable glycaemic control.

Introduction

Balanced nutrition is essential for health, wellbeing and recovery from illnesses. Alongside pharmacological therapy, a healthy diet and good nutrition are essential for the management of diabetes in older people. However, older people are vulnerable to malnutrition due to age-related physiologic decline, reduced access to nutritious food and comorbidities.

Care of Older People with Diabetes: A Manual for Healthcare Practice, First Edition.
Edited by Alan J. Sinclair and Ahmed H. Abdelhafiz.

Companion website: www.wiley.com/go/sinclair/1e

In addition to age, diabetes increases the risk of malnutrition and micronutrients deficiencies. Malnutrition, as described by the World Health Organization, refers to deficiencies, excesses or imbalances in a person's intake of energy and/or nutrients [1]. Malnutrition incorporates both undernutrition (reduced protein, energy and micronutrients intake) and over-nutrition (increased intake, overweight and obesity). This chapter reviews nutritional challenges, with a focus on nutritional deficiencies as a cause of malnutrition in older people with diabetes.

Nutritional Deficiencies

Protein–energy malnutrition is an independent predictor of mortality [2]. Malnutrition tends to become more common as functional and health status worsen. The reported prevalence rates of malnutrition varies significantly according to the criteria employed. In older individuals who live independently, these rates are less than 10%. On the other hand, in acute care and rehabilitation centres, the prevalence of malnutrition can reach up to two thirds of older people [3, 4]. Multiple risk factors may coexist in the older population, causing decreased oral intake and subsequent malnutrition. Older people face a risk of malnutrition when they consume less than 50% of their nutritional needs for more than three consecutive days. This can occur due to increased nutritional demands, such as during acute illness, or reduced dietary intake associated with cognitive disorders and difficulties with chewing and swallowing [5]. Decreased caloric intake will lead to loss of body fat, while decreased protein intake will lead to sarcopenia, which is associated with frailty. Micronutrients deficiencies are particularly common in older people who are institutionalised and can have a significant impact on their health and quality of life.

Causes of Malnutrition in the Elderly

The decline in food intake is very common in older people, which can be due to several causes:

- Loss of appetite may result from a decreased sense of smell and psychosocial factors such as separation, widowhood, loneliness, moving to an care-home facility and depression, as well as systemic illness and adverse effects of medications [6].

- Difficulty in chewing is common and is related to a reduction in salivary production as well as poor oral health secondary to dental and gum disease. It will significantly affect food intake [7].
- Difficulty in swallowing is present in up to 33% of older people, and may be related to stroke or other neurological disorders such as Alzheimer's and Parkinson's diseases [8]. Sarcopenia causes weakness in the muscles responsible for swallowing, which subsequently leads to a further decrease in food consumption setting a negative vicious cycle.
- Polypharmacy can significantly affect appetite and weight. It is one of the potentially modifiable factors of malnutrition in high-risk older people. Several classes of medications can have a negative effect on nutrition through different mechanisms:
  - Antipsychotic drugs such as chlorpromazine, haloperidol and risperidone can affect the swallowing reflex with their anticholinergic properties and can also cause extrapyramidal symptoms, which limit mouth and tongue movements. This can result in difficulty in chewing, forming a food bolus and passing it through the pharynx [9].
  - Xerostomia is a known adverse effect of diabetes medications (e.g. glucagon-like peptide-1 receptor agonists, GLP-1RAs), antidepressants, antipsychotics and urological medications.
  - Metformin may cause weight loss with or without diarrhoea. The chronic use of metformin can also lead to vitamin B_{12} deficiency and low serum folate concentration [10].
  - GLP-1RAs suppress appetite, resulting in early satiety and weight loss. In contrast to young overweight patients, this is a disadvantage in frail older people. In addition, adverse effects such as nausea, vomiting and diarrhoea are not uncommon. This group of medications is therefore best avoided in frail older people with diabetes.

Recommendations

ESPEN (the European Society for Clinical Nutrition and Metabolism) guidelines offer general recommendations for nutrition in the older population, which include the following: [5]

- Recommended energy intake is 30 kcal/kg/day with 50–55% coming from carbohydrates.
- Recommended protein daily intake amounts are between 1.0–1.2 g/kg/day for healthy older people, going up to 2 g/kg/day in severe illness.
- Hydration with 1.6–2 l is recommended including milk, fortified drinks and juices.
- For those on enteral nutrition, 25–30 g of dietary fibre is required.
- If there is no specific deficiency, micronutrients should be delivered according to the recommendation of the European Food Safety Authority.
- All older people should be screened for malnutrition routinely, using a validated tool to identify those at risk of malnutrition.

Specific Recommendations for Older People with Diabetes

- In older people with diabetes mellitus, restrictive diets should be avoided to prevent malnutrition and accompanying functional decline.
- Management of malnutrition is far more important than the possible complications of hyperglycaemia.

Practical Steps for Nutritional Care in the Elderly

Nutritional screening for the risk of malnutrition is important for early identification and assessment of malnutrition along with adequate and timely intervention.

Screening

Nutritional screening is the first step in identifying patients at nutritional risk. It can help to identify patients who would benefit from nutritional intervention. It should be a quick and simple procedure that can be completed by all clinical staff on the first contact with the patient so that clear guidelines for action can be implemented and appropriate advice provided. ESPEN recommends three screening tools to be used in different settings:

1. Nutritional Risk Screening 2002 for patients in hospitals.
2. Malnutrition Universal Screening Tool (MUST) for ambulatory settings (community).
3. Mini Nutritional Assessment for institutionalised older people.

MUST is the most commonly used screening tool in all settings in the United Kingdom. The tool was developed in 2003 and is valid, reliable and easy to use for all adults. It can detect both over- and under-nutrition and is linked to a nutritional care plan. It is not designed to detect deficiencies or excessive intake of vitamins and minerals.

Assessment

Once screening is completed and a risk of malnutrition has been identified, the following assessments should be determined to plan interventions:

- anthropometric measures such as height, weight, body mass index, grip strength, mid-upper arm circumference and skin fold
- oedema/hydration status
- nutritional deficits from detailed diet history
- causes of malnutrition.

Further evaluation may be necessary to determine the presence of micronutrient deficiencies (e.g. blood tests for full blood count, iron studies, folate, vitamin B_{12}, vitamin D, calcium and magnesium levels).

Intervention

- Identify causes of malnutrition, if present (Table 14.1).
- Supportive interventions, (e.g. mealtime assistance and adaptation of environmental factors) should be put in place.
- Dietary modifications may include individualised meal plans, additional snacks, finger food, nourishing drinks, fortification and texture modification.
- Diabetes-specific dietary counselling and education should be provided for patients and families, including information on glycaemic index and suitable snacks.
- Regular support and follow-up from professionals with expertise in diabetes and nutrition.

Table 14.1: Causes of malnutrition and suggested interventions.

Cause	Intervention
Chewing problems	Oral care, dental treatment, texture-modified diet
Dysphagia	Swallowing training (speech and language therapy team), texture-modified diet
Impaired upper-limb function	Help with feeding (e.g. cutting food, hand feeding, finger foods), provision of feeding aids
Cognitive impairment	Supervision, help with meals
Depression, loneliness, social isolation	Eating and drinking with others, shared meals, social visits by charity groups
Adverse effects of medications (e.g. xerostomia, apathy)	Replace or stop medications
Restricted diets	Revision and liberalisation of dietary restrictions

According to ESPEN guidelines, when dietary counselling and food fortification are not sufficient to achieve nutritional goals, the following should be considered:

- Oral nutritional supplements should be offered to older people with malnutrition or at risk of malnutrition for at least one month. These supplements should provide at least 400 kcal/day, including ≥ 30 g of protein per day.
- Enteral nutrition should be started if oral intake is expected to be impossible for more than three days or is expected to be below half of energy requirements for more than one week. A nasogastric tube is used if the expected duration of enteral nutrition is less than four weeks; for longer periods, a percutaneous endoscopic gastrostomy (PEG) tube is recommended.
- Parenteral nutrition should be considered if oral and enteral nutrition are not possible and/or the person is in gastrointestinal failure.

Phosphate, magnesium, potassium and thiamine will need to be monitored and supplemented even in cases of mild deficiency.

Enteral Nutrition

Types of Enteral Tubes

A nasogastric tube can be used temporarily, typically for less than 30 days, in individuals with insufficient oral intake or those who have experienced sudden difficulties in swallowing, such as after a stroke.

A gastrostomy tube (PEG) is used for patients who require long-term enteral feeding exceeding 30 days, such as those with neuromuscular disorders, oesophageal pathologies, head and neck cancers and other conditions.

Types of Feeds

A variety of standard feeds are offered to cater for the individual needs of patients, such as whole protein, predigested protein, disease-specific and reduced sodium feeds [11].

Enteral Feed Delivery Options

Bolus intermittent feeding (using a syringe or pump) involves delivering feeds over shorter periods, mimicking normal eating pattern and is more commonly used in ambulatory settings or at home.

Continuous feeding (using a pump) is delivered slowly over extended durations at a reduced rate. The duration of feed can range from 14 to 18 hours but can last up to 24 hours, depending on the patient's tolerance. For more convenience, feed can be provided overnight. Continuous/extended feeds are suitable for bedridden individuals, but certain precautions should be undertaken to minimise the risk of aspiration such as positioning during and after the feed.

The medical team in charge of a person with diabetes needs to clarify the type, pattern and duration of feeds for each patient, to be able to interpret the blood glucose readings and adjust the antidiabetic medications and insulin accordingly (Figure 14.1).

Management of Blood Glucose

For people with diabetes on prolonged enteral feeds, capillary blood glucose (CBG) should be monitored every four to six hours. The target CBG is 6–12 mmol/l, as advised by the Joint British Diabetes Societies guidance [12]. For individuals with type 2 diabetes, liquid metformin is

Normal feeding	• **Population:** healthy • **Feed:** individualised meal plans, additional snacks, finger food, nourishing drinks, fortification and texture modification • **Glucose management:** routinely, target 6–12 mmol/l
Enteral feeding	• **Population:** swallowing difficulty • **Feed:** Bolus intermittent feeding using a syringe or continuous feed using a pump. • **Glucose management:** 4- to 6-hourly, target 6–12 mmol/l
Parenteral feeding	• **Population:** gastrointestinal failure • **Feed:** provided continuously or cyclically through a central venous catheter over a period of 12–24 hours • **Glucose management:** 4- to 6-hourly, target 7.8–10.0 mmol/l

Figure 14.1: Feeding patterns in different populations and suggested blood glucose targets.

the only antidiabetic medication that can be delivered through nasogastric tubes. It can be used as a sole treatment or as an adjunct to insulin. Those who are not achieving targets on metformin alone will require insulin. Individuals with type 1 diabetes on enteral feeding will require a basal/bolus regimen. If insulin is required for the management of poorly controlled type 2 diabetes, one of the following regimens can be chosen:

- isophane insulin twice daily
- premixed human insulin (30/70) twice daily
- basal/bolus as in type 1 diabetes.

For those with type 1 diabetes, continue basal insulin (e.g. glargine or detemir) and add boluses of short-acting insulin, depending on the feed regimen (Table 14.2). If hypoglycaemia develops, 60 ml of Glucojuice® (BBI Healthcare, Pencoed, Wales) can be used for patients on nasogastric or PEG feeding.

Parenteral Nutrition

Parenteral nutrition is a method of nutrition that bypasses the gastrointestinal tract. It is generally indicated when there is impaired gastrointestinal function and contraindications to enteral nutrition.

Table 14.2: Glucose monitoring and insulin administration during enteral and parenteral feeding.

Type of feed	Glucose monitoring	Insulin administration	
		T1DM	T2DM
Bolus	Pre-feed 2 hours post feed	Basal + bolus before feed	Premixed insulin before breakfast and evening meals. Basal + bolus before feed
Continuous (12–24 hours)	Pre-feed 4–6 hours during and 2 hours post feed (if <24 hours)	Basal + bolus at 0/6/12 hours[a]	Premixed (30/70) or neutral protamine Hagedorn at start and midpoint of feed. Basal + bolus at 0/6/12 hours[a]

[a] Bolus can be given at 0 , 6 , 12 and 18 hours if blood glucose is >12 (depending on length of feed).

It is sometimes combined with oral or enteral nutrition. Parenteral nutrition typically comprises glucose, fats and amino acids. Electrolytes, vitamins and trace elements may be incorporated into the feed or provided separately. The feed itself can be provided continuously or cyclically through a central venous catheter over a period of 12–24 hours. Individuals with diabetes can use the same parenteral nutrition formula, provided that blood glucose levels can be effectively regulated with insulin. Alternatively, the parenteral nutrition content can be modified for better blood glucose control.

Management of Blood Glucose

Approximately 50% of hospitalised patients receiving parenteral nutrition develop hyperglycaemia. The recommended blood glucose range for this group is between 7.8 and 10.0 mmol/l [13]. Insulin can be delivered via the subcutaneous or intravenous route for patients on parenteral nutrition.

In critical care, intravenous insulin infusion is the preferred route of delivery as the rate can be adjusted more rapidly to keep glucose levels within target. CBG is monitored at least every two hours. For stable patients in the wards, subcutaneous insulin is used in preference to intravenous insulin in most patients on parenteral nutrition. The insulin regimen can vary depending on the duration of the parenteral nutrition, CBG monitoring and whether any enteral nutrition or oral feeds are provided to the patient. Generally, for those on continuous parenteral nutrition, a basal insulin is combined with correction boluses of quick-acting insulin as for continuous enteral nutrition. Monitoring of CBG four- to six-hourly is required to guide insulin adjustments (Table 14.2).

General Considerations for Patients on Nutritional Support

- Diabetes inpatient specialist nurses should be involved in the management of patients who require insulin while on enteral or parenteral nutrition.
- Variable rate intravenous insulin infusion should not be used routinely in patients on enteral or parenteral nutrition [12]. It is required for patients with type 1 diabetes if they remain nil by mouth or if feeding is stopped for more than two hours. It is also required if CBG rises significantly in the absence of ketonaemia.
- If a feed is interrupted while a patient is on basal insulin, CBG should be monitored hourly.
- Continuous glucose monitoring and closed-loop insulin delivery have shown favourable outcomes in inpatients receiving nutritional support [14]. The diabetes inpatient team should be consulted to decide whether or not the use of this technology is suitable for individual patients.

Summary

Adequate nutrition is an important aspect of diabetes management. In older people with diabetes, malnutrition is common due to both ageing and diabetes-related risk factors. Therefore, regular screening, assessment and timely intervention are important to avoid the development of malnutrition in this vulnerable population. In addition, dietary restriction should be avoided; adequate nutrition should be prioritised over glycaemic control, especially in frail and malnourished older people with diabetes.

Clinical Practice Questions

Mary is an 81-year-old woman who lives in a care home. She has Alzheimer's disease and long-standing type 2 diabetes. A stroke two years ago left her with unilateral weakness, and she has frequent lower urinary tract infections. Mary is currently on a level 6 diet (soft and bite-sized pieces) and level 0 fluids (thin fluids like water and juice). She has lost over 15 kg in weight since her stroke and her body mass index is currently 17.5 kg/m^2. She is currently on metformin 1 g twice a day, linagliptin 5 mg once a day and humulin M3 10 units at breakfast and 10 units at her evening meal. She often has episodes of hypoglycaemia. Her most recent haemoglobin A1c is 47 mmol/mol.

Q1. What nutritional screening tool would be appropriate to use?
- **A.** Malnutrition Universal Screening Tool
- **B.** Mini Nutritional Assessment
- **C.** Both are appropriate

Q2. What first-line intervention would you consider?
- **A.** Diabetes-specific dietary counselling and education
- **B.** Assistance with meals
- **C.** Enteral nutrition

Q3. What would be considered suitable blood glucose targets for this patient?
- **A.** 4–7 mmol/l
- **B.** 7–12 mmol/l
- **C.** 10–15 mmol/l

Q4. What medications may require adjusting?
- **A.** Insulin and metformin
- **B.** Linagliptin and metformin
- **C.** Linagliptin

Fred is an 86-year-old man who has been admitted to hospital from his own home with pneumonia. He has had type 2 diabetes for 25 years. It is decided that a nasogastric feed would be appropriate on this admission, because of his poor oral intake and clinical condition. He is currently taking metformin 1 g twice a day and humulin M3, 12 units with breakfast and evening meals. The team has decided that his nasogastric feed is to run for 20 hours as he is currently unable to eat or drink orally.

Q5. How frequently should his capillary blood glucose be monitored?
  A. Every 6 hours
  B. Every 2 hours
  C. Hourly

Q6. What would his capillary blood glucose targets be while he is in hospital?
  A. 4–7 mmol/l
  B. 6–12 mmol/l
  C. 10–15 mmol/l

Q7. Is his current insulin regimen suitable for continuous feed?
  A. No; start on isophane insulin at the beginning and 10 hours after the start of the feed.
  B. No; start on variable rate intravenous insulin infusion.
  C. No; start on short-acting insulin every 4 hours.

References

Key references only are listed here. For a full list of references visit: `https://www.wiley.com/go/sinclair/1e`.

1. World Health Organization (2023). Malnutrition. `https://www.who.int/news-room/fact-sheets/detail/malnutrition` (accessed 10 January 2024).
3. Kaiser, M.J., Bauer, J.M., Rämsch, C. et al. (2010). Frequency of malnutrition in older adults: a multinational perspective using the mini nutritional assessment. *J. Am. Geriatr. Soc.* 58: 1734–1738.
4. Cereda, E., Pedrolli, C., Klersy, C. et al. (2016). Nutritional status in older persons according to healthcare setting: a systematic review and meta-analysis of prevalence data using MNA®. *Clin. Nutr.* 35: 1282–1290.
5. Volkert, D., Beck, A.M., Cederholm, T. et al. (2019). ESPEN guideline on clinical nutrition and hydration in geriatrics. *Clin. Nut.* 38: 10–47.
8. Thiyagalingam, S., Kulinski, A.E., Thorsteinsdottir, B. et al. (2021). Dysphagia in older adults. *Mayo Clin. Proc.* 96: 488–497.
9. Kose, E., Wakabayashi, H., and Yasuno, N. (2021). Polypharmacy and malnutrition management of elderly perioperative patients with cancer: a systematic review. *Nutrients* 13: 1961.
10. Wakeman, M. and Archer, D.T. (2020). Metformin and micronutrient status in type 2 diabetes: does polypharmacy involving acid-suppressing medications affect vitamin B12 levels? *Diabetes Metab. Syndr. Obes.* 13: 2093–2108.

12. Roberts, A.W., Penfold, S., and Diabetes Societies (JBDS) for Inpatient Care (2018). Glycaemic management during the inpatient enteral feeding of people with stroke and diabetes. *Diabet. Med.* 35: 1027–1036.
13. Schönenberger, K.A., Reber, E., Dürig, C. et al. (2022). Management of hyperglycemia in hospitalized patients receiving parenteral nutrition. *Front. Clin. Diabetes Healthc.* 3: 829412.
14. Boughton, C.K., Bally, L., Martignoni, F. et al. (2019). Fully closed-loop insulin delivery in inpatients receiving nutritional support: a two-centre, open-label, randomised controlled trial. *Lancet Diabetes Endocrinol.* 7: 368–377.

15 Sexual Health

Pann Ei Hnynn Si[1] *and Ahmed H. Abdelhafiz*[2]

[1] *Sheffield Kidney Institute, Sheffield Teaching Hospitals, Sheffield, UK*

[2] *Department of Geriatric Medicine, Rotherham General Hospital, Rotherham, UK*

Key Points

- Sexual dysfunction is common in people with diabetes and tends to be under-reported, especially in women.
- Diabetes-related neurovascular diseases, in addition to psychological factors, are the main cause of sexual dysfunction in both genders.
- Routine discussion of sexual health should be part of the annual reviews for older people with diabetes.
- Providing education for patients and healthcare professionals is the basis for successful management of sexual dysfunction.
- A holistic and patient-centred approach will have a positive impact on quality of life in managing sexual dysfunction in older people.

Introduction

Diabetes mellitus is a systemic disease that affects several body functions, including sexual health. Sexual dysfunction may be a presenting manifestation of undiagnosed diabetes as well as a complication of the already established disease. Sexual problems in older people with diabetes is associated with increasing age, duration of diabetes and comorbidity burden [1]. Although previous studies have focused on the effects of diabetes on male sexual function, diabetes also affects women's sexual health but women may be less likely to discuss this

Care of Older People with Diabetes: A Manual for Healthcare Practice, First Edition.
Edited by Alan J. Sinclair and Ahmed H. Abdelhafiz.

Companion website: www.wiley.com/go/sinclair/1e

issue with healthcare professionals [2]. Failure to recognise and treat sexual dysfunction among older people with diabetes may lead to failure to cope with disease burden and poor quality of life. Untreated sexual dysfunction may also lead to marital conflicts, restricted lifestyle, depression and social isolation. Regular screening for potentially treatable sexual dysfunction in older people with diabetes may improve diabetes care and enhance quality of life. This chapter reviews sexual problems in older people with diabetes and ways of early detection and treatment.

Ageing and Sexual Function

Normal ageing brings physiological changes sexual organs, which may lead to sexual dysfunction. In men, the main changes are erectile and ejaculatory dysfunction. Most of the changes occur after the age of 70 years and are related to psychological and physiological factors but are exacerbated by the presence of obesity, smoking, diabetes, cardiovascular disease and depression [3]. In postmenopausal women, reduced oestrogen secretion and vulvovaginal atrophy can cause reduction in vaginal lubrication with increased thinning of vaginal epithelium, which may lead to painful intercourse or dyspareunia [4]. Despite these changes, older people are still sexually active, and the trend of sexual activity is increasing over time. A Swedish study of 1506 people aged 70 years, followed up between 1971 and 2001, reported an increase in sexual intercourse in all groups studied, from 52% to 68% in married men, 38% to 56% in married women, 30% to 54% in unmarried men and 0.8% to 12% in unmarried women [5].

Diabetes and Sexual Dysfunction

Diabetes has been associated with sexual dysfunction in both men [12–14] and women [15–17]. Diabetes is an established risk factor for sexual dysfunction in men; a threefold increased risk of erectile dysfunction was documented in men with diabetes compared with those without [12, 18]. Among women, the evidence regarding the association between diabetes and sexual dysfunction is less conclusive [19, 20], although most studies have reported a higher prevalence of sexual dysfunction in women with diabetes compared with those without diabetes [15, 16, 21].

Persistent hyperglycaemia, as a determinant of atherosclerosis, may be the main contributing risk factor for diabetes-related sexual dysfunction but other diabetes-associated risk factors such as hypertension, obesity, depression, smoking, alcohol excess, metabolic syndrome and dyslipidaemia may also play a significant role.

Sexual Dysfunction in Men

Aetiology and Pathogenesis

Sexual dysfunction is three times more common and occurs 10–15 years earlier in men with diabetes compared to those without diabetes. Erectile dysfunction is the most common sexual dysfunction in men with diabetes, and is associated with cardiovascular risk. Erectile dysfunction increases with increasing age, sedentary lifestyle, duration of diabetes, obesity, hypertension, cardiac autonomic neuropathy, cardiovascular disease, distal sensorimotor polyneuropathy, non-alcoholic fatty liver disease, depression and hypogonadotropic hypogonadism (Box 15.1) [6]. Erectile dysfunction is more common in type 2 compared with type 1 diabetes, especially in patients with severe insulin resistance [6]. It can be a manifestation of undiagnosed diabetes and a marker of an undiagnosed cardiovascular disease. Erectile dysfunction has been shown to affect up to 52.5% of men with diabetes as reported in a meta-analysis of 145 studies, including 88 577 men with diabetes [7].

Erectile dysfunction in diabetes is caused by multifactorial factors, including nervous, vascular and muscular impairments. Vascular disease and endothelial dysfunction lead to less bioavailability of the vasodilator nitric oxide and reduced relaxation of the smooth muscles of the corpora cavernosa. In addition, autonomic neuropathy leads to reduced parasympathetic activity required for the relaxation of the smooth muscles of the corpus cavernosa. Several medications such as beta-blockers, thiazide diuretics, spironolactone and antidepressants can worsen erectile dysfunction in people with diabetes. Testosterone deficiency is another cause of sexual dysfunction in older men with diabetes (Figure 15.1).

Box 15.1: Risk Factors for Erectile Dysfunction in Older Men with Diabetes Mellitus

- Increasing age
- Increased duration of diabetes
- Overweight
- Obesity
- Sedentary lifestyle
- Smoking
- Alcohol excess
- Non-alcoholic fatty liver disease
- Hypertension
- Dyslipidaemia
- Cardiovascular disease
- Peripheral vascular disease
- Cardiac autonomic neuropathy
- Distal sensorimotor polyneuropathy
- Autonomic neuropathy
- Depression
- Anxiety
- Stress
- Hypogonadotropic hypogonadism
- Polypharmacy
- Local penile disorders such as Peyronie's disease, balanitis and phimosis
- Testosterone deficiency
- Psychological factors
- Social factors

Diagnosis

Detailed history is the first step in diagnosing sexual dysfunction. Standard questionnaires such as the International Index of Erectile Function can aid in diagnosis. Physical examination may help to identify vascular, neurological, hormonal, anatomical, drug-induced or psychogenic factors involved in the aetiology. Diagnosis of testosterone deficiency can be suspected by the presence of symptoms such as low sexual desire and loss of early morning erections, which can

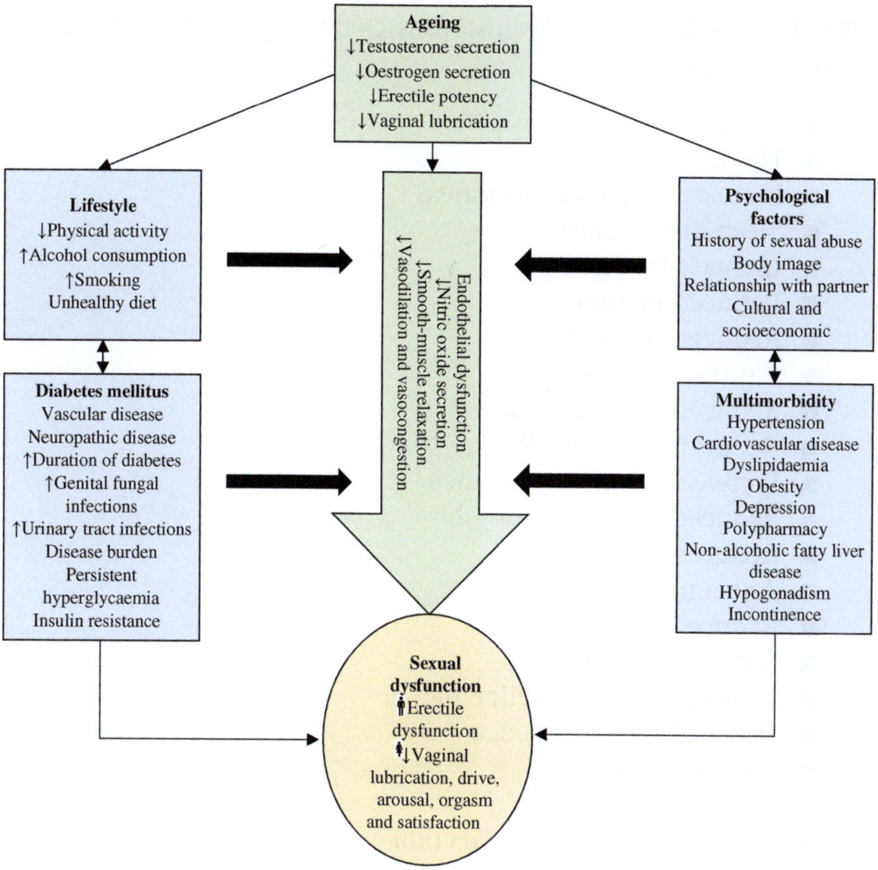

Figure 15.1: Aetiology and pathogenesis of sexual dysfunction in older people with diabetes mellitus.

be confirmed by low serum testosterone levels (Box 15.2). Specialised diagnostic tests, such as penile doppler ultrasound or nocturnal penile tumescence, may be useful in diagnosis.

Treatment

Management starts by addressing modifiable risk factors such as stopping smoking, reducing alcohol consumption, eating a healthy diet, achieving ideal body weight, taking physical exercise, avoiding stress, achieving glycaemic control and treatment of hypertension and dyslipidaemia.

Box 15.2: Symptoms of Testosterone Deficiency in Older Men with Diabetes Mellitus

- General fatigue
- Hot flushes
- Increased daytime sleepiness
- Sleep disturbance
- Increased irritability
- Reduced memory
- Reduced concentration
- Central obesity
- Reduced muscle mass
- Reduced bone density
- Increased insulin resistance
- Reduced physical strength
- Reduced energy
- Anaemia
- Reduced motivation
- Depressed mood
- Reduced sense of wellbeing
- Reduced self confidence
- Low sexual desire
- Erectile dysfunction
- Loss of early morning erection
- Body and facial hair loss
- Reduced sperm count
- Gynaecomastia

Lifestyle modification will help to reduce sexual dysfunction by improving insulin-resistance and endothelial dysfunction and reducing chronic inflammation. Glycaemic control, through reducing long-term microvascular disease, may improve sexual function.

Phosphodiesterase 5 (PDE5) inhibitors such as sildenafil, vardenafil and tadalafil are the first-line treatments for erectile dysfunction. They work by inhibiting the PDE5 enzyme, which leads to prolonged action of cyclic guanosine monophosphate in corpora cavernosa smooth muscles. This maintains smooth-muscle relaxation and improves penile blood supply, which prolongs duration of erections [8]. PDE5 inhibitors should be used with caution in patients with ischaemic heart disease,

Table 15.1: Advantages and cautions of testosterone therapy.

Advantages	Cautions
Improves sexual function and activity	Cardiovascular disease
Increases lean muscle mass, muscle strength and bone density	Prostate cancer
Reduces fat mass	Gynaecomastia and breast cancer
Improves physical function and performance	Polycythaemia and risk of thrombosis
Improves glycaemic control, lipid profile and increases haemoglobin	Peripheral oedema
Improves mood and cognition	Sleep apnoea
Increases lean muscle mass, muscle strength and bone density	Hepatic dysfunction
	Behavioural changes
	Acne

unstable angina, recent myocardial infarction, poorly controlled blood pressure or concomitant use of nitrate therapy.

Another cause of sexual dysfunction is testosterone deficiency, which affects up to 33% of men with diabetes [9]. Testosterone replacement therapy can be used in patients who are less responsive to PDE5 inhibitors (Table 15.1). In addition to its independent efficacy, testosterone replacement therapy can be adjuvant therapy to improve response to PDE5 inhibitors compared with PDE5 inhibitors alone [10]. Routes of administration include patches, gels, tablets, implants and injections.

Non-pharmacological interventions for erectile dysfunction include vacuum erection devices, which provide passive enlargement of corpora cavernosa, low-intensity extracorporeal shock wave therapy, which stimulates penile neovascularisation and intracavernosal or intrapenile injection of prostaglandin E_1. Antioxidants such as L-arginine may increase nitric oxide availability and improve smooth-muscle relaxation of corpora cavernosa. These modalities of therapy can be used concomitantly with PDE5 inhibitors to have a better effect. Surgical interventions include penile prosthesis implants, arterial bypass or venous ligation procedures. Stem cell therapy is a promising novel therapy under investigation (Figure 15.2).

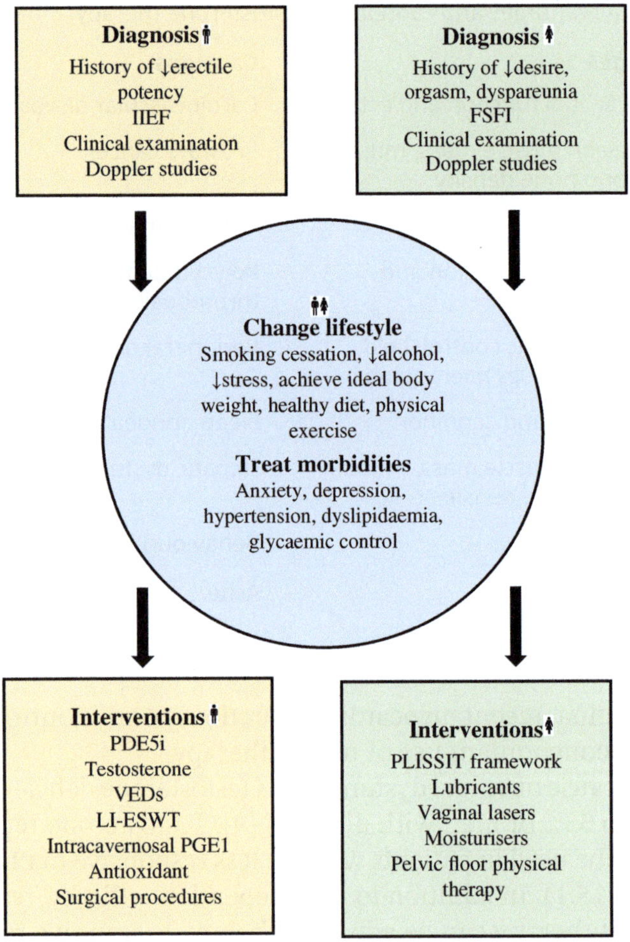

Figure 15.2: Management of sexual dysfunction in older people with diabetes. IIFE, International Index of Erectile Function; FSFI, Female Sexual Function Index; PDE5i, phosphodiesterase 5 inhibitors; VEDs, vacuum erection devices; LI-ESWT, low-intensity extracorporeal shock wave therapy; PGE1, prostaglandin E_1; PLISSIT, permission, limited information, specific suggestions, intensive therapy.

Sexual Dysfunction in Women

Aetiology and Pathogenesis

As in men, sexual response in women is a neurovascular-dependent event. Adequate blood and nerve supply to female genital area is required for healthy sexual function, which can be affected by diabetes-related vascular and neuropathic disease. All phases of the sexual cycle response, including desire, arousal, lubrication, orgasm and satisfaction are impaired in women with diabetes. Sexual dysfunction is about twofold more in women with diabetes compared with those without diabetes, especially those with a higher body mass index or depression [11]. Genital fungal infection, urinary tract infection and urinary incontinence reduce libido, increase vaginal dryness and cause dyspareunia [12]. Increased prevalence of depression in women with diabetes may reduce sexual desire. Body image problems, such as arising from wearing medical devices, skin scars and insulin-related lipohypertrophy, can play a role in sexual dysfunction. In addition, self-care tasks including the need to pretest for blood glucose prior to sexual activity may affect the spontaneity of having sex. Other factors such as relationship with partner or partner-related sexual function may affect sexual health in women. Psychological or behavioural factors such as history of sexual abuse, multimorbidities, socioeconomic and cultural factors may also play a key role (Figure 15.1).

Diagnosis

Sexual dysfunction is under-reported in women with diabetes, so regular discussion in clinical practice initiated by healthcare professionals or self-reported questionnaires such as the use of Female Sexual Function Index (FSFI), may help early detection. Three main categories in the *Diagnostic and Statistical Manual of Mental Disorders* V can be used for the diagnosis of sexual dysfunction in women with diabetes. First is reduced sexual arousal or interest in having sex, second is disorder with orgasm, such as delayed or absent orgasm, and third is dyspareunia associated with sexual intercourse. These symptoms should be present for at least 75% of the time for a minimum of six months to make the diagnosis. This is to distinguish diabetes-related sexual dysfunction from transient stress-related disorders [13]. Doppler ultrasonography is an objective and non-invasive technique that can be used to provide a real-time assessment of anatomy and blood flow of female genitalia.

Treatment

Physical and psychological assessments are required to treat relevant comorbidities such as hypertension, obesity, anxiety or depression, which may improve sexual function. For example, the Look AHEAD study reported improvement in sexual function in women with obesity participating in the intensive lifestyle intervention compared with the placebo group [14]. Although PDE5 inhibitors may increase clitoral blood flow and improve sexual function, they are not licensed, as the evidence for their use in women is not yet conclusive. Hormone replacement therapy reduces the menopausal symptoms but it also it increases the risk of breast cancer and cardiovascular events and is not suitable in older women with diabetes. Similarly, although testosterone therapy may have some positive effects on sexual function, it is not yet licensed for routine use as substantial evidence of benefit is still lacking. Psychological interventions such as the framework of 'PLISSIT' (permission [giving patient permission to raise sexual issues], limited information [giving information about treatment], specific suggestions [giving suggestions based on evaluation of presenting complaint] and intensive therapy [giving patient variety of therapies]) can be used, but has limited effects in women with diabetes [15]. Non-pharmacological interventions such as lubricants, vaginal lasers, moisturisers and pelvic floor physical therapy may be of help (Figure 15.2).

Summary

There is an unmet need for treating sexual dysfunction in older people with diabetes. Multidisciplinary team involvement is required for a holistic management of sexual dysfunction addressing physical and psychological multimorbidities. Future research is still needed to explore novel and effective therapy.

Clinical Practice Questions

Q1. A 71-year-old man with a history of type 2 diabetes mellitus, hypertension and dyslipidaemia. His haemoglobin A1c is 8.1 mmol/mol, total cholesterol 5.7 mmol/l, body mass index 32 kg/m^2 and average home blood pressure reading is 160/87 mmHg. He is an ex-smoker but drinks 44 units of alcohol/week. His medications include metformin 1 g twice a day, atorvastatin 20 mg once a day and ramipril 10 mg once a day. He visited his general practitioner complaining of difficulty in maintaining erections.

Choose the most appropriate response:

A. Increase his hypoglycaemic, hypotensive and cholesterol lowering medications.
B. Start him on a phosphodiesterase 5 inhibitor.
C. Check his testosterone level.
D. Advise him to reduce his alcohol intake.
E. Refer him to an intensive lifestyle programme and review his medications.

Q2. A 66-year-old woman known to have diet-controlled type 2 diabetes mellitus and hypertension. Her haemoglobin A1c is 7.5 mmol/mol and average blood pressure reading is 156/77 mmHg. She takes ramipril 2.5 mg once a day. She recently visited her general practitioner complaining of a lack of energy and reduced ability to do her daily activities. Her partner mentioned that she is also feeling lonely and has lost interest in sexual activity.

Choose the most appropriate response:

A. Start metformin therapy.
B. Organise counselling for the partner.
C. Screen her for depression.
D. Increase ramipril to 5 mg once a day.
E. She needs social support.

References

Key references only are listed here. For a full list of references visit: `https://www.wiley.com/go/sinclair/1e`.

1. Bhasin, S., Enzlin, P., Coviello, A., and Basson, R. (2007). Sexual dysfunction in men and women with endocrine disorders. *Lancet* 369: 597–611.
2. Lindau, S.T., Tang, H., Gomero, A. et al. (2010). Sexuality among middle-aged and older adults with diagnosed and undiagnosed diabetes: a national, population-based study. *Diabetes Care* 33: 2202–2210.
3. Krzastek, S.C., Bopp, J., Smith, R.P., and Kovac, J.R. (2019). Recent advances in the understanding and management of erectile dysfunction. *F1000Res* 8: 102.
4. Thomas, H.N., Neal-Perry, G.S., and Hess, R. (2018). Female sexual function at midlife and beyond. *Obstet. Gynecol. Clin. North Am.* 45: 709–722.
5. Beckman, N., Waern, M., Gustafson, D., and Skoog, I. (2008). Secular trends in self reported sexual activity and satisfaction in Swedish 70 year olds: cross sectional survey of four populations, 1971–2001. *BMJ* 337: a279.

6. Maalmi, H., Herder, C., Bönhof, G.J. et al. (2022). Differences in the prevalence of erectile dysfunction between novel subgroups of recent-onset diabetes. *Diabetologia* 65: 552–562.
7. Kouidrat, Y., Pizzol, D., Cosco, T. et al. (2017). High prevalence of erectile dys- function in diabetes: a systematic review and meta-analysis of 145 studies. *Diabetes Med.* 34: 1185–1192.
8. Francis, S.H. and Corbin, J.D. (2011). PDE5 inhibitors: targeting erectile dysfunction in diabetics. *Curr. Opin. Pharmacol.* 11: 683–688.
9. Dhindsa, S., Prabhakar, S., Sethi, M. et al. (2004). Frequent occurrence of hypogonadotropic hypogonadism in type 2 diabetes. *J. Clin. Endocrinol. Metab.* 89: 5462–5468.
10. Corona, G., Isidori, A.M., Buvat, J. et al. (2014). Testosterone supplementation and sexual function: a meta-analysis study. *J. Sex. Med.* 11: 1577–1592.

16a

Special Issues in Old Age: Frailty

Alan J. Sinclair[1,2] *and Ahmed H. Abdelhafiz*[3]

[1] *King's College London, London, UK*
[2] *Foundation for Diabetes Research in Older People, Droitwich Spa, UK*
[3] *Department of Geriatric Medicine, Rotherham General Hospital, Rotherham, UK*

Key Points

- Diabetes and frailty have a reciprocal relationship and share a common pathogenic pathway.
- Frailty accelerates diabetes-related adverse outcomes.
- Frailty in diabetes is a heterogenous metabolic spectrum, which starts from a sarcopenic obese phenotype at one end and an anorexic malnourished phenotype at the other end.
- The sarcopenic obese phenotype is associated with increased insulin resistance and accelerated diabetes trajectory while the anorexic malnourished phenotype is associated with reduced insulin resistance and decelerated diabetes trajectory.
- The metabolic phenotypes of frailty should be considered in decision making in diabetes management.

Introduction

The global prevalence of diabetes mellitus is around 10.5% in adults aged 20–79 years and is expected to increase by 46% in 2045, due to increased life expectancy [1]. The prevalence peaks at 24% in older people aged between 75–79 years; about 50% of people with diabetes are 65 years of age or older [1]. In addition to the traditional diabetes-related micro- and macrovascular diseases, frailty is emerging as a new

Care of Older People with Diabetes: A Manual for Healthcare Practice, First Edition.
Edited by Alan J. Sinclair and Ahmed H. Abdelhafiz.

Companion website: www.wiley.com/go/sinclair/1e

complication category, affecting about 32–48% of older people with diabetes [2–5]. Frailty is a state of increased vulnerability to physical or psychological stressors due to decreased physiological reserve at multiple organ levels, which leads to a limited capacity to maintain homeostasis [6]. Although the prevalence of frailty increases with increasing age, frailty is neither an inevitable part of growing old nor a synonymous with ageing [7, 8].

Frailty has significant clinical consequences on older people and healthcare systems. For example, frail older people are at increased risk of injurious falls, fractures and dementia, which lead to disability, poor quality of life and premature mortality [9–14]. Frailty increases the risk of incident disability independent of comorbidities [15]. These adverse effects are associated with an increased burden on healthcare systems, such as increased emergency department visits, hospitalisation and care-home admissions [16]. Therefore, healthcare costs for frail older people are several-fold higher than non-frail individuals [17]. This chapter reviews the inter-relationship between frailty and diabetes in older people, the impact of each condition on the other and ways of prevention and management.

Frailty–diabetes Inter-relationship

The causes of diabetes-associated frailty are likely to be multifactorial, such as diabetes-associated comorbidities and diabetes-related complications. Although comorbidity and frailty are distinct conditions, they overlap and the terms are sometimes used interchangeably. Frailty is the clinical manifestation of the gradual and progressive physiological decline of multiple organ systems because of the accumulation of diseases over the years. Fundamental to this process is the multiorgan dysfunction concept, which leads to vulnerability of the individual to stressors and progression to frailty. While the clinical manifestation of multimorbidity will reflect the underlying comorbid diseases, frailty is characterised by multiple manifestations that include weakness, weight loss, wasting, lack of endurance, reduced mobility, balance disturbance, tendency to falls and slowness in performing activities of daily living. Frailty, therefore, is a syndrome of symptoms characterised by weakness, which is not part of comorbidity [18]. Both frailty and morbidity follow the disablement process model pathway, which incorporates four sequential stages from disease to impairment to functional decline then to disability [19]. The multimorbidity mediator effect to frailty appears to be synergistic when more than one morbidity coexist with diabetes. For example, the Mexican Health and Nutrition Survey of 7164 older people, mean age 70.6 years (standard deviation [SD] 8.1 years), has shown that diabetes was independently associated with frailty (coefficient 0.28, $p < 0.001$) [20]. The association was incremental when hypertension (0.63, $p < 0.001$) or any diabetic complication was also present (0.55, $p < 0.001$) [20]. Similarly, a Japanese cross-sectional study that included 9606 participants (≥ 65 years), demonstrated an increased risk of frailty (odds ratio [OR] 1.83, 95% confidence interval [CI] 1.01–3.45) in participants with renal impairment (estimated glomerular filtration rate [eGFR] < 30.0 ml/minute/1.73 m^2) compared with participants with better renal function (eGFR ≥ 60.0 ml/minute/1.73 m^2). Individuals with a history of hypertension or diabetes mellitus showed a higher risk of frailty and the risk increased further when both hypertension and diabetes coexisted (OR 3.67, 95% CI 1.13–14.05) [21]. Comorbidities such as cerebrovascular disease, ischaemic heart disease and chronic kidney disease are more common in people with diabetes compared with those without and may increase the risk of frailty [22]. In addition, hormonal factors and vitamin D deficiency are more common in older people with diabetes and may accelerate the development of frailty [23, 24]. Geriatric syndromes (cognitive impairment, depressive symptoms, falls, urinary incontinence and pain), which are common in diabetes, are associated with increased risk of frailty and disability as opposed to other chronic conditions [25]. Other factors common in older people include inadequate nutrition, especially poor protein intake, reduced physical exercise and decline in neuromuscular junction. These factors may also contribute to muscular weakness and development of frailty [26]. Patients with diabetes and weak muscles are at increased risk of falls, fractures and further deterioration in physical functions, which may establish a vicious circle of frailty [27]. Reciprocally, diabetes prevalence is higher in frail compared with non-frail patients [28], so it appears that diabetes and frailty are interrelated and may have a common pathogenic pathway. For example, chronic low-grade inflammation is link or a contributing factor to the occurrence of chronic diseases such as diabetes and frailty [29]. Furthermore, diabetes and frailty have been shown to share a common cardiovascular risk factors pathway as reported in the Whitehall II Prospective Cohort Study [30].

Effect of Diabetes on Frailty

Diabetes may directly increase the risk of frailty due to diabetes-associated loss of skeletal muscle mass, weakness, reduced muscle quality, reduced muscle strength, decline in gait speed, diminished functional capacity and accelerated ageing process [31–36] (Figure 16a.1). Hyperglycaemia has been shown to be associated with poor muscle quality, muscle mass loss and reduced physical performance in a dose-response manner [37, 38]. The risk of frailty appears to increase proportionally with increasing blood glucose levels. For example, the Beijing Longitudinal Study of Ageing II, which included 10039 subjects, mean age 70.5 years (SD 7.8 years) at baseline, reported that the prevalence and incidence of frailty was higher in people who had diabetes compared with those who did not (19.3% vs 11.9% and 12.3% vs 7.0%, respectively). People with prediabetes had a similar prevalence (11.43%) but slightly higher incidence of frailty (8.7%) than people without diabetes, suggesting that prediabetes may mediate the risk of frailty [39]. Several studies showed association of hyperglycaemia with frailty (Table 16a.1) [40–42]. Hypoglycaemia has also been shown to increase the risk of incident frailty in patients with a new-onset diabetes. These patients had fewer morbidities, suggesting that the effect of hypoglycaemia on frailty is independent of diabetes-related complications, diabetes-associated comorbidities or the duration of diabetes [43]. The association of hypoglycaemia and frailty has also been shown in other studies (Table 16a.1) [44, 45]. Zaslavsky et al. found a U-shaped association between blood glucose/haemoglobin A1c (HbA1c) levels and incident frailty, confirming that both hyper- and hypoglycaemia may be involved in the development of frailty in older people with diabetes [46]. Although the risk of frailty due to hyperglycaemia may be due to its association with chronic inflammatory state, microvascular and macrovascular disease or skeletal muscle mitochondrial dysfunction, the risk of frailty due to hypoglycaemia is less explained [47–49]. Frailty risk associated with hypoglycaemia may be related to a variability in glucose levels, which contributes to endothelial damage, or other unknown factors associated with low blood glucose [50]. Indeed, variability of blood glucose levels has been shown to increase the risk of frailty [51]. Other factors may be related to the fact that hypoglycaemia increases the risk of other conditions that are associated with frailty, such as dementia and stroke [52, 53].

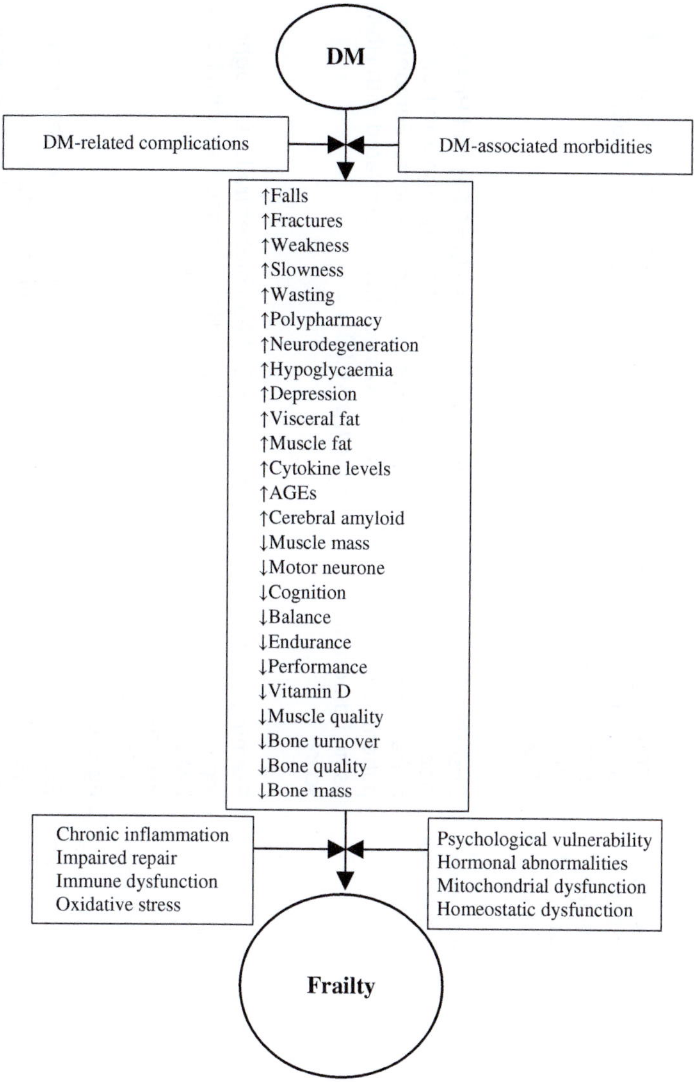

Figure 16a.1: Effects of diabetes mellitus (DM) on frailty. Diabetes leads to widespread systemic complications that increases the risk of frailty. AGEs, advanced glycation end products.

Effects of Frailty on Diabetes

As diabetes increases the risk of frailty, the development of frailty will have significant consequences on diabetes. Theses consequences impact on the adverse outcomes and on the metabolic trajectory of diabetes (Figure 16a.2).

Table 16a.1: Studies investigating glycaemic effects on frailty.

Study	Type, Country	Patients	Aims	Main findings
Kong et al. 2021 [40]	Cross-sectional, China	291 community-dwelling older people, median age 69 years (IQR 67–72 years) with type 2 DM	Identify predictors of frailty among Chinese community-dwelling older people with type 2 DM	Higher HbA1c was a significant predictor of frailty (OR 1.434, 95% CI 1.045–1.968)
Bilgin et al. 2020 [41]	Cross-sectional, Turkey	101 patients with DM (41 frail, 60 not frail), mean age 64.2 years (SD 8.0 years) frail, 62.2 years (SD 7.0 years) non-frail	Observe clinical and laboratory indices of frail and non-frail patients with DM using Edmonton frail score	Fasting blood glucose ($p = 0.02$) and HbA1c ($p = 0.04$) were significantly higher in frail compared with non-frail patients. Edmonton frail score was positively correlated with HbA1c ($r = 0.44$, $p < 0.001$)
Aguayo et al., 2019 [42]	Prospective, UK	5377 participants, median age 70 years (IQR 65, 77 years), follow-up 10 years	Examine whether individuals with DM or high HbA1c experience different frailty trajectories with ageing	People with DM had higher frailty throughout later life. Higher HbA1c associated with frailty ($b = 4.2$, 95% CI 2.5–5.9)
Chao et al. 2020 [43]	Prospective, Taiwan	2119 patients with and 8432 without hypoglycaemia, mean age 65.9 years (SD 14 years)	Examine whether hypoglycaemia increases risk of frailty	After 2.68 years offollow-up, 172 patients with hypoglycaemia developed incident frailty (HR 1.60, 95% CI 1.14–2.42). The risk of frailty persisted despite confounder adjustment (1.44, 1.01–2.05)

MacKenzie et al. 2020 [44]	Retrospective, Canada	400 patients, mean age 81.4 years (SD 8.1 years) acutely hospitalised, assessed by geriatrician	Investigate association of diabetes and frailty (assessed by CFS) with hospital outcomes	Mean admission glucose decreased with increasing frailty ($p = 0.003$), with mean admission glucose of 13.0 mmol/l (SD 8.4 mmol/l) for mildly, 9.0 mmol/l (SD 3.4 mmol/l) for moderately and 8.6 mmol/l (SD 3.4 mmol/l) for patients who are severely frail, respectively; 9 patients had hypoglycaemia on admission and all were frail
Yanagita et al. 2018 [45]	Cross sectional–prospective, Japan	132 patients hospitalised with diabetes, mean age 78.3 years (SD 8.0 years)	Evaluate frailty risk factors including HbA1c using CFS for frailty assessment	HbA1c significantly lower, mean 7.13 (SD 0.99) in frail compared with non-frail, 7.27 (SD 1.04) group, $p < 0.001$. Values of HbA1c inversely correlated with values of CFS ($r = -0.31$, $p < 0.01$). In multiple regression analysis, HbA1c independently predicted frailty ($\beta = -0.367$, $p < 0.01$)
Zaslavsky et al. 2016 [46]	Prospective, United States	Total 1848 participants, 200 with and 1648 without diabetes	Examine association of blood glucose level and frailty	In patients with diabetes, U-shaped relation between HbA1c and frailty risk, compared with a reference HbA1c 7.6%: (A) lower HBA1c: HR 1.41, 95% CI 1.12–1.78 for HbA1c 6.9% and 1.10 (1.0–1.20) for HbA1c 7.2%; (B) higher HbA1c: HR 1.08, 95% CI 1.0–1.17 for HbA1c 7.9% and 1.30 (1.08–1.56) for HbA1c 8.2%

CFS, clinical frailty scale; CI, confidence interval; HbA1c, haemoglobin A1c; HR, hazard ratio; IRR, incidence rate ratio; SD, standard deviation.

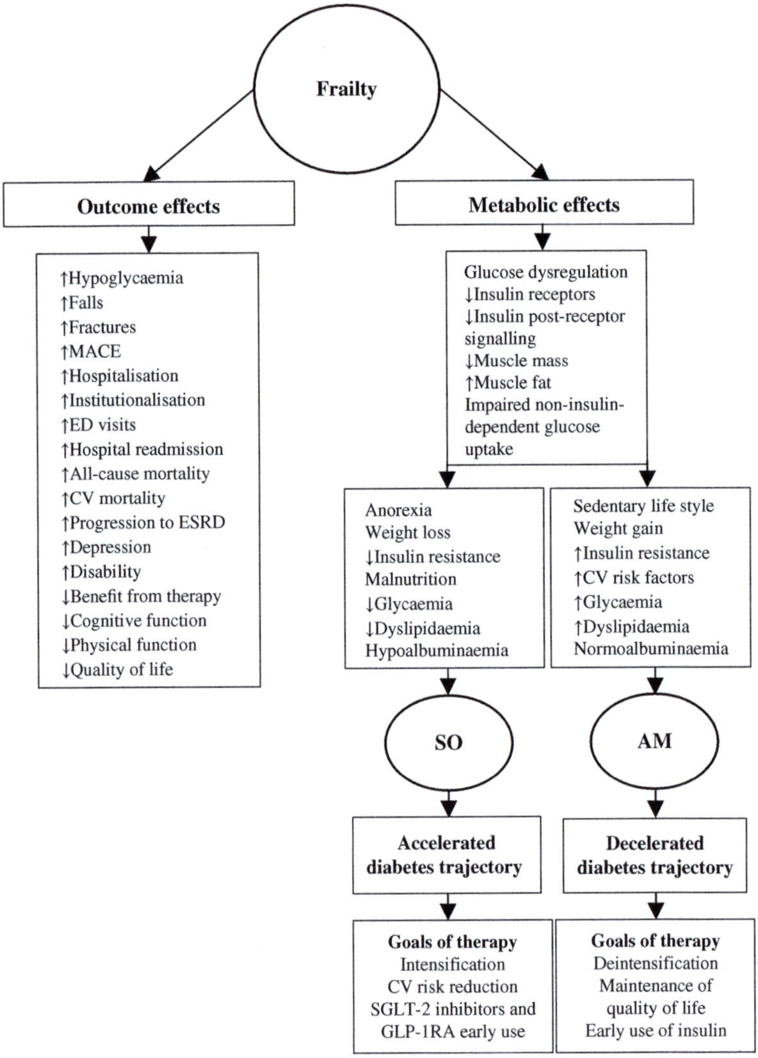

Figure 16a.2: Effects of frailty on diabetes. Frailty increases adverse outcomes of diabetes and affects the metabolic profile in older people with diabetes, which will have impact of their management. AM, anorexic malnourished; CV, cardiovascular; ED, emergency department; ESRD, end stage renal disease; GLP-1RA, glucagon like peptide receptor agonists; MACE, major cardiovascular adverse events; SGLT-2, sodium glucose transporter; SO, sarcopenic obese.

Outcome Effects

The development of frailty in older people with diabetes accelerates the occurrence of adverse outcomes compared with non-frail patients with diabetes. In a large UK Biobank data study (20 566 participants), frailty measures were associated with mortality, major adverse cardiovascular events, hypoglycaemia and falls or fractures [54]. The ADVANCE study showed that frailty increased risk of vascular events, all-cause and cardiovascular mortality and hypoglycaemia. In addition, frailty attenuated the benefits from blood-pressure lowering and intensive glycaemic therapy [55]. After eight-years of follow-up in the Look AHEAD study, the increase in frailty incidence was associated with poor cognitive function, physical function and mortality [56]. Frailty, independent of morbidity, was associated with all-cause hospitalisation and mortality [57]. Frailty was associated with increased risk of hospitalisations, institutionalisation, emergency department visits, fractures and mortality in older people with diabetes [58]. Among patients with diabetic kidney disease, frailty accelerated the progression to end-stage renal disease on a dose-response manner [59]. Low health-related quality of life, depression and higher numbers of healthcare visits in people with diabetes and chronic kidney disease was reported in a cross-sectional analysis [60]. In a very old (≥ 80 years) cohort of patients with diabetes and acute coronary syndrome, frailty was associated with increased incidence of death or six-month hospital readmission [61]. Frailty was associated with all-cause mortality and disability in older people with mild diabetes [62]. Frailty, as well as pre-frailty, were associated with increased cardiovascular events, healthcare service use, hospitalisation and mortality [63]. Frailty was associated with increased hospitalisation while both pre-frailty and frailty were associated with increased emergency department visits [64]. Frailty led to disability potentiated by cognitive impairment and both increased risk of mortality (Table 16a.2) [65].

Metabolic Effects

The development of frailty will have a significant metabolic effect in older people with diabetes. Frailty is associated with significant skeletal muscle loss or sarcopenia. Skeletal muscle is responsible for about 80% of the total blood glucose uptake [66]. Skeletal muscle tissue consists mainly of type I and type II muscle fibres. Type II fibres are less

Table 16a.2: Studies investigating frailty effects on diabetes adverse outcomes.

Study	Study type, country	Patients	Aim	Main findings
Hanlon et al. 2021 [54]	Longitudinal cohort, United Kingdom	UK Biobank, 20 566 with type 2 DM aged 40–72 years	Assess implications of frailty/multimorbidity in middle/older-aged people with type 2 DM using 2 morbidity and 2 frailty measures	(A) 42% of participants were frail or multimorbid by at least 1 measure, 2.2% by all 4 measures. (B) Each measure was associated with mortality, MACE, hypoglycaemia, fall or fracture. (C) Mortality risk was higher in older vs younger participants with a given level of frailty (1.9%, and 9.9% in men 45 years and 65 years, respectively), or multimorbidity (1.3% and 7.8% in men with 4 morbidities, aged 45 years and 65 years, respectively)
Nguyen et al. 2021 [55]	Retrospective, multicentre	11 140 with type 2 DM, mean age 65.78 years (SD 6.39 years)	Explore effect of frailty on intensive glycaemic and blood pressure control	(A) Frailty increased risk of combined macro- and microvascular events (HR 1.03, 95% CI 0.90–1.19, $p = 0.02$) and all-cause mortality (1.11, 0.92–1.34). (B) Severe hypoglycaemia was higher in frail, 8.39 (6.15–10.63) vs 4.80 (3.84–5.76) in non-frail ($p < 0.001$). (C) No significant difference in discontinuation of BP treatment due to hypotension/dizziness between frail and non-frail
Espeland et al. 2021 [56]	Prospective, United States	3842 with type 2 DM aged 45–76 years at baseline, follow-up 8 years	Examine effect of multimorbidity and frailty on cognition, physical function and mortality	Increases in both multimorbidity and frailty index were associated with poor composite cognitive function and how long it takes for patient to walk 400 metres, and increased risk for death (all $p < 0.001$)

Ferri-Guerra et al. 2020 [57]	Retrospective, United States	763 with DM, mean age 72.9 years (SD 6.8 years)	Determine association of frailty with all-cause hospitalisations and mortality	Frailty was associated with higher all-cause hospitalisations, HR 1.71 (95% CI 1.31–2.24), $p < 0.0001$ and greater mortality, HR 2.05, (95% CI 1.16–3.64), $p = 0.014$
Sable-Morita et al. 2021 [58]	Retrospective, Japan	477 with DM, mean age 74.2 years (SD 6.2 years)	Assess whether frailty and DM-related factors could predict occurrence of adverse events	Microvascular complications and frailty were significant predictors of adverse event incidence, respective OR 1.403 (95% CI 1.11–1.78) per additional complication, OR 2.419 (95% CI 1.33–4.40) for frailty; both $p < 0.05$)
Chao et al. 2019 [59]	Retrospective, Taiwan	165 461 with DKD, aged > 20 years	Examine effect of frailty on DKD progression to ESRD, mortality, and adverse episodes	(A) Patients with 1, 2, and ≥3 on FRAIL scale had increased risks of ESRD and mortality HR 1.13, 1.18, and 1.2 and 1.25, 1.41, and 1.34, respectively. (B) frailty increased risk of CV events and ICU admission in a dose–response manner
Adame Perez et al. 2019 [60]	Cross-sectional, Canada	41 with DM and CKD, median age 70 years (range 65–74 years)	Compare differences in body composition, HRQoL, mental health, cognition and vitamin D status with healthcare service use by frail and non-frail	Frail, compared with non-frail had lower lean body mass, lower HRQoL scores, more depression ($p =< 0.05$) and higher numbers of health visits ($p < 0.05$). No differences in healthcare visit types or vitamin D status were noted between frail and non-frail participants

(*Continued*)

Table 16a.2: Continued

Study	Study type, country	Patients	Aim	Main findings
Gual et al. 2019 [61]	Prospective, Spain	532 with ACS, 212 with DM, mean age 83.7 years (SD 5.0 years)	Evaluate impact of DM on mortality or 6-month readmission according to frailty status	Association of DM and incidence of clinical outcomes was significant only in patients with established frailty (HR 1.72, 1.05–2.81) compared with non-frail patients
Kitamura et al. 2019 [62]	Prospective, Japan	1271, 174 with DM, mean age 71.0 years (SD 5.6 years), follow-up 8.1 years	Clarify risks of death and disability in diabetes, frailty, both or neither	(A) Compared with non-frail without diabetes, those with diabetes and frailty had higher risks of mortality, HR 5.0, 95% CI 2.4–10.3) and incident disability (HR 3.9, 2.1–7.3). (B) Non-frail with diabetes did not have a significant increased risk of mortality, but a tendency for disability compared with non-frail without diabetes
Chao et al. 2018 [63]	Longitudinal cohort, Taiwan	560 795 with type 2 DM, mean age 56.4 SD 13.8 years), 3.14-year follow-up	Examine frailty impact on long-term mortality, CV risk, all-cause hospitalisation, and ICU admission	Pre-frailty (1, 2 FRAIL scale) and frailty (≥3) increased risk of: (A) mortality, HR 1.05, 1.13, and 1.25 (95% CI 1.02–1.07, 1.08–1.17 and 1.15–1.36, respectively); (B) CV events, HR 1.05, 1.15, and 1.13 (95% CI 1.02–1.07, 1.1–1.2 and 1.01–1.25, respectively); (C) hospitalisation, HR 1.06, 1.16, and 1.25 (95% CI 1.05–1.07, 1.14–1.19 and 1.18–1.33, respectively); (D) ICU admission, HR 1.05, 1.13 and 1.17 (95% CI 1.03–1.07, 1.08–1.14 and 1.06–1.28, respectively) compared with non-frail

Li et al. 2018 [64]	Cross-sectional, Taiwan	3203, 719 with DM, aged ≥65 years	Investigate prevalence of frailty and its relationship with healthcare	A. Frailty, but not pre-frailty, significantly associated with hospitalisation, OR 5.31, 95% CI 1.87–15.10). B. Pre-frail and frail significantly associated with emergency department visits (OR 2.64, 95% CI 1.35–5.17 and OR 4.05, 95% CI 1.31–12.49, respectively)
Thein et al. 2018 [65]	Prospective, Singapore	2696, 486 with DM, mean age 67.3 years (SD 7.5 years)	Investigate effect of frailty and cognitive impairment on functional and mortality outcomes	(A) Frailty associated with higher prevalence of IADL disability, OR 6.72, 95% CI 1.84–24.5. (B) Frailty and cognitive impairment associated with highest prevalence of IADL (OR 17.8, 95% CI 3.66–8.68) and ADL disabilities (OR 93.8, 95% CI 23.6–372.4). (C) Cognitive impairment (HR 2.72, 95% CI 1.48–5.01), frailty (4.30, 1.88–9.82) and cognitive impairment with frailty (HR 8.41, 95% CI 3.95–17.9) associated with mortality

ACS, acute coronary syndrome; ADL, activities of daily living; CHD, coronary heart disease; CI, confidence interval; DFUs, diabetic foot ulcers; DKDF, diabetic kidney disease; DM, diabetes mellitus; ESRD, end stage renal disease; HF, heart failure; HR, hazard ratio; HRQoL, health-related quality of life; IADL, instrumental ADL; ICU, intensive care unit; IRR, incidence rate ratio; LDL, low density lipoprotein; MACE, major adverse cardiovascular events; MI, myocardial infarction; NDCMP, national diabetes care management program; OR, odds ratio; SBP, systolic blood pressure; SD, standard deviation.

oxidative and more glycolytic, which is associated with more insulin resistance than type I fibres [67]. With increasing age, there is a predominance of loss of type II muscle fibres over type I fibres and this loss is accelerated by the development of frailty, which will have a significant impact on glucose metabolism in frail older people with diabetes [68, 69]. Although weight loss is one of the frailty criteria, it is not a prerequisite for frailty diagnosis. Obesity can be associated with physical function decline and frailty. There is a U-shaped relationship between body mass index and frailty [70]. Frail older people with diabetes will have a metabolic spectrum that starts from a sarcopenic obese (SO) phenotype at one end and an anorexic malnourished (AM) phenotype at the other end.

Sarcopenic Obese Phenotype

Sarcopenia and obesity are the main characteristics of this phenotype. Sarcopenic obesity is associated with frailty, (OR 2.00, 95% CI 1.42–2.82) and disabilities in activity of daily living (1.58, 1.12–2.24) and instrumental activity of daily living (1.36, 1.05–1.76) [71]. The sarcopenic obese (SO) phenotype is associated with unfavourable metabolic profile, with increased insulin resistance and dyslipidaemia [72, 73]. Obesity is associated with fewer type I muscle fibres and more type II muscle fibres [74]. This leads to lower oxidative capacity, increased fat storage, increased insulin resistance and hyperglycaemia [75–77]. In addition, the surplus of energy is stored as ectopic muscular adipose tissue, increasing insulin resistance further. Therefore, although the predominant loss of type II muscle fibres associated with frailty and sarcopenia may have a positive effect on glucose metabolism, the presence of obesity attenuates this benefit and shifts the balance into unfavourable metabolism with an overall increased insulin resistance.

Anorexic Malnourished Phenotype

Anorexia and malnutrition dominate in the anorexic malnourished (AM) phenotype and lead to significant weight loss. Anorexia of ageing is the reduction of appetite and food intake in older people, which leads to increased risk of weight loss and the subsequent development of frailty [78]. Anorexia is more common in institutionalised individuals than those living in the community [79]. The prevalence of anorexia seems to match that of frailty linking both conditions together. Anorexia affects up to 30% and frailty up to 28% of older people [79, 80]. Older people with anorexia are at increased risk to progress to frailty when they develop acute illness [81]. This frailty phenotype is associated with a predominant loss of the insulin-resistant type II muscle fibres, which may improve insulin sensitivity, spontaneous resolution of hyperglycaemia and normalisation of HbA1c [82]. In addition to the type of skeletal muscle fibre loss, altered blood glucose–insulin homeostasis may be another factor that explain the resolution of hyperglycaemia in this frailty phenotype. It has been shown that insulin resistance is demonstrated in frail older people only when abdominal obesity is present, while insulin resistance is the same in non-obese frail compared with healthy older persons [83].

Prevention and Management

Non-pharmacological therapy of lifestyle interventions with a focus on the maintenance of muscle mass and muscle strength, in addition to pharmacological therapy, is the mainstay in the prevention and management of frailty in older people with diabetes. In addition, metabolic phenotypes of frailty in older people with diabetes should be taken into consideration when choosing the most suitable regimen of non-pharmacological and pharmacological therapy, as well as on the decision making of the overall glycaemic goals.

Screening

Screening for frailty should be part of holistic diabetes care due to the significant impact of frailty on diabetes management. In addition, early detection of pre-frailty and frailty will help to tailor interventions that may reduce the risk of progression to disability [84]. Holistic assessment should include multiple domains such as nutritional status along with physical, and cognitive functions [85, 86]. Multiple frailty assessment tools are available but two conceptual frames comprise the basics for understanding frailty. The Fried criteria of unintentional weight loss, exhaustion, slowness, weak hand grip and low activity is the most commonly used tool to screen for frailty in older people with diabetes [87]. Presence of one to two criteria diagnose pre-frail status, while three or more criteria indicate frailty. Those who do not meet any of the criteria are classified as robust.

The Rockwood cumulative deficit model is defined by the presence of deficits that accumulate with increasing age and progress over time to a vulnerability level that becomes incompatible with living independently [88]. This conceptual framework is represented in a frailty index that describes the health status of the individual and the progression of frailty over time in a quantitative way, which includes multiple domains including cognitive, physical, nutritional, health perception, balance, strength, mobility, activities of daily living, sleep, morbidities and social aspects. The frailty index is calculated as a ratio of the observed deficits to the total number of possible deficits. Although other frailty tools exist, there is marked heterogeneity between studies and, as yet, there is no optimal tool to assess frailty in older people with diabetes specifically [54]. Comprehensive Geriatric Assessment (CGA), a multidimensional evaluation across interrelated domains, which include physical, cognitive, psychological, functional and social aspects, is central in any tool to assess frailty and tailoring the care needs of older people with diabetes.

Non-pharmacological Therapy

Adequate nutrition and exercise are the main interventions to prevent or delay the development of frailty [90]. In addition, such multidisciplinary programmes that focus on nutrition and exercise training may also improve the overall functional capacity [90]. Malnutrition is associated with a decline in physical function and is more common in older people with compared with those without diabetes and frailty [91]. Nutritional management is mainly based on reaching ideal body weight and, at the same time, reducing muscle mass loss. Insufficient dietary protein intake is associated with reduced lean body mass and frailty [92, 93]. For example, hypoalbuminaemia is associated with chronic inflammation and serum albumin levels are inversely related to frailty [94, 95]. Higher daily protein intake may be required in older people due to reduced protein absorption or the anabolic resistance associated with old age [96]. A daily protein intake of 1–1.2 g/kg may enhance muscle mass and function [97]. Few data are available on the quality of protein supplements, although the inclusion of the essential amino acids in the diet seems reasonable, especially leucine-enriched essential amino acids (whey protein) [98]. Weight loss via energy restriction alone should be avoided because it may cause simultaneous loss of muscle mass. In addition, vitamin B_{12} deficiency has been shown in older people with diabetes, especially those taking metformin, which may be associated with neurological disorders, muscle weakness, recurrent falls and increased risk of frailty [99]. Vitamin D supplementation may increase muscle strength and reduce the frequency of falls, especially in older people with low vitamin D levels [100, 101]. Both resistance and aerobic exercise are useful, although a combination of both has been shown to be superior to either of them alone [90]. During exercise, protective myokines such as interleukin-6, are released by muscle contractions, which may inhibit the activity of the proinflammatory cytokines such as TNF-α, which may reduce the chronic low-grade inflammation associated with frailty [102]. Resistance exercise improves muscle mass while aerobic exercise reduces obesity. Resistance training may result in improvements in physical capacity, muscle quality, fat-free mass and gait speed in a short period of time [103]. Aquatic exercise may be a useful modality to help compliance and adherence, and is also suitable for patients with arthritis [104]. Other exercise modalities which may be suitable in disabled people, such as whole-body electromyostimulation, vibration, yoga and tai-chi, may have some benefits and can be considered as an alternative in these patients [105, 106]. Whole-body electromyostimulation has shown a favourable metabolism in sarcopenic obese phenotypes, which may be considered an effective and safe technology in those who are unable or unwilling to exercise conventionally [105]. Diet, combined with exercise, appears to be the best strategy for improving metabolic profile and preservation of lean muscle mass [107]. The combination of resistance training and protein supplementation has been shown to reduce fat mass and to improve lean muscle mass and strength in frail older people than exercise alone [108]. A structured multimodal intervention, which included nutrition, resistance exercise training and optimal diabetes care, led to a clinically relevant and cost-effective improvement in the functional status of older frail and pre-frail participants with type 2 diabetes mellitus [109].

Pharmacological Therapy

There are no hypoglycaemic agents specifically designed for the prevention of frailty in older people with diabetes. Metformin is the most studied hypoglycaemic agent to show a positive effect on frailty. Metformin has been shown to improve muscle function [110].

Sulfonylureas, especially glibenclamide, and glinides may be associated with muscle atrophy in humans [111]. In a cohort study of 2415 veterans, 307 (12.7%) on metformin and 2108 (87.3%) on sulfonylurea therapy, mean age 73 years (SD 5.2 years), metformin reduced the risk of frailty (OR 0.66, 95% CI 0.61–0.71, $p < 0.0001$) compared with sulfonylureas [112]. In addition, metformin was shown to delay the development of age-related comorbidities such as dementia, depression and frailty in a large prospective study of 41 204 men with type 2 diabetes, mean age 74.6 years (SD 5.8 years), followed up for over nine years [113]. In participants with a high risk of frailty, metformin reduced the risk of frailty-related diseases by 23.8%, depression by 15.6%, dementia by 3.8%, as well as the odds of mortality (OR 0.39, 95% CI 0.35–0.43) [113]. Metformin also improved the gait speed of 120 pre-frail older (≥ 60 years) people without diabetes after 16 weeks of therapy, in a small Indonesian double-blind randomised controlled study compared with placebo [114]. In the follow-up phase of the study of osteoporotic fractures, which included a total of 2864 community dwelling older women, mean age 78.5 years (SD 3.6 years), insulin sensitiser treatment (metformin/glitazones) had preserved walk speed compared with non-insulin sensitiser treatment ($p < 0.05$) [115]. In a Japanese study that included 194 patients with diabetes, mean age 65.7 years, the prevalence of patients with a high risk of falling (defined as a weaker hand grip and a shorter duration of standing on one leg) was significantly higher in those treated with glucagon like peptide-1 receptor agonists (GLP-1RA) compared with other hypoglycaemic medications (45.7% vs 27.5%). This might suggest that GLP-1RA may increase the risk of frailty, but further studies are needed [116]. Studies on the sodium glucose transporter (SGLT-2) inhibitors luseogliflozin and canagliflozin have shown a reduction of skeletal muscle mass and suggested that SGLT-2 therapy may increase the risk of sarcopenia and frailty [117–119]. However, another study showed that dapagliflozin did not reduce muscle mass [120]. On the other hand, it has been reported that SGLT-2 inhibitors improve muscle quality rather than muscle mass which may have an overall positive effect [121]. Dipeptidyl peptidase-4 (DPP-4) inhibitors, through improvement of muscular blood supply, may have a beneficial effect on the reduction of lean muscle loss, although there are no clinical trials yet available [122]. Insulin stimulates muscle protein synthesis only in younger but not in older people, and has not been shown to reduce muscle atrophy in diabetes [123].

Special Considerations

With the development of frailty and its metabolic impact on diabetes, special considerations should be taken into account, such as glycaemic control, choice of hypoglycaemic agents and overall glycaemic goals.

Glycaemic Control

Target HbA1c ranges between <7.5% and 9.0% (<59–75 mmol/mol) have been suggested in guidelines for older people with diabetes, depending on their overall function [124–128]. Lower end of HbA1c is recommended for independent and physically well older people, with gradual relaxation of targets in proportion to physical function decline [124–128]. Targets are driven from the effects of HbA1c on cardiovascular or renal outcomes and mostly extrapolated from studies conducted on younger age groups. The reduction of HbA1c to less than 7.0% (53 mmol/mol) may reduce long-term microvascular complications with no clear effect on cardiovascular outcomes [129–132]. There is little literature on the effect of glycaemic control on physical function or frailty. The results of the available studies are conflicting. For example, some studies shown that low HbA1c (<7.0%; 53 mmol/mol) to be beneficial on lower extremity performance and high HbA1c (>8.0%, 63.9 mmol/mol) to increase functional disability, while other studies shown that low HbA1c to increase the risk of hypoglycaemia, falls and fractures with no benefit on physical function [133–135]. For non-frail older people with diabetes, a U-shaped relationship has been reported between HbA1c and the risk of frailty with an HbA1c of 7.6% (59.6 mmol/mol) to be associated with the lowest risk [46]. A systematic review of clinical studies that included frail older people with diabetes (defined as significantly or severely impaired by cut-off scores of assessment instruments on frailty, activities of daily life or physical functional impairment) reported that HbA1c less than 7.0% (53 mmol/mol) with low variability to be associated with preservation of physical function in community-dwelling older people with diabetes [136]. On the other hand, an HbA1c of 8.0–8.9% (63.9–73.8 mmol/mol) was associated with a reduction in the composite outcome of death or functional decline in those who needed skilled assistance. Those who needed skilled assistance are likely to be the most frail participants in the cohort, which may support the current guidelines that a higher HbA1c is more appropriate as physical function declines. However, studies included in this latter review were at high risk of bias to conclude specific Hba1c targets for each category of patients [136]. The current guideline recommendation on glycaemic target in proportion to physical function seem reasonable, considering the limited available evidence in this group of patients.

Choice of Hypoglycaemic Agent

The choice of hypoglycaemic agent should be determined by the frailty metabolic phenotype [137].

Sarcopenic Obese Phenotype

SGLT-2 inhibitors and GLP-1RA should be considered early in the SO phenotype because of their weight losing properties and their favourable effect on the metabolic profile. The SO phenotype is at increased risk of cardiorenal adverse outcomes and these therapies are appropriate in significantly reducing this risk, which includes reductions in major adverse cardiovascular events, stroke, myocardial infarction, hospitalisation for heart failure, mortality, albuminuria and progression to end-stage renal disease [138]. These therapies also improve liver function and histological features and reduce liver fat content in patients with non-alcoholic fatty liver disease and non-alcoholic steatohepatitis [139–141]. These protective effects occur within few months of therapy and independent of tight glycaemic control. Therefore, frail older people with an SO phenotype will benefit from such therapies, even if they have short life expectancy or are at risk of hypoglycaemia. Another advantage is the reduction of polypharmacy, which is associated with negative consequences such as adverse effects of medication and non-compliance. People with an SO phenotype are likely to have associated multiple comorbidities of the metabolic syndrome, and the use of the new therapies may reduce the burden of other medications, such as diuretics and antihypertensives [142]. Insulin should be a last resort in the SO frailty phenotype due to insulin-associated weight gain and the increased insulin resistance in this phenotype.

Anorexic Malnourished Phenotype

Insulin therapy should be considered early in the AM frailty phenotype due to its weight gain effect. The AM phenotype is likely to be more prevalent in the advanced aged population with multiple comorbidities, poor multiple organ dysfunction and intolerance to oral therapy. In addition, insulin has anabolic properties through increasing glucose uptake, glycogenesis, lipogenesis and skeletal muscle protein synthesis [143, 144]. Previous studies have shown the anabolic properties of insulin to be more prominent in younger people and blunted with increasing age [145, 146]. However, more recent studies have shown that endogenous insulin to be positively correlated with skeletal muscle mass, low insulin levels to be associated with sarcopenia and insulin therapy to improve skeletal muscle index, muscle mass and delayed the progression of sarcopenia [147–150]. The parenteral route of administration and the risk of hypoglycaemia are the main disadvantages of insulin therapy. Long-acting insulin analogues are a suitable choice in the AM frail phenotype because of their convenient once-daily administration, simplicity of their regimen and their low risk of hypoglycaemia due to their peakless blood levels and long duration of action. Long-acting insulin analogues have been shown to be more effective and safer than intermediate-acting human insulins [151–154]. For example, insulin analogues reduced the gross variations in blood glucose levels, achieved better glycaemic control, reduced hypoglycaemia-related hospitalisation or emergency department visits and improved quality of life compared with intermediate-acting human insulins [151–154]. Oral hypoglycaemic therapy can be adjuvant to insulin therapy but the new SGLT-2 inhibitors and GLP-1RA are not suitable in this frailty phenotype because of the significant weight loss, risk of dehydration, hypotension, falls and fractures [155].

Goals of Therapy

The goals of therapy should be tailored according to metabolic phenotypes. The SO phenotype is associated with increased insulin resistance, unfavourable metabolic profile, accelerated diabetes trajectory and increased risk of major adverse cardiovascular events. Although clinical guidelines suggest relaxed targets based on function, patients with an SO frail phenotype are likely to benefit from therapies such as SGLT-2 inhibitors and GLP-1RA based on their metabolic profile rather than their function [134]. Therefore, an approach that aims at intensification of therapy to improve metabolic profile, reduce insulin resistance and cardiovascular risk is appropriate. In addition, pharmacological therapy of cardiovascular risk factors such as antihypertensives, cholesterol-lowering agents and antiplatelet therapies help to reduce cardiovascular risk. The AM phenotype is associated with significant weight loss, reduced insulin resistance and decelerated trajectory of diabetes. In addition, due to reduced oral intake and anorexia, these patients are likely to need less hypoglycaemic therapy. Therefore, an approach that aims at deintensification of therapy to avoid the risk of hypoglycaemia is appropriate. Furthermore, complete withdrawal of hypoglycaemic agents may be required in certain patients with this phenotype who have severe weight loss [156, 157]. A Maintenance of quality of life in this phenotype is required with a focus on maintenance of blood glucose levels in comfortable zone to avoid severe fluctuations of blood glucose levels that leads to decompensations and unnecessary hospitalisations.

Summary

Diabetes prevalence is increasing, especially in the older age group, due to increased life expectancy. Frailty is a newly recognised diabetes-related complication. Diabetes and frailty appear to share a common pathogenic pathway and have a reciprocal relationship. The development of frailty increases the risk of diabetes-related adverse outcomes and exerts metabolic changes that lead to different metabolic phenotypes. The metabolic phenotypes of frailty changes diabetes trajectory and should be considered in decision making regarding glycaemic control, choice of hypoglycaemic agents and determining overall goals of therapy.

Future Perspectives

Frailty has not been a common outcome target in diabetes clinical trials. Future studies are still required to investigate whether glycaemic control reduces the risk of frailty. Similarly, hypoglycaemic therapy is designed mainly to reduce blood glucose levels with fewer adverse effects, especially hypoglycaemia. Novel therapies with extraglycaemic effects, such as improvement of muscle function and prevention of frailty are needed. Identification of the aberrant molecular pathways of sarcopenia and frailty and the possible hormonal disturbance may help to develop novel agents that target this imbalance. Myostatin antibodies may decrease body fat, increase muscle mass and improve physical function in older people with sarcopenia, although this still needs to be confirmed [158]. Hormonal therapies, such as growth hormone, growth hormone-releasing hormone analogues, hormone replacement in postmenopausal women and androgen receptor agonists in men, are experimental [159, 160]. Selective androgen receptor modulators are under development, which may reduce muscle wasting, stimulate muscle growth and improve sarcopenia without the adverse effects of hormonal therapy [161]. There is some evidence to suggest that they may also improve physical function and ability to climb stairs in older people [162]. The characteristics of frail older people with diabetes are still not well defined in clinical trials as well as their metabolic profile.

We have suggested that frail older people with diabetes have at least two metabolic profiles, the SO and AM phenotype, which are likely to have significant metabolic characteristics that will affect diabetes trajectory, choice of hypoglycaemia agents and goals of therapy. Therefore, full exploration of the metabolic spectrum of frailty still needs future exploration. The association of dysglycaemia with frailty can be explained by the presence of two rather than one metabolic phenotype of frailty, which will need future confirmation [163]. Further investigation in this area is required to accurately substratify frailty associated with diabetes, to identify which hypoglycaemic agent is suitable in each phenotype and to guide precise medical practice. The extraglycaemic benefits of SGLT-2 inhibitors and GLP-1RA of improving cardiorenal outcomes, cognitive function and Parkinson's disease may have a potential to reduce the risk of degenerative diseases and frailty in older people [164]. The potential anabolic effects of insulin therapy on muscle function needs further study, especially with the possible introduction of once-weekly insulin analogue, which is a more convenient regimen in frail older people with diabetes [165].

Clinical Practice Question

An 87-year-old man with a history of type 2 diabetes mellitus for the past 34 years lives in a care home. He takes metformin 1 g twice a day, together with linagliptin 5 mg once a day. He was admitted to hospital with recurrent falls of no obvious cause. His haemoglobin A1c was 39 mmol/mol, creatinine 42 µmol/l, haemoglobin 110g/l, albumin 23 g/l and cholesterol 2 mmol/l. According to the care-home staff, his appetite has declined and he has lost weight. His body mass index is 17.3kg/m^2.

Q1. What is the possible cause of his falls?
Choose all the options that apply.
- **A.** Underlying frailty.
- **B.** Recurrent hypoglycaemia.
- **C.** He is likely to be in the anorexic malnourished frail phenotype.
- **D.** Old age.
- **E.** Low haemoglobin A1c.

Q2. What actions need to be taken?
Choose all the options that apply.
- **A.** Deintensification of hypoglycaemic therapy is appropriate.
- **B.** A dietician review is beneficial.
- **C.** Stop all hypoglycaemic therapy.

References

Key references only are listed here. For a full list of references visit: `https://www.wiley.com/go/sinclair/1e`.

1. Sun, H., Saeedi, P., Karuranga, S. et al. (2022). IDF diabetes atlas: global, regional and country-level diabetes prevalence estimates for 2021 and projections for 2045. *Diabetes Res. Clin. Pract.* 183: 109119.
2. Sinclair, A.J., Abdelhafiz, A.H., and Rodríguez-Mañas, L. (2017). Frailty and sarcopenia – newly emerging and high impact complications of diabetes. *J. Diabetes Complications* 31: 1465–1473.
3. Assar, M.E., Laosa, O., and Rodríguez, M.L. (2019). Diabetes and frailty. *Curr. Opin. Clin. Nutr. Metab. Care* 22: 52–57.
4. Collard, R.M., Boter, H., Schoevers, R.A., and Oude Voshaar, R.C. (2012). Prevalence of frailty in community-dwelling older persons: a systematic review. *J. Am. Geriatr. Soc.* 60: 1487–1492.
5. Sinclair, A.J. and Rodriguez-Mañas, L. (2016). Diabetes and frailty: two converging conditions? *Can. J. Diabetes* 40: 77–83.
6. Bergman, H., Ferrucci, L., Guralnik, J. et al. (2009). Frailty: an emerging research and clinical paradigm-issues and controversies. *J. Gerontol. A Biol. Sci. Med. Sci.* 62A: 731–737.

7. Collard, R.M., Boter, H., Schoevers, R.A. et al. (2012). Prevalence of frailty in community-dwelling older persons: a systematic review. *J. Am. Geriatr. Soc.* 60: 1487–1492.
8. Clegg, A., Young, J., Iliffe, S. et al. (2013). Frailty in elderly people. *Lancet* 381: 752–762.
9. Kojima, G. (2015). Frailty as a predictor of future falls among community-dwelling older people: a systematic review and meta-analysis. *J. Am. Med. Dir. Assoc.* 16: 1027–1033.
10. Kojima, G. (2016). Frailty as a predictor of fractures among community-dwelling older people: a systematic review and meta-analysis. *Bone* 90: 116–122.

16b Special Issues in Old Age: Multimorbidity

Alan J. Sinclair[1,2] *and Ahmed H. Abdelhafiz*[3]

[1] *King's College London, London, UK*
[2] *Foundation for Diabetes Research in Older People, Droitwich Spa, UK*
[3] *Department of Geriatric Medicine, Rotherham General Hospital, Rotherham, UK*

Key Points

- Multimorbidity is a predicting factor for adverse outcomes in older people with diabetes.
- Discordant morbidity such as mental health disorders significantly augments the adverse outcomes predicted by multimorbidity.
- Prospective clinical trials are still required to investigate whether interventions to reduce multimorbidity would improve outcomes.

Introduction

About 50% of people diagnosed with type 2 diabetes are 65 years of age or older and the trend is likely to increase further towards older age groups due to ageing of the population. With increasing life expectancy, the prevalence of older people living with diabetes will continue to increase. Because diabetes-related complications are duration dependent, most people with diabetes will develop diabetes-related complications at an older age. In addition, with increasing age, most older people will also develop age-related comorbidities. Older people with diabetes are therefore likely to have multimorbidity compared with the ageing population without diabetes. Multimorbidity affects more that 80% of patients with diabetes and the number increases proportionally with increasing age and duration of diabetes. For example, in one study, multimorbidity increased with age of people with diabetes, four or more

Care of Older People with Diabetes: A Manual for Healthcare Practice, First Edition.
Edited by Alan J. Sinclair and Ahmed H. Abdelhafiz.

Companion website: www.wiley.com/go/sinclair/1e

morbidities were observed in 25.3% of patients aged less than 65 years, 42.4% in patients 65–74 years and 48.5% in those 75 years and above [1]. Multimorbidity is a clinical marker that can distinguish biological from chronological age and can be predictive of downstream adverse clinical outcomes. This chapter reviews the current literature of the role of multimorbidity as a clinical marker of adverse outcomes in older people with diabetes and explores its impact on diabetes management.

Multimorbidity

Multimorbidity is more than two illnesses or diseases occurring in the same person at the same time [2]. Multimorbidity is closely linked and increases proportionally with increasing age. Multimorbidity reflects the impact of multiple illnesses or diseases on the physiological function or physiological reserve of the individual. To reflect this concept, other terms are used to describe multimorbidity, such as morbidity burden (the overall impact of different diseases taking into account their severity) and patient complexity (the overall impact of the different diseases taking into account their severity and other health-related attributes such as socioeconomic, cultural, environmental and patient behaviour characteristics) [3]. Several tools have been developed to measure multimorbidity in a single scale (Table 16b.1). The Charlson

Table 16b.1: Commonly used multimorbidity scales.

Scale	Population	Function
Charlson Comorbidity Index	Several populations, such as elderly, care-home residents and cancer patients	Correlates with mortality, disability, readmissions and length of hospital stay
Index of Coexisting Disease	Care-home residents and patients with hip replacements	Predicts mortality and disability
Incalzi	Several populations, including elderly	Predicts mortality
Cumulative Illness Rating Scale	Several populations, including elderly, care-home residents and cancer patients	Correlates with ADL, IADL and age
Kaplan Index	Patients with diabetes mellitus and those with breast cancer	Predicts mortality

Comorbidity Index (CCI) is the most widely studied multimorbidity tool, which positively correlates with various outcomes such as mortality, disability, readmissions and length of hospital stay [4].

Multimorbidity–Frailty Interaction

Although multimorbidity and frailty are distinct conditions, they overlap, and the terms are sometimes used interchangeably. Frailty can be viewed as the clinical manifestation of the progressive accumulation of physiological decline of multiple organ systems. This starts with subclinical decline in various organ systems until organ dysfunction becomes clinically detectable. Fundamental to this process, is the multiorgan dysfunction concept, rather than a single organ, which leads to vulnerability to stressors and progression to frailty. While multimorbidity will present with signs and symptoms that reflect the underlying conditions, frailty is characterised by multiple manifestations that include weakness, wasting, weight loss, loss of endurance, reduced mobility, lack of balance, tendency to fall and slowness in performing activities. Similar to a clinical syndrome, no single manifestation is enough or essential to diagnose frailty. These characteristics are unique to frailty, and it has been reported that weakness does not appear to be associated with multimorbidity [5]. Both frailty and multimorbidity lead to disability and eventually mortality. However, multimorbidity and frailty may be overlapping and not interchangeable risk factors for adverse outcomes in older people with diabetes.

Multimorbidity Effects on Diabetes

Multimorbidity is common in older people with diabetes due to the development, over time, of diabetes-related complications and the coexistence of diabetes-associated morbidities. Multimorbidity negatively affects diabetes outcomes. Multimorbidity plays a mediator role to the development to frailty when more than one diabetes-related complication is present especially the coexistence of renal impairment and hypertension [6]. Multimorbidity is associated with adverse outcomes in older people with diabetes, such as difficulties in achieving metabolic targets, poor self-rated health, increased hospitalisation, high risk of recurrent hypoglycaemia, progression to disability, reduced quality of life and increased mortality. Certain multimorbidity

Box 16b.1: Adverse Outcome Predicted by Multimorbidity in Older People with Diabetes

- Cognitive dysfunction
- Physical dysfunction
- Disability
- Poor quality of life
- Poor self-rated health
- Increased hospital emergency visits
- Increased hospitalisation due to hypoglycaemia
- Increased all-cause hospitalisation
- Increased risks of falls and fractures
- Adverse cardiovascular outcomes
- Cardiac mortality
- All-cause mortality

combinations such as those including depression, hypertension and arthritis may increase the risk of disability in older people with diabetes while cardiovascular multimorbidity may increase the risk of subsequent cardiovascular events, all-cause mortality and cardiovascular mortality [7]. Adverse effects of multimorbidity on diabetes outcomes are summarised in Box 16b.1.

Clusters of Multimorbidity

Multimorbidity can be either concordant (diabetes related) or discordant (diabetes unrelated). Both concordant and discordant multimorbidity are significantly associated with mortality, however the hazard ratios are largest for the concordant multimorbidity, especially cardiovascular and renal diseases [8]. It is not clear how chronic conditions form distinct groups and patterns of coexistence that clusters in older people with type 2 diabetes. The most common multimorbidity clusters with diabetes are: (1) cardiometabolic diseases such as obesity, hypertension and dyslipidaemia; (2) vascular conditions such as macrovascular disease, microvascular disease, atrial fibrillation and chronic kidney disease; and (3) mental health conditions such as depression, anxiety and substance abuse [9]. However, with increasing age and longer duration of diabetes, the disease burden increases, as well as the prevalence of all morbidities, with diversification of conditions as diabetes progresses. In other words, the number and heterogeneity of clusters in the advanced diabetes depart from the original distinct patterns found in the early period of diabetes [10]. The impact of multimorbidity clusters on outcome may thus be more prominent in younger age groups with short duration of diabetes while in older people with longer duration of diabetes the high multimorbidity burden, rather than the specific clusters, will have more impact on outcomes especially in patients with advanced diseases and multiple end-organ damage.

Clinical Implications

The development of multimorbidity will increase the risk of adverse outcomes in older people with diabetes. In addition, multimorbidity will impact on the effect of management to achieve the metabolic targets. Clinical interventions targeted at improving multimorbidity are likely to be associated with less burden on healthcare resources and better health-related quality of life for older people with diabetes. However, data from the Look AHEAD study suggest that the improvement in gait speed was independent of improvement in multimorbidity and the beneficial effect of intensive lifestyle intervention on multimorbidity did not translate into improvements in the risks of cognitive impairment or mortality [11]. The authors suggested that the magnitude of benefits in multimorbidity was too small to have a measurable effect on outcomes. Other possibilities, intensive lifestyle intervention such as weight loss may have a differential effect across age groups. For example, with advanced age and a decline in health, the intervention of weight loss may have a reverse benefit. Therefore, the impact of interventions targeting multimorbidity to reduce the risks of adverse outcomes are not yet clear. Higher prevalence of multimorbidity is observed in populations living in more deprived areas, which highlights the need to address health inequalities [10]. Although current healthcare services focus on the prevention of cardiovascular and other physical health conditions, the growing burden of mental health disorders will need service and workforce review and restructure [10]. The relationship between multimorbidity and glycaemic control appears to be mixed. In addition, the increased mortality predicted by multimorbidity is not linked to haemoglobin A1c (HbA1c) [12]. Observational studies showed that tight glycaemic control is only beneficial for diabetes-related outcomes in older people with low to moderate comorbidity burden but the benefit is less in those with higher level of multimorbidity [13]. This suggests that immediate and intensive treatment for newly diagnosed patients with diabetes and low level of morbidity may be necessary to avoid irreversible long-term risk for diabetes-related complications. In other words, tighter glycaemic control in newly diagnosed diabetes is appropriate for reducing adverse outcomes, while in people with multimorbidity and longer duration of diabetes the benefit is less clear and a relaxed target is more suitable (Figure 16b.1). However, better understanding of the implications of multimorbidity on glycaemic control is still required. With increasing prevalence of multimorbidity in older people with diabetes and their association with adverse outcomes, the clinical guidelines should move from a disease-specific to a patient-centred holistic care. The holistic approach should include the care of discordant diseases, particularly mental health conditions, in addition to the care of traditional concordant cardiometabolic diseases. Guidelines also provide little direction

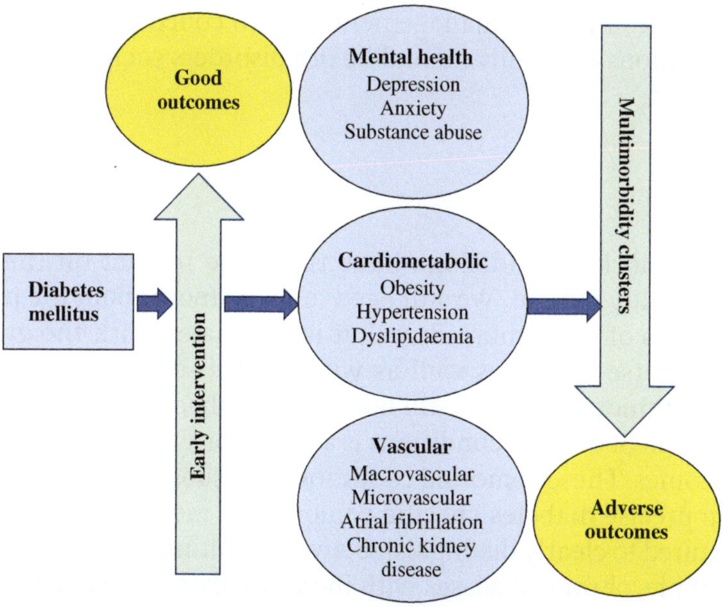

Figure 16b.1: Impact of multimorbidity on diabetes management. Early intervention is important to improve the outcomes in older people with diabetes with low burden of multimorbidity. The establishment of multimorbidity reduces the benefits of interventions and leads to adverse outcomes.

for self-care in the presence of other chronic conditions. It has been shown that diabetes-concordant comorbidities are more associated with higher adherence to diabetes self-care compared with discordant conditions, so guidelines should integrate diabetes self-care among patients with multimorbidity, especially discordant conditions to optimise clinical outcomes [14].

Summary

Multimorbidity is prevalent in older people with diabetes and is associated with a wide range of adverse outcomes, including disability and mortality. Multimorbidity reduces the benefit of glycaemic control however, the relationship between multimorbidity and HbA1c needs further exploration. The clustering of morbidities may have some effect on adverse outcomes prediction, although this may be attenuated with increasing age and duration of diabetes. Discordant conditions such as mental health disorders increase the risk of adverse outcomes. Therefore, comprehensive guidelines that incorporate a holistic approach that includes screening and management of both concordant and discordant conditions especially mental health disorders such as depression are required.

Future Perspectives

Not all comorbid conditions have the same impact on the total multimorbidity burden. We still need to know more about the pattern and clusters of multimorbidity that is associated with the greatest risk of adverse events as well as whether this effect differs across different ethnic groups. It is still not clear whether the effect of certain combination of chronic conditions is additive or synergistic in predicting outcomes. These comorbid conditions can subsequently be used to develop precise diabetes-specific comorbidity measures. Research is still required to clearly distinguish between multimorbidity and frailty. For example, chronic diseases with increased catabolic state that constitute multimorbidity may have similar symptoms to frailty such as fatigue, weight loss and exhaustion. Longitudinal studies that include frail participants with multimorbidity are needed to investigate the independent effect of each condition on adverse outcomes.

Clinical Practice Question

Q1. A 76-year-old man known to have type 2 diabetes mellitus has been on oral hypoglycaemic therapy for 16 years. Insulin was introduced over the past two years for better control of his diabetes. He also suffers from hypertension and osteoarthritis. Over the past six months, he became more withdrawn with reduced appetite. He finds it difficult to sleep at night and has lost a half stone in weight. Which of these statements are appropriate?

A. Screen for depression.
B. He is at risk of progression to disability.
C. Reduce insulin dose given history of weight loss.
D. Multidisciplinary follow-up.
E. He is at risk of less adherence to self-care.

References

Key references only are listed here. For a full list of references visit: `https://www.wiley.com/go/sinclair/1e`.

1. Iglay, K., Hannachi, H., Joseph Howie, P. et al. (2016). Prevalence and co-prevalence of co- morbidities among patients with type 2 diabetes mellitus. *Curr. Med. Res. Opin.* 32: 1243–1252.
2. Feinstein, A.R. (1970). The pre-therapeutic classification of comorbidity in chronic disease. *J. Chronic Dis.* 23: 455–468.
3. Valderas, J.M., Starfield, B., Sibbald, B. et al. (2009). Defining comorbidity: implications for understanding health and health services. *Ann. Fam. Med.* 7: 357–363.
4. Charlson, M.E., Pompei, P., Ales, K.L. et al. (1987). A new method of classifying prognostic comorbidity in longitudinal studies: development and validation. *J. Chronic Dis.* 40: 373–383.
5. Rivera-Almaraz, A., Manrique-Espinoza, B., Ávila-Funes, J.A. et al. (2018). Disability, quality of life and all-cause mortality in older Mexican adults: association with multimorbidity and frailty. *BMC Geriatr.* 18: 236.
6. Lee, S., Lee, S., Harada, K. et al. (2016). Relationship between chronic kidney disease with diabetes or hypertension and frailty in community-dwelling Japanese older adults. *Geriatr. Gerontol. Int.* 17: 1527–1533.
7. Sinclair, A.J. and Abdelhafiz, A.H. (2022). Multimorbidity, frailty and diabetes in older people-identifying interrelationships and outcomes. *J. Pers. Med.* 12: 1911.

8. Chiang, J.I., Hanlon, P., Li, T.C. et al. (2020). Multimorbidity, mortality, and HbA1c in type 2 diabetes: a cohort study with UK and Taiwanese cohorts. *PLoS Med.* 7: e1003094.
9. Cicek, M., Buckley, J., Pearson-Stuttard, J. et al. (2021). Characterizing multimorbidity from type 2 diabetes: insights from clustering approaches. *Endocrinol. Metab. Clin. North Am.* 50: 531–558.
10. Nowakowska, M., Zghebi, S.S., Ashcroft, D.M. et al. (2019). The comorbidity burden of type 2 diabetes mellitus: patterns, clusters and predictions from a large English primary care cohort. *BMC Med.* 17: 145.

16c Special Issues in Old Age: Type 1 Diabetes Mellitus

Alex M. Summerbell[1] *and Ahmed H. Abdelhafiz*[2]

[1] *Leeds Teaching Hospitals NHS Trust, Leeds, UK*
[2] *Department of Geriatric Medicine, Rotherham General Hospital, Rotherham, UK*

Key Points

- The prevalence of type 1 diabetes mellitus in older people is increasing due to increased life expectancy.
- Insulin replacement therapy is the main treatment in older people with type 1 diabetes.
- Continuous glucose monitoring is ideal in older people with type 1 diabetes, which allows timely intervention to extreme blood glucose levels.
- Insulin pumps and the hybrid closed loop system are increasingly used in older people with type 1 diabetes, which improves glycaemic control and reduces risk of hypoglycaemia.
- Glycaemic targets and goals of therapy should be regularly reviewed to match patients' changing physical and cognitive functions.

Introduction

The population of older people with type 1 diabetes mellitus (T1DM) is increasing due to the increase in life expectancy and the improved diabetes care. In addition, although T1DM commonly occurs in children, the incidence of adult-onset T1DM is increasing. Furthermore, new-onset T1DM is increasingly recognised in older people [1]. Childhood-onset disease may commonly present with acute complication such as

Care of Older People with Diabetes: A Manual for Healthcare Practice, First Edition.
Edited by Alan J. Sinclair and Ahmed H. Abdelhafiz.

Companion website: www.wiley.com/go/sinclair/1e

diabetic ketoacidosis (DKA) due to insulin deficiency. In older people, however, DKA presentation is less frequent due to the presence of residual beta cells with some insulin production. Therefore, in addition to the care-needs of people growing old with T1DM, clinicians should be aware of the increased prevalence of new-onset diabetes in old age, to avoid a delay in diagnosis and start of appropriate therapy. This chapter reviews the different aspects of care for older people with T1DM.

Epidemiology and Diagnosis

The prevalence of T1DM is increasing by 2–5% per year worldwide. Although it is known as a childhood disease, adult-onset T1DM is increasingly more common than childhood-onset [2]. Worldwide, it is likely that over half of all new-onset cases of T1DM occur in adults. Although childhood T1DM is associated with the presence of serum autoantibodies against beta-cell antigens, in adult-onset disease, multiple diabetes-associated autoantibodies tend to be less prevalent with increasing age at diagnosis. Serum glutamic acid decarboxylase autoantibodies remain positive and are useful as a predictor of T1DM in adults [3], so diabetes thought to be caused by autoimmune destruction of beta cells should be classified as type 1. However, the absence of autoantibodies does not rule out the possibility of a diagnosis of T1DM. C-peptide at diagnosis is higher in adults than in children due to higher body mass index, and adults are more likely to have residual insulin-producing beta cells. C-peptide level alone cannot distinguish between type 1 or type 2 diabetes and must be interpreted within the context of other clinical and laboratory features. A random non-fasting C-peptide paired with a blood glucose in the same sample is considered the gold standard assessment of insulin secretory function in established T1DM [4]. Factors leading to difficulties in diagnosing T1DM in older age and aids of diagnosis are summarised in Boxes 16c.1 and 16c.2.

Management

Management of T1DM in older people is challenging because diabetes in this age group is likely to be of long duration and associated with diabetes-related complications, diabetes-associated morbidities, increased prevalence of geriatric syndromes and increased risk of hypoglycaemia. In addition, there is an increased need

Box 16c.1: Difficulties in Diagnosis of Type 1 Diabetes Mellitus in Older People

- Lack of awareness of older age onset of type 1 diabetes mellitus
- Type 1 diabetes is largely pathophysiologically rather than clinically defined
- Most of diabetes diagnosis in older age is type 2
- The phenotype of obesity or metabolic syndrome has poor discriminatory value
- Increased prevalence of obesity biases towards type 2 diabetes diagnosis
- Slow progression of type 1 in old age mimics type 2 diabetes
- Less availability of biomarkers testing in the diagnosis of diabetes types
- Type 1 diabetes in older age presents less acutely (e.g. less metabolic decompensation with diabetic ketoacidosis complication)

Box 16c.2: Diagnostic Aids for Type 1 Diabetes Mellitus in Older People

- Check islet cell antibodies in all patients who are clinically suspected to have type 1 diabetes mellitus
- Trial of non-insulin therapy in patients with negative islet cell antibodies
- Check C-peptide after three years in patients tested negative for islet cell antibodies
- Routine islet cell antibodies testing is not required in patients with clear features of type 2 diabetes mellitus
- Consider C-peptide and islet cell antibodies testing in patients diagnosed with type 2 diabetes mellitus but required insulin therapy in a short period (< 3 years after diagnosis)
- Repeat C-peptide testing in patients with uncertain classification: low C-peptide levels (< 200–300 pmol/l) suggest type 1, while higher levels (> 600 pmol/l) indicate type 2 diabetes mellitus

for social support due to difficulties in performing self-care tasks because of physical and cognitive dysfunction and associated frailty. Figure 16c.1 outlines the characteristics and management of T1DM in older people.

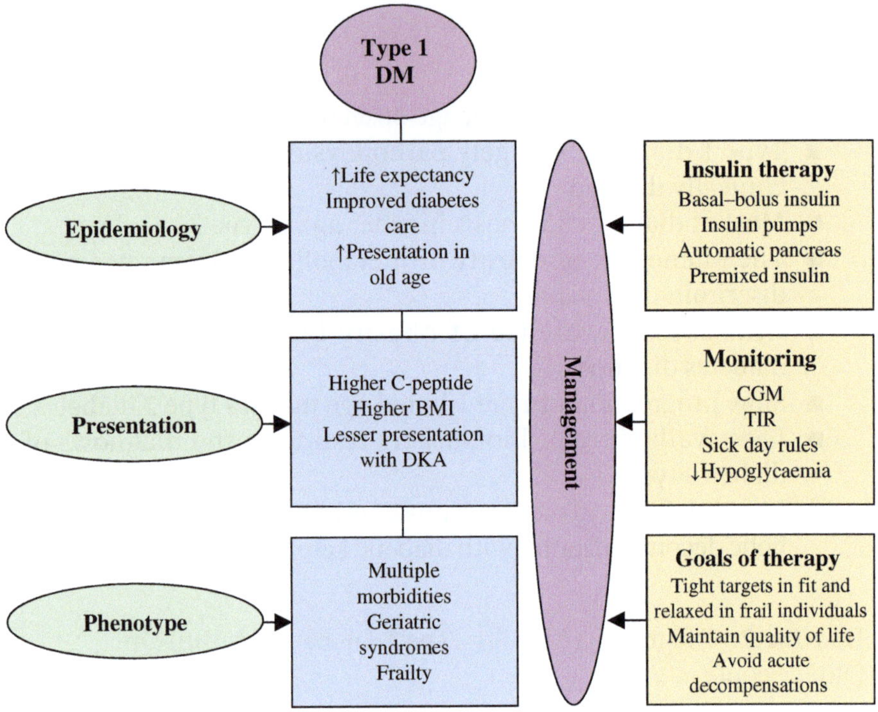

Figure 16c.1: Characteristics and management of type 1 diabetes mellitus in older people. DM, diabetes mellitus; BMI, body mass index; CGM, continuous glucose monitoring; TIR, time in range.

Insulin Therapy

All older people with T1DM will require insulin replacement therapy. Insulin therapy consists of basal–bolus regimen or continuous pump infusion with the aim of achieving the best possible glycaemic control, measured as haemoglobin A1c (HbA1c) or percentage of time in range (TIR), and at the same time avoiding hypoglycaemic events. A simplified insulin regimen such as a fixed premeal short-acting insulin or a premixed insulin can be used but have the disadvantage of the need for patient's compliance with a fixed amount of carbohydrate consumption and little room for flexibility on meal times. Smart pens (Bluetooth-enabled) can record time and dose of the insulin delivered, which may help patients and clinicians to keep track of insulin administration and identify any challenges with adherence to therapy. Insulin pumps are increasingly used in older people with T1DM and appear to be safe and reduce the risk of severe hypoglycaemia and hospitalisation

Box 16c.3: Competences for Successful Insulin Therapy in Older People with Type 1 Diabetes Mellitus

- Physical ability to administer injections
- Mental ability to understand concepts of insulin therapy
- Healthy and regular eating pattern
- Physically active
- Able to monitor blood glucose levels
- Compliance with medications
- Recognition and awareness of hypoglycaemia
- Ability to adjust insulin dosages to variable blood glucose levels
- Able to react to extreme blood glucose levels to reduce the risk of acute decompensations
- Understanding and compliance with the sick day rules

as much as in younger people [5]. The hybrid closed loop (HCL) system or automatic pancreas works by sensing glucose readings from continuous glucose monitoring (CGM) and uses an algorithm to tell an insulin pump how much insulin to deliver to mitigate both hyper- and hypoglycaemia. It has been used in older people and has shown improved glycaemic control [6]. Successful insulin therapy will depend on the older person's ability to administer insulin, adjusting the insulin dose according to the amount of carbohydrate consumed each meal, and the continuous monitoring of their blood glucose level (Box 16c.3). In individuals with severe cognitive impairment and erratic or unpredictable eating pattern, a basal–bolus regimen with a bolus dose based on the amount of carbohydrate intake given after meal consumption is more appropriate to reduce the risk of hypoglycaemia when patients eat less than expected [7]. Ultrafast-acting insulin analogue, which can be administered up to 20 minutes after a meal, is another option to reduce postprandial glucose peaks [8].

Monitoring

Time in range of blood glucose, defined as time of the day spent between 3.9–10 mmol, provides more accurate clinical information than HbA1c alone. The TIR target should be at least 50% or above in older people compared with 70% or above in younger people with diabetes. Achieving this range may reduce the number of episodes of both hyper- and hypoglycaemia and is associated with a low incidence of microvascular complications [9]. CGM improves glycaemic control and is increasingly used in older people with T1DM, which shows details of TIR and time above and below range in an illustrated format easy to follow by patients and their carers. In addition, CGM devices equipped with alarms can transmit data to carers or healthcare professionals to help monitoring of extreme blood glucose readings and to take timely and appropriate actions to avoid glycaemic decompensations and unnecessary hospitalisations. CGM is superior to intermittent monitoring as it can detect episodes of asymptomatic hypoglycaemia even in patients with relaxed HbA1c targets [10]. In addition, the use of an HCL system may reduce the burden of self-monitoring of blood glucose, multiple insulin injections and improve TIR [6]. Monitoring during acute illnesses is necessary to adjust insulin dosages affected by medication adverse effects, such as the use of steroid therapy or the reduced oral intake during illness, which may increase the risk of hypoglycaemia. Patients should have an up to date glucagon emergency kit, which is easy to use in emergencies. Moreover, patients should be aware of sick day rules to avoid dehydration, have access to ketone bodies testing, not to stop insulin when they are ill, to seek medical advice and have sick day rules card to help adjust their medications during sick days.

Reducing Hypoglycaemia

Hypoglycaemia is the main barrier to achieve good glycaemic control in older people with T1DM. Severe episodes of hypoglycaemia are common in this age group and are associated with acute cardiovascular risks, including mortality. Repeated episodes may lead to cognitive impairment and physical dysfunction, including frailty [11]. It appears that the number and severity of hypoglycaemic episodes has a detrimental effect, together with pre-existing poor glycaemic control and elevated systolic blood pressure, on the speed of cognitive function decline in older people with T1DM. The combined effect of the presence of these three risk factors is the equivalent to an additional 9.4 years of age [12]. Repeated hospital admissions due to frequent episodes of hypoglycaemia are associated with further deterioration in patients' general health, which eventually leads to frailty, disability and poor outcomes. The decline in cognitive function, associated with hypoglycaemia increases the risk of frailty in a reciprocal relationship. Hypoglycaemia unawareness is a risk factor for severe and recurrent hypoglycaemic episodes. With ageing and long duration of diabetes, counter-regulatory responses to hypoglycaemia are impaired, as the glycaemic threshold at which autonomic symptoms occur is lowered and reaction time for these responses is prolonged [13]. Therefore, symptoms of hypoglycaemia in this age group may not be specific leading to delayed diagnosis. Early recognition and treatment of hypoglycaemia are therefore an essential part of the management of older people with T1DM (Box 16c.4).

Box 16c.4: Reducing Hypoglycaemia in Older People with Type 1 Diabetes Mellitus

- Recognition of atypical presentation such as dizziness, reduced balance, poor coordination, falls, delirium, weakness and reduced communication.
- Educational programmes should be available to patients and their cares that suit their cognitive abilities.
- Awareness that severe hypoglycaemia is more common in the presence of microvascular complications, depression, polypharmacy and lower socioeconomic status.
- Awareness that patients with dementia are unable to communicate their feelings or symptoms.
- Awareness that hypoglycaemia in this age group has little warning and patients have little autonomic symptoms.
- Identification of high risk group, which includes older age, long duration of diabetes, low body weight, malnutrition, anorexia, multiple morbidities, frailty, renal or hepatic impairment, haemodialysis, gastroparesis and advanced malignancy.
- Glycaemic targets and pharmacologic interventions need to be re-adjusted with the progression of cognitive dysfunction.
- Simplification of insulin regimens and deintensification of therapy in frail patients with tight glycaemic control.
- Patients with advanced dementia and limited life expectancy will require an approach that focuses on comfort and symptom control.

Goals of Therapy

Continuous education for patients and their carers, which is regularly reviewed to match their cognitive and physical abilities, is required to insure compliance with self-care tasks and reduce acute glycaemic decompensations. In addition, glycaemic targets and goals of therapy should be regularly reviewed to match their progressive decline in physical and/or cognitive function. Integrated services that incorporate regular diabetes aspects of care, neuropsychological testing for early detection of cognitive decline and physical assessment of self-care competencies are the ideal. Prevention of hypoglycaemia is a priority when older people with T1DM develop cognitive dysfunction and frailty and glycaemic targets should be relaxed and the focus is to maintain quality of life and avoid unnecessarily hospitalisations. An initial target HBA1c of 7.5% (58.5 mmol/mol) is appropriate for fit individuals, which should be relaxed to around 8% (63.9 mmol/mol) in patients with mild cognitive impairment and 8.5% (69.4 mmol/mol) in those with dementia and/or frailty. In addition to HbA1c, avoiding gross fluctuations in blood glucose levels is important to avoid adverse effects on cognitive function.

Summary

The prevalence of T1DM in older people is increasing due to increased life expectancy. CGM and the HCL insulin system are ideal in older people with T1DM for better glycaemic control and the reduction of the risk of hypoglycaemia. Older age is associated with increased prevalence of morbidities, reduction in function and the need for social support, so glycaemic targets and goals of therapy should be regularly reviewed according to the patient's overall function.

Clinical Practice Question

Q1. An 83-year-old woman with type 1 diabetes for the past 71 years is on a basal–bolus insulin regimen. She regularly monitors her blood glucose levels, which normally range between 6 and 13 mmol/l. Previously, she counted carbohydrates and adjusted her short-acting insulin dosage accordingly. However, she has found this increasingly difficult with wide variations noted in her blood glucose. She has also lost a few pounds in weight and her food consumption is becoming inconsistent. Which of the following is the most appropriate intervention for managing her diabetes? You may select more than one answer.

A. Carer education and involvement to help correct extreme blood glucose readings.
B. Change the bolus doses to after meals rather than before meals.
C. Change to a premixed insulin regimen.
D. Reduce the bolus doses and increase the basal dose.
E. Start using continuous glucose monitoring equipped with an alarm system.

References

Key references only are listed here. For a full list of references visit: `https://www.wiley.com/go/sinclair/1e`.

1. LeRoith, D., Biessels, G.J., Braithwaite, S.S. et al. (2019). Treatment of diabetes in older adults: an Endocrine Society Clinical Practice Guideline. *J. Clin. Endocrinol. Metab.* 104: 1520–1574.
2. Thomas, N.J., Jones, S.E., Weedon, M.N. et al. (2018). Frequency and phenotype of type 1 diabetes in the first six decades of life: a cross-sectional, genetically stratified survival analysis from UK Biobank. *Lancet Diabetes Endocrinol.* 6: 122–129.
3. Muñoz, C., Floreen, A., Garey, C. et al. (2019). Misdiagnosis and diabetic ketoacidosis at diagnosis of type 1 diabetes: patient and caregiver perspectives. *Clin. Diabetes* 37: 276–281.
4. Hope, S.V., Knight, B.A., Shields, B.M. et al. (2016). Random non-fasting C-peptide: bringing robust assessment of endogenous insulin secretion to the clinic. *Diabet. Med.* 33: 1554–1558.
5. Matejko, B., Cyganek, K., Katra, B. et al. (2011). Insulin pump therapy is equally effective and safe in elderly and young type 1 diabetes patients. *Rev. Diabet. Stud.* 8: 254–258.
6. Boughton, C.K., Hartnell, S., Thabit, H. et al. (2022). Hybrid closed-loop glucose control compared with sensor augmented pump therapy in older adults with type 1 diabetes: an open-label multicentre, multinational, randomised, crossover study. *Lancet Healthy Longev.* 3: e135–e142.
7. Hopkins, R., Shaver, K., and Weinstock, R.S. (2016). Management of adults with diabetes and cognitive problems. *Diabetes Spectr.* 29: 224–237.

8. Nally, L.M., Sherr, J.L., Van Name, M.A. et al. (2019). Pharmacologic treatment options for type 1 diabetes: what's new? *Expert Rev. Clin. Pharmacol.* 12: 471–479.
9. Battelino, T., Danne, T., Bergenstal, R.M. et al. (2019). Clinical targets for continuous glucose monitoring data interpretation: recommendations from the international consensus on time in range. *Diabetes Care* 42: 1593–1603.
10. Munshi, M.D., Slyne, C., Segal, A.R. et al. (2017). Liberating A1C goals in older adults may not protect against the risk of hypoglycaemia. *J. Diabetes Complications* 31: 1197–1199.

16d Special Issues in Old Age: Cognitive Health Agility, Cognitive Dysfunction, Dementia and Diabetes

Tali Cukierman-Yaffe[1,2]

[1] Center For Successful Aging With Diabetes, Division of Endocrinology and Metabolism, Sheba Medical Center, Ramat Gan, Israel
[2] Epidemiology Department, School of Public Health, Faculty of Medicine, Herczeg Institute on Aging, Tel-Aviv University, Tel Aviv, Israel

Key Points

- Cognitive dysfunction is a long-term complication of diabetes.
- Cognitive dysfunction impedes self-care capacity, a cornerstone of diabetes treatment.
- There is evidence to suggest a cognitive protective effect of insulin and glucagon-like peptide-1 receptor analyst.
- Assessment of cognitive function (cognitive health agility) as part of routine care of older people with diabetes is recommended by many professional organisations and is imperative to tailor treatment plan and introduce early preventive strategies.

Care of Older People with Diabetes: A Manual for Healthcare Practice, First Edition.
Edited by Alan J. Sinclair and Ahmed H. Abdelhafiz.

Companion website: www.wiley.com/go/sinclair/1e

Introduction

The risk of diabetes is increased by age. It is estimated that approximately 30% of people over the age of 65 years have a diagnosis of type 2 diabetes mellitus (T2DM) [1, 2]. Studies from the past 20–30 years have demonstrated that diabetes is a risk factor for cognitive dysfunction, an accelerated rate of cognitive decline and the development of dementia. Cognitive dysfunction may thus be considered a long-term complication of diabetes that is increasingly prevalent with the ageing of the population.

Cognitive decline is a process starting from normal cognitive function progressing to cognitive dysfunction without dementia and, at the tip of the iceberg, 'dementia'– a form of cognitive impairment that is accompanied by functional impairment. Preceding the onset of dementia is a phase of cognitive dysfunction without functional impairment, often termed minimal cognitive impairment (MCI). It is estimated that 3–20% of individuals over the age of 65 years have MCI. These individuals have a 5–10% annual progression rate to dementia compared with 1–2% in age-matched individuals without MCI [3, 4].

In this chapter, the relationship between diabetes and cognitive dysfunction is explored and possible explanations for the relationship are presented. The chapter elaborates on the complex relationship between cognitive dysfunction and self-care capacity, the need for screening and surveillance as part of routine care and other implications for patient care. Ways of assessing cognitive function in older people with diabetes are presented. Finally, prevention and treatment options are discussed, including the effect of current diabetes pharmacological agents on this diabetes complication.

Population Studies Demonstrating the Relationship Between Cognitive Dysfunction, Dementia and Diabetes

Many prospective studies and systematic reviews have demonstrated that individuals with diabetes have an increased risk for dementia, MCI and an accelerated rate of cognitive decline. Thus, in a systematic review that included 144 studies, pertaining to approximately a million individuals, with follow-up ranging from 1.5–32 years, people with diabetes compared with those without had a 1.42 (95% CI 1.33–1.53) greater risk for the development of all-cause dementia, 1.43 (95% CI 1.25–1.62) greater risk for the development of Alzheimer's dementia and a 1.91 (95% CI 1.61, 2.25) greater risk for vascular dementia. They also had a 1.49 (95% CI 1.26–1.77) greater risk for the development of MCI and a 1.25 (95% CI 1.2–1.39) greater risk for an accelerated rate of cognitive decline in global cognitive function, as well as a 1.44, 1.5, 1.6, 1.27 greater risk for an accelerated rate of cognitive decline in executive function, processing speed attention and reasoning and memory, respectively [5].

There are also data to suggest that people with type 1 diabetes mellitus (T1DM) have a higher risk of developing dementia. [6]. The cognitive domains affected in T1DM are slightly different than those in T2DM. The 30-year long-term follow-up of the Diabetes Control and Complications Trial provides important insights in this respect. The trial reported that those with T1DM experienced an accelerated rate of cognitive decline in psychomotor and mental efficiency as well as delayed recall and immediate memory [7].

In summary, there is strong evidence demonstrating that cognitive dysfunction is a complication of diabetes, with a 1.5–2 fold greater risk for the development of dementia, MCI and an accelerated rate of cognitive decline.

Implications of the Relationship Between Diabetes and Cognitive Dysfunction

The relationship between diabetes and cognitive dysfunction has several implications (Figure 16d.1). First, self-care is an important aspect of diabetes management. Self-care is affected by cognitive function, so should be considered when devising a treatment plan for older people with diabetes [8]. Second, as cognitive dysfunction is a complication of diabetes, it is important to elucidate the effect of the different diabetes pharmacological agents on this complication. Third, like other diabetes complications, for example in the eye, measuring and staging (screening and surveillance) the preclinical stages of the complication may be a first stage in slowing its progression.

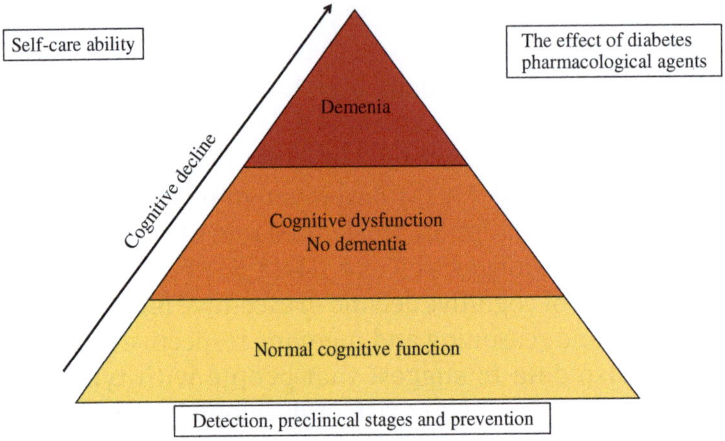

Figure 16d.1: Effects of cognitive decline.

The Effect of Cognitive Dysfunction on Self-care Capacity in Older People with Diabetes

Self-care is a cornerstone in diabetes management and prevention of its long-term complications. Adherence to self-care management in diabetes is complex and multifaceted. It involves a variety of health-promoting behaviours such as diet, physical activity, behavioural changes, self-inspection, glucose monitoring, adherence to oral and insulin injection treatment regimens. It also entails understanding how differing life situations affect glucose and how to treat and prevent hypoglycaemia. However, all these behaviours require intact cognitive function (better termed 'cognitive health agility'). Specifically, executive function, which includes behaviours such as judgement, problem solving, starting new behaviours or stopping old ones, is especially important in management of diabetes. Many studies have demonstrated the relationship between cognitive dysfunction and reduced self-care ability. In the ACCORD MIND study, 3000 individuals with T2DM were followed for a median of 3.25 years. Hypoglycaemia requiring medical assistance (i.e. hospital admission, emergency department or assistance from medical personnel). The cohort was divided into tertiles according to baseline Digit Symbol Substitution Test score. Those in the higher compared with the lower tertile had an almost 50% lower risk for hypoglycaemia requiring medical assistance [9]. Other studies and a systematic review have shown that people with cognitive impairment compared with those without impairment had more difficulty in checking glucose levels, following a meal plan, exercising, inspecting feet, problem solving when to adjust insulin dose and making decisions regarding insulin dosing and severe hypoglycaemia prevention [10].

Self-management in T1DM is even more demanding and complex. Mismanagement can result in hypo- and hyperglycaemia. In a study conducted in individuals with T1DM from the type 1 exchange programme, a battery of non-parametric tests and functional assessments were conducted, including a measure of diabetes-specific self-management skills; the diabetes numeracy test, in which the participant is asked to make calculations with respect to every day diabetes tasks such as the number of insulin units before a certain meal, number of units for corrections, and so on. A higher severity of cognitive deficits was associated with diminished numeracy skills. The model also included age, which accounted for 30% of the variance in the numeracy score. Specifically, the domains that were highly correlated with the numeracy score were memory and complex speeded attention [11]. The effects of cognitive dysfunction on self-care capacity in older people with diabetes are summarised in Box 16d.1.

Box 16d.1: Summary of the Effects of Cognitive Dysfunction on Self-care Capacity in Older People with Diabetes

- Self-care capacity, a corner stone of diabetes management
- Self-care impaired in individuals with cognitive dysfunction
- There is strong evidence demonstrating that older individuals with diabetes and cognitive dysfunction have difficulties in insulin dosing and preventing hypoglycaemia, as well as adherence to exercise, self-inspection and nutritional recommendations
- This results in a higher risk for emergency department admissions and hospitalisations related to hypo- and hyperglycaemia
- It is now well recognised that cognitive assessment should be part of the routine assessment of older people with diabetes, as recommended by many professional organisations across the world
- Assessment of cognitive function in this population enables tailoring of an appropriate treatment plan

Assessment of Cognitive Health Agility in Older People with Diabetes

Many professional organisations across the world recommend performance of cognitive assessment as part of the routine care of older people with diabetes, to conduct screening and surveillance that may allow adapting treatment regimen accordingly and enable introduction of preventive strategies (discussed further in Chapter 16e). Measurement of cognitive health agility is also important in clinical trials of older people with diabetes, to assess the effects of different treatment modalities in this complication of diabetes. Previous studies have tested the feasibility of using several cognitive screening tools in older people with diabetes. The Montreal Cognitive Assessment (MoCA) and Mini-Mental Status Examination (MMSE) are the most common cognitive screening tools worldwide. Among individuals with diabetes, the MoCA appears to be a better screening tool than MMSE for detecting MCI [12] Two additional cognitive assessment self-administered paper and pencil tools, the Test Your Memory and the Self-Administered Gerocognitive Examination (SAGE), were tested on older individuals with diabetes. In a study including 225 individuals, sensitivity for cognitive impairment was superior to the MMSE, and the SAGE questionnaire demonstrated the highest diagnostic accuracy [13]. Novel methods for diagnosis and monitoring of cognitive function in older people with diabetes have emerged recently; for example, the diabetes-specific dementia risk score and retinal microperimetry. Several of the diabetes cardiovascular clinical trials published in recent years have implemented paper and pencil cognitive assessments. Among tests widely used were the MMSE, MOCA, the digital symbol substitution test (DSST) and the trail making test [14–17].

Despite the availability of these tests, existing data and recommendations from many professional organisations, cognitive testing is rarely conducted in the primary care or diabetes clinic setting. This may be due to the time-consuming and labour-intensive nature of cognitive assessments [18].

The Sheba Medical Center has recently developed and validated a digital version of the DSST, which exhibits excellent correlation with the paper and pencil version (publication in preparation). This type of a tool may provide the means for enabling conduction of cognitive assessment in the busy clinic setting as well as in clinical trials.[1]

Paper and pencil cognitive screening tests	Digital cognitive screening tests	Other cognitive screening tests
Mini mental state examination (MMSE)	Digital symbol substitution test (DSST)	Retinal microperimetry
Montreal cognitive assessment (MOCA)	Montreal cognitive assessment (MOCA)	
Test you memory (TYM)		
Self-administered gerocognitive examination (SAGE)		
Digital symbol substitution test (DSST)		
Diabetes specific dementia risk score (DSDRS)		

Prevention and Treatment of Cognitive Dysfunction in Older People with Diabetes

The Effect of Current Diabetes Pharmacological Agents on Cognitive Dysfunction

Not many of the cardiovascular outcome trials conducted in people with diabetes have included cognitive assessment. In the next several paragraphs, the cognitive outcomes that have been reported from trials in people with T2DM are presented (Table 16d.1).

[1] The Sheba Medical Center has recently developed and validated a digital version of the DSS. If you are interested in trying to use this in your clinic, please email: tcukierm@gmail.com.

Table 16d.1: Diabetes-specific interventions in cognitive decline.

Intervention	Trial/prospective data	Effect on cognitive dysfunction
Glycaemic control	ACCORD-MIND trial	No effect on cognitive function, intensive group vs. standard of care less of a reduction in total brain volume
Insulin	ORIGIN trial	Post hoc analysis reduction in CS-SCI in those treated with Glargine vs. standard of care group
DPP-4 inhibitors	CARMELINA, CAROLINA trials	No difference between the groups
GLP-1RA	REWIND trial	Reduction in CS-SCI in those treated with dulaglutide vs. standard of care group
GLP-1RA	Combined analysis from several trials	Post hoc analysis of adverse events reduction in dementia incidence in liraglutide/semaglutide vs. standard of care
Multidisciplinary intervention	FINGER trial	Multidisciplinary intervention (30% people with diabetes) reduction in the rate of cognitive decline with prominent effect on executive function

CS-SCI, Country Standardised Substantive Cognitive Impairment; DPP-4, dipeptidyl peptidase-4; GLP-1RA, glucagon-like peptide-1 receptor analyst.

Glucose Control

Glucose control has been tested in the ACCORD-MIND trial and in the ADVANCE trial. The ACCORD-MIND trial tested the effect of very intensive glucose control (haemoglobin A1c [HbA1c] 6.4%) compared with standard control (HbA1c 7.5%) on cardiovascular outcomes. The cognitive substudy assessed the effect of these interventions on the rate of cognitive decline as measured by four cognitive instruments (MMSE, DSST, Stroop test, Rey Auditory Verbal Test). It also included a sub-study in which participants underwent structural magnetic resonance imaging (MRI). Unfortunately, the study was terminated early, so sample size assumptions were not met; thus, a high chance of a beta type error exists (i.e. that no difference between the groups was detected despite the existence of such a difference). An analysis including the 20- and 40-month data failed to show an effect on the change in the cognitive test scores. However, in the subgroup that underwent brain MRI, a significant difference was noted in the change in total brain MRI volumes, with the intensively treated group experiencing less of a reduction than the conventional group [14]. The ADVANCE trial also assessed the effect of an intensive glucose control regimen (HbA1c 6.5%) using gliclazide compared with standard care (HbA1c 7.3%) on cardiovascular outcomes. The MMSE was administered to participants and incident dementia was assessed. During a median follow-up of five years, there was no difference between the groups in the rate of cognitive decline as assessed by the MMSE or in incident dementia rates [19].

Insulin

The ORIGIN trial was a 12 500-person multicentre international randomised trial that studied the effects of glargine-insulin mediated normoglycaemia compared with standard care, and omega-3 polyunsaturated fatty acids compared with placebo on the risk of cardiovascular events in people with diabetes and pre-diabetes with a median follow-up of 6.2 years. The cognitive substudy tested the effect of this intervention on the rate of decline in two cognitive instruments, the DSST and MMSE, and incident probable cognitive impairment (defined as incident MMSE <24) or reported dementia was assessed. Both groups experienced a decline in cognitive test scores over time. There was, however, no difference between the groups in the rate of decline. When a categorical outcome was used, there was numerical difference between the groups but it did not reach statistical significance [15].

On a methodological level, these differences in the continuous compared with categorical outcomes have provided important insights into how to best define cognitive dysfunction in future randomised controlled trials (RCTs). Indeed, in a recent publication using a dichotomous country standardised definition for the cognitive outcome, the Country Standardised Substantive Cognitive Impairment (CS-SCI), a 9% reduction in the cognitive outcome was noted in those who were treated with basal insulin compared with those who were not, with no effect for the omega-3 fatty acid–placebo comparison [20].

Dipeptidyl Peptidase-4 Inhibitors

The CAROLINA study tested the effect of linagliptin compared with glimepiride in people with T2DM and suboptimal glucose control at high cardiovascular risk and a MMSE score of above 24. The primary cognitive outcome was accelerated cognitive decline, defined as a regression-based index less than 16 percentile points on the MMSE or a composite measure of attention and executive function (based on the study population). Over the median follow-up of 6.1 years in the 3163 individuals included in the study, there was no difference between the groups in the primary cognitive outcome [21].

The CARMELINA trial assessed the effect of linagliptin compared with placebo in 6979 individuals with T2DM and cardiorenal disease. Over a median follow-up of 2.5 years, there was no difference between the groups in incident accelerated cognitive decline [17].

Glucagon-like Peptide-1 Receptor Agonists

The REWIND trial included people with diabetes and cardiovascular disease (CVD) or cardiovascular risk factors and assessed the effect of dulaglutide compared with placebo. The primary prespecified cognitive outcome for this trial was CS-SCI. Country standardisation was conducted by subtracting a person's score at any time point from the mean baseline country-specific score and dividing it by the mean standard deviation (SD) of that country baseline score. Substantive cognitive impairment was defined as the first occurrence of a score on either MOCA or DSST scores equal or lower than 1.5 SD from the baseline mean for that country. Over a median of 5.4 years, in 8825 individuals, those treated with dulaglutide compared with placebo had a 12% lower risk for the development of the primary cognitive outcome [16].

A combined analysis using the data collected for dementia as an adverse event from three RCTs of glucagon-like peptide-1 receptor analyst (GLP-1RA; (liraglutide, semaglutide, $N = 15\,820$) reported a 64% reduction in dementia among those allocated to the GLP-1RA compared with placebo [22]. The SOUL trial is testing the CV effect of oral semaglutide compared with placebo in individuals aged 50 years or older with T2DM and CVD or renal disease [23]. Cognitive assessments

(MOCA) were conducted at several time points in the study. Results will be published in the next several years.

In conclusion, not many of the large cardiovascular outcome trials conducted in people with T2DM have included cognitive assessments or provided data with respect to cognitive outcomes. There are some data to suggest that insulin may have cognitive protecting properties. Supporting this hypothesis is the post hoc analysis of the ORIGIN trial, which showed a 9% reduction in the primary cognitive outcome in those treated with basal insulin. There is even stronger evidence supporting the hypothesis that the GLP-1RA possess cognitive protective properties. Data from one large RCT demonstrates that dulaglutide a GLP-1RA reduced incident cognitive dysfunction by 12%. There are also post hoc combined analyses from other GLP-1RA trials and prospective studies that further support this hypothesis.

The Multidomain Approach

The Finnish Geriatric Intervention Study to Prevent Cognitive Impairment and Disability (FINGER) trial was the first RCT to demonstrates that it is possible to slow the rate of cognitive decline using a multidomain intervention among older people at high risk for CVD, 30% of whom had diabetes. The two-year intervention targeted multiple cognitive dysfunction risk factors and included a personalised physical, cognitive, nutritional treatment plan, some parts of which were conducted in groups. It also included maximal risk factor reduction (including glucose, blood pressure and lipids) [24]. Following the impressive results of the trial, a FINGER trial network was established and there are currently several multi-domain trials being conducted across the globe. The Center for Successful Aging with Diabetes, Sheba Medical Center), conducts multi-domain assessments and offers a case manager-led multidisciplinary intervention (medical, cognitive, nutritional, physical) to those in need [25, 26].

Implementing such a model in busy healthcare systems in a challenge. Technology may have a role in enabling implementation in busy healthcare systems, by providing a means for remote, passive assessment of physical and cognitive status and integrating it with a technology-enabled case-manager system. The Center is currently in the process of building and testing such a system.

Summary, Knowledge Gaps and Future Research

Cognitive dysfunction is yet another long-term complication of diabetes that is becoming increasingly important with the ageing of the population and the large number of older people with diabetes. It is important to recognise that cognitive dysfunction impairs self-care capacity and thus it is important to assess cognitive function as part of the routine care of older people with diabetes as recommended by the American Diabetes Association and other professional organisations. For this field to move forward, to be able to slow the progression of this diabetes complication, there is need for a way to detect, diagnose and stage the preclinical stages of the complication, possibly taking the retinopathy model. On a clinical level, this would allow development of cognitive rehabilitation strategies and support systems to aid older people with diabetes and cognitive dysfunction, exclusion of secondary causes, early introduction preventive strategies and, on a research and drug development level, would enable inclusion of cognitive dysfunction as an outcome. In this respect, CS-SCI may be an attractive novel way of defining cognitive dysfunction in an international RCT.

Clinical Practice Question

A 75-year-old man who is a retired engineer. Medical history: hypertension, atrial fibrillation, abnormal gait, recurrent falls. Brain MRI shows lacunar infarcts. He has had type 2 diabetes since 2007, with variable glucose control. He started insulin in 2021. Diabetes complications include nephropathy (microalbuminuria). Hypoglycaemia neuroglycopenic symptoms, no adrenergic symptoms. No serious event requiring the aid of another. Currently taking long-acting insulin, glucagon-like peptide-1 receptor analyst, sodium glucose transporter-2, metformin, short-acting insulin at larger meals. Last haemoglobin A1c 8%.

Cognitive health agility assessment: Montreal Cognitive Assessment 25–30; standardised digital symbol substitution test 9 (raw 46). Physical health agility assessment: grip strength: normal; sit to stand normal; 10-minute walk normal; time to up and go 10.5 seconds; six-minute walk 464 metres.

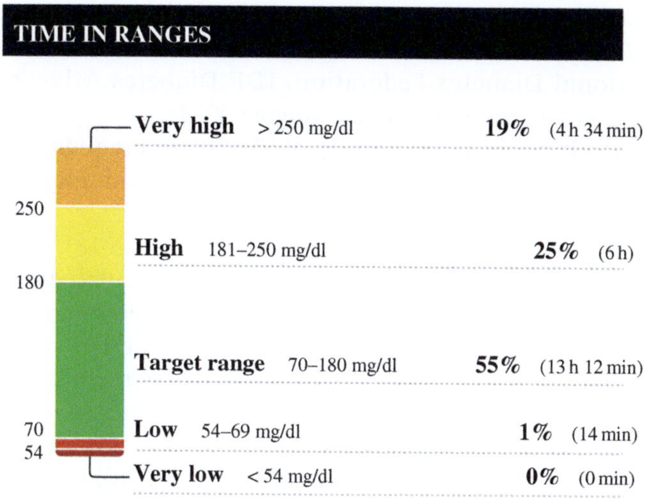

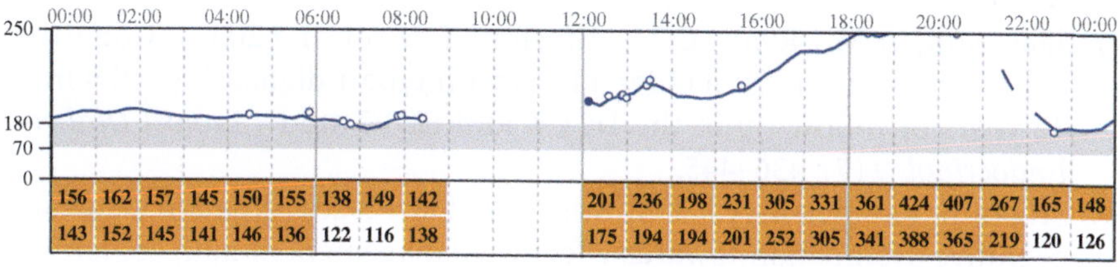

What are the treatment goals for this individual?

A. Adapt glucose control to cognitive health agility status.
B. Implement cognitive, physical and nutritional interventions to prevent further deterioration.
C. Monitor continuing cognitive health agility status and adapt glucose control accordingly.
D. Insulin and glucagon-like peptide-1 receptor analysts may have a beneficial cognitive effect.
E. All of the above.

References

Key references only are listed here. For a full list of references visit: https://www.wiley.com/go/sinclair/1e.

1. Kirkman, M.S., Briscoe, V.J., Clark, N. et al. (2012). Diabetes in older adults. *Diabetes Care* 35 (12): 2650–2664.
2. International Diabetes Federation. IDF Diabetes Atlas. https://diabetesatlas.org (accessed 6 August 2024).
3. Manly, J.J., Tang, M.X., Schupf, N. et al. (2008). Frequency and course of mild cognitive impairment in a multiethnic community. *Ann. Neurol.* 63 (4): 494–506.
4. Pal, K., Mukadam, N., Petersen, I., and Cooper, C. (2018). Mild cognitive impairment and progression to dementia in people with diabetes, prediabetes and metabolic syndrome: a systematic review and meta-analysis. *Soc. Psychiatry Psychiatr. Epidemiol.* 53 (11): 1149–1160.
5. Xue, M., Xu, W., Ou, Y.N. et al. (2019). Diabetes mellitus and risks of cognitive impairment and dementia: a systematic review and meta-analysis of 144 prospective studies. *Ageing Res. Rev.* 55: 100944.
6. Kuo, C.L., Lu, C.L., Chang, Y.H., and Li, C.Y. (2018). Population-based cohort study on dementia risk in patients with type 1 diabetes mellitus. *Neuroepidemiology* 50 (1–2): 57–62.
7. Jacobson, A.M., Ryan, C.M., Braffett, B.H. et al. (2021). Cognitive performance declines in older adults with type 1 diabetes: results from 32 years of follow-up in the DCCT and EDIC study. *Lancet Diabetes Endocrinol.* 9 (7): 436–445.
8. Srikanth, V., Sinclair, A.J., Hill-Briggs, F. et al. (2020). Type 2 diabetes and cognitive dysfunction-towards effective management of both comorbidities. *Lancet Diabetes Endocrinol.* 8 (6): 535–545.
9. Punthakee, Z., Miller, M.E., Launer, L.J. et al. (2012). Poor cognitive function and risk of severe hypoglycemia in type 2 diabetes: post hoc epidemiologic analysis of the ACCORD trial. *Diabetes Care* 35 (4): 787–793.
10. Santos, T., Lovell, J., Shiell, K. et al. (2018). The impact of cognitive impairment in dementia on self-care domains in diabetes: a systematic search and narrative review. *Diabetes Metab. Res. Rev.* 34 (6): e3013.

16e Special Issues in Old Age: Depression

Sara-Louise Wylie

General Practice, Clinical Commissioning Group, Sheffield, UK

Key Points

- Diabetes mellitus increases the risk of depression and the relationship is bidirectional.
- Depression in older people presents with physical more than emotional symptoms.
- Depression increases the risk of cognitive and physical dysfunction and mortality in people with diabetes and the risk is particularly high in older people.
- Regular screening and early diagnosis of depression is an important part of holistic diabetes care.
- A multifaceted intervention that includes lifestyle change, pharmacological and psychological therapy in a collaborative care setting is the best approach for care of comorbid depression and diabetes.

Introduction

Diabetes in old age is associated with diabetes-related complications and diabetes-associated comorbidities. Due to the interplay between metabolic dysfunction, vascular disease, increasing age and age-related disorders, diabetes in older people can be a disabling condition. In addition to physical dysfunction, psychological complications and mood disorders such as depression are common. Unlike

Care of Older People with Diabetes: A Manual for Healthcare Practice, First Edition.
Edited by Alan J. Sinclair and Ahmed H. Abdelhafiz.

Companion website: www.wiley.com/go/sinclair/1e

other chronic conditions, diabetes care is dependent upon patients' ability to perform self-care tasks. The presence of depression may lead to lethargy and less compliance in undertaking these self-care responsibilities, which may lead to further long-term complications [1]. Therefore, early recognition and treatment of depression in older people with diabetes may improve outcomes. This chapter reviews the association and the impact of depression on older people with diabetes and explores the management challenges in this group of complex patients.

Depression and Diabetes

Ageing-related metabolic changes and age-related risk factors increase the risk of both diabetes mellitus and depression (Figure 16e.1). Depression is more common in people compared with those without diabetes and the relation is likely bidirectional. The knowledge of diabetes diagnosis, its complications and the burden of its treatment may lead to patients feeling helpless and hopeless, which may result in depression. On the other hand, the increased rate of obesity-promoting health behaviours, such as physical inactivity and poor dietary habits in people with depression or the increased rate of insulin resistance associated with depressive symptoms, may increase the risk of incident diabetes [2]. The development of depression in older people with diabetes will have negative consequences, such as less compliance with self-care tasks, diet and medication, which causes poor glycaemic control. In addition, depression can accelerate cognitive decline, as shown in the ACCORD-MIND study, which may further compromise patients' self-care [3]. Depression is also associated with reduced physical function and poor quality of life in a dose–response manner [4]. Furthermore, depression increases the risk of mortality in people with combined diabetes and depression compared with those with only diabetes; the effect of depression on mortality is most significant in older people [5].

Presentation

Older people are less likely to report depressive symptoms than younger people. When they do report symptoms, those symptoms often manifest differently with a predominance of physical more than emotional symptoms (Table 16e.1).

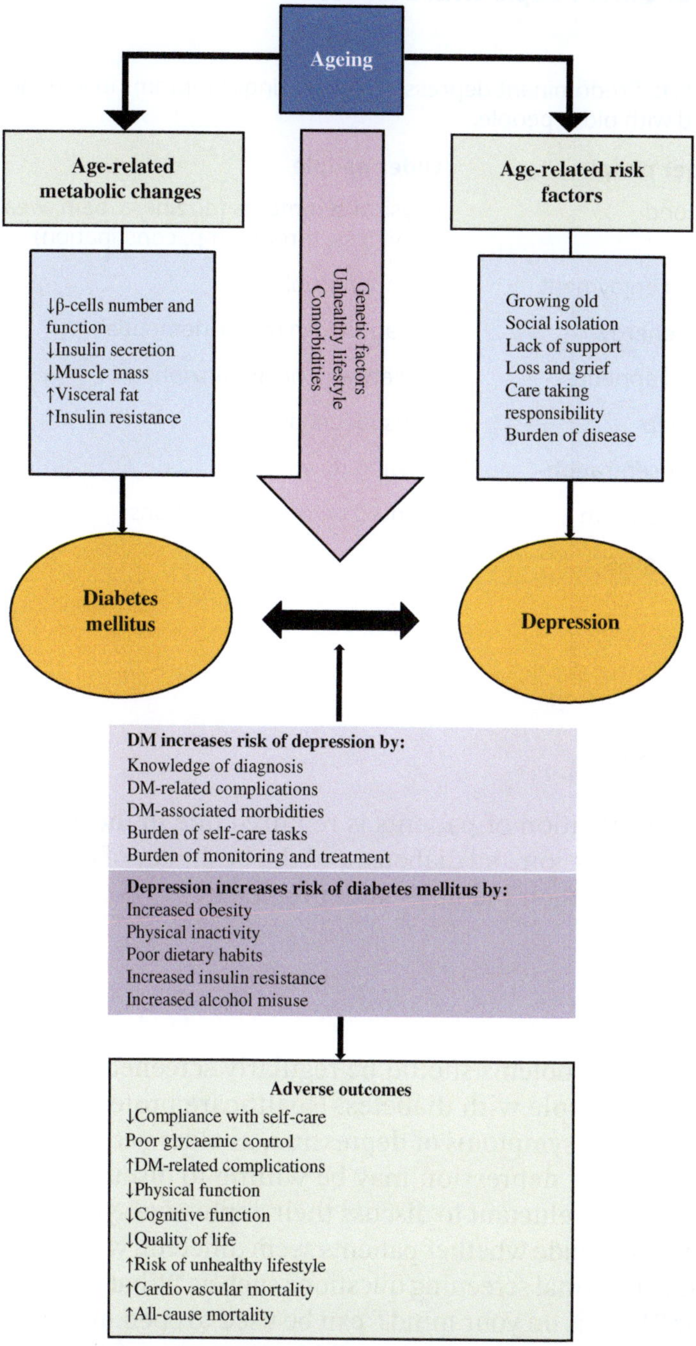

Figure 16e.1: Relationship between ageing, diabetes mellitus and depression. Age-related metabolic changes and accumulation of risk factors increase the risk of both diabetes and depression. The relationship between diabetes mellitus and depression is bidirectional and associated with adverse outcomes.

Table 16e.1: Predominant depression presenting symptoms in younger compared with older people.

Younger people	Older people
Low mood	Physical symptoms (dizziness, pain, weakness, heaviness, throat lump, constipation)
Reduced enjoyment	Memory problems
Lack of energy	Agitation (can mimic dementia)
Reduced appetite	Anxiety and health anxieties
Poor sleep	Unusual behaviour
Poor concentration	Slowing down
Low self-esteem	Blunted emotional reactions
Hopelessness	
Guilt	

Evaluation

A holistic evaluation of patients is required due to the complexity of comorbid depression and diabetes and the hesitancy of older people to complain about their mental health problems.

Screening

Psychological problems should be regularly screened for when evaluating older people with diabetes. Healthcare professionals should actively look for symptoms of depression, as older people with comorbid diabetes and depression may be willing to discuss their glycaemic control but reluctant to discuss their depressive symptoms. Initial assessments include whether patients seem different, withdrawn or disinterested. Informal screening questions such as 'What is troubling you now?' or 'What is on your mind?' can be used to open up conversation. Inquiry about what they think could be the cause of their symptoms may uncover some hidden ideas and point towards underlying depression. Factors that indicate that patients may be at high risk are summarised in Box 16e.1.

Box 16e.1: Factors Indicating Patients at High Risk of Depression

- Physical health problems
- Loss of independence
- Social isolation
- Loss of purpose
- Bereavement
- Female gender
- Medication adverse effects

Diagnosis

The *Diagnostic and Statistical Manual of Mental Disorders*, fifth edition, outlines the criteria for making a diagnosis of depression (Box 16e.2). The individual must be experiencing five or more symptoms during the same two-week period and at least one of the symptoms should be either depressed mood or loss of interest or pleasure [6]. Diagnostic difficulties are common in people with concomitant cognitive impairment.

Box 16e.2: Criteria for Depression Diagnosis

- Depressed mood most of the day, nearly every day.
- Markedly diminished interest in all or almost all activities, most of the day, nearly every day.
- Significant unintentional weight loss, or ↑ or ↓ in appetite nearly every day.
- Slowing of thought and reduced physical movement (observed by others not self-reported).
- Fatigue or loss of energy nearly every day.
- Feeling of worthlessness, excessive or inappropriate guilt nearly every day.
- Diminished ability to think or concentrate or indecisiveness, nearly every day.
- Recurrent thoughts of death, or suicidal ideation without suicide attempt or a specific plan for committing suicide.

Diagnostic and Statistical Manual of Mental Disorders, 5th edition.

Box 16e.3: Barriers to Patients at Risk of Depression Accessing Healthcare

- Frailty
- Stigma of mental health issues
- Perceived hopelessness
- Not wanting to be a burden
- Difficulty navigating appointment system
- Lack of social or family support
- Lack of awareness of available services
- Ethnic and cultural differences

Symptoms of depression and dementia may overlap; however, speech and word-finding difficulties are more often seen in dementia than in depression. In addition, depressive symptoms, such as fatigue and reduced appetite, may also be mistaken for symptoms of uncontrolled diabetes or normal ageing process resulting in under-diagnosis. For example, doctors detected only 43% of nursing home residents with depression [7]. Furthermore, general practitioners failed to diagnose up to 50% of older patients with depression [8]. In a study to investigate whether diabetes specialist nurses and endocrinologists would recognise depression in 175 patients with diabetes, only 43.5% of patients with depression were detected by staff. The only significant predictor of detection was the severity of depressive symptoms [9]. Awareness of barriers to accessing healthcare allows us to tackle these barriers both in primary and secondary care, with the aim of early diagnosis of depression (Box 16e.3).

Assessment

Several formal depression assessment tools can be used for initial screening, assessment of severity and then monitoring of response to treatment of depression. Shorter tools are usually used for screening and longer versions can then be used for detailed assessment whenever screening is positive. Simple scales can be self-reported by patients, while other detailed tools will need administration by clinicians. Examples of the main depression screening scales are summarised in Table 16e.2. Following history taking and making a probable diagnosis of depression, it is important to document a mental state examination,

Table 16e.2: Depression screening tools.

Tool	Criteria	Advantage
Geriatric Depression Scale, short forms	15, 10, and 4-point scales that focus on psychiatric symptoms. 4-point better for screening, longer forms better for assessing clinical severity of depression and monitoring treatment	Questions are a yes or no, easy to understand, suitable for older people who may suffer from cognitive dysfunction
Patient Health Questionnaire-9	9-point scale to screen for how often patients suffer from symptoms that may suggest underlying depression over the past 2-week period	It can also measure severity, a score of 5, 10, 15, and 20 suggest mild, moderate, moderately severe and severe depression, respectively
Beck Depression Inventory	21-point scale that provides a quantitative assessment of the intensity of depression	Can be self or interviewer reported and takes only 10 minutes to be administered
Centre for Epidemiologic Studies Depression Scale	20-item scale that measures major dimensions of depression experienced over the preceding week	Self-reported, can be used in primary care settings
Hamilton Depression Rating Scale (HAM-D)	21-item scale administered by health care professional and takes 15–20 minutes to complete	Can be used in clinical practice for assessment of severity of depression, changes in its severity over time and efficacy of treatment
Montgomery–Asberg Depression Rating Scale	10-item scale designed to measure severity of depression and can be completed in 20–30 minutes	It is an adaptation of the HAM-D scale with a greater sensitivity of change in depression severity over time
Quick Inventory of Depressive Symptomatology	16-item scale that is available in both self-report and clinician-rated formats	Highly acceptable in clinical practice and takes only 5–7 minutes to complete

(*Continued*)

Table 16e.2: Continued

Tool	Criteria	Advantage
Life Satisfaction Rating	5-point scale that measures life satisfaction in older people >50 years old	Measures wellbeing and successful ageing and takes only 10 minutes to complete
Cornell Scale for Depression in Dementia	19-item scale based on depressive signs and symptoms during the week prior to interview, takes 30 minutes to complete	Designed to screen for depression among patients with dementia
Self-Rating Depression Scale	20-item scale that covers affective, psychological and somatic symptoms associated with depression	Self-reported, takes only 10 minutes to complete, can be used in primary care

paying special attention to cognition and insight (Box 16e.4). This examination aids in the diagnosis but can also allow monitoring of progress. Physical examination is also important for patients presenting with physical symptoms. It is also important to assess the severity of depression and identify patients with severe symptoms especially those at risk of suicide (Box 16e.5).

Box 16e.4: Mental State Examination

- Appearance: unkempt, self-neglect.
- Behaviour: tearful, aggressive, body language cues, eye contact.
- Speech: rate, quantity, tone, volume.
- Mood and affect: what they report mood as, what affect, are they congruent?
- Thoughts: any unusual thoughts, delusions, thought possession?
- Perception: any hallucinations?
- Cognition: are they orientated, any cognitive issues?
- Insight: are they aware of situation, do they understand?
- Risk: assess risk to self and others.

Box 16e.5: Patients at High Risk of Suicide

- Severe current depression
- History of depression
- Male gender
- Being widowed
- Increasing age
- Social isolation
- Physical illness
- Pain
- Alcohol misuse

Management

As depression in diabetes is associated with negative impact on psychological as well as physical functions, management should be directed towards improving both psychological and physical outcomes. Remission of depressive symptoms may help to improve physical functioning and medical outcomes, such as glycaemic control, vascular complications and mortality. For the best outcome, depression should be treated with a combination of lifestyle changes, pharmacological therapy and psychotherapy in a collaborative care setting, which looks after the comorbid depression and diabetes. Electroconvulsive therapy is another safe mode of therapy in severe cases of depression not responding to conventional therapy, and it is effective and well tolerated even in frail older people (Figure 16e.2). Referral to an older people's mental health service may be required due to diagnostic difficulty, the presence of psychotic symptoms, suicidal thoughts, suspicion of underlying cognitive impairment, inadequate response to treatment and need for advice on medication in complex patients or the rise of crisis.

Lifestyle

Healthy lifestyle, which includes reduction of alcohol misuse and regular exercise, will contribute to the treatment of both diabetes and depression. For example, in the look AHEAD (Action for Health in Diabetes) study, intensive lifestyle intervention significantly reduced the incidence of depressive symptoms (hazard ratio 0.85, 95% confidence

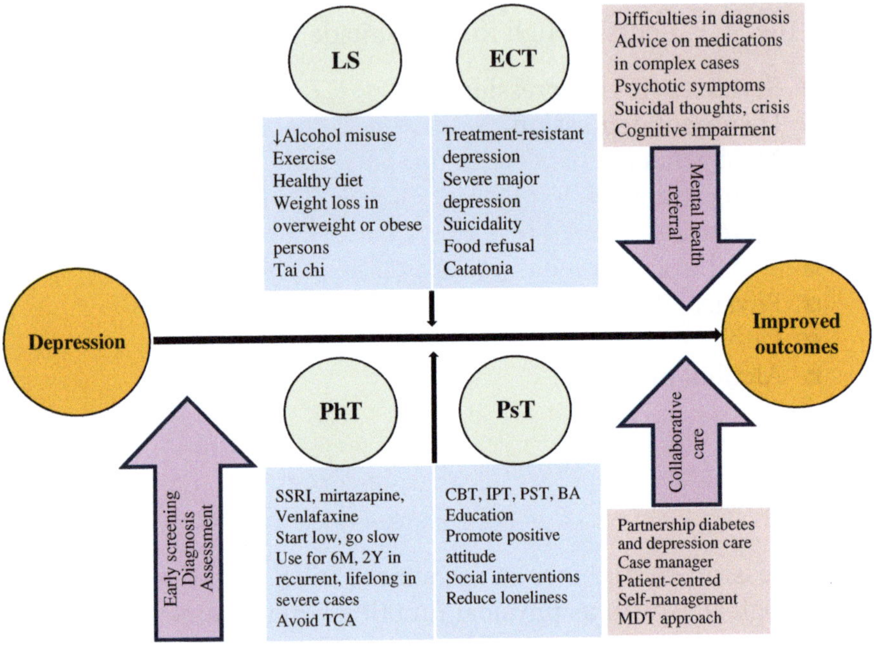

Figure 16e.2: Management of depression in older people with diabetes mellitus. Early diagnosis and multifaceted interventions are crucial in improving outcomes. BA, behavioural activation and pleasant activity scheduling; CBT, cognitive behavioural therapy; ECT, electroconvulsive therapy; IPT, interpersonal psychotherapy; LS, lifestyle; M, months; MDT, multidisciplinary team; PhT, pharmacotherapy; PsT, psychotherapy; TCA, tricyclic anti-depressants; Y, years.

interval 0.75–0.97, $p = 0.02$) and preserved better function compared with usual care [10]. Tai chi, which involves a series of slowly performed, dance-like postures that flow into one another, together with mental concentration, physical balance and muscle relaxation, is emerging as a form of mind and body exercise that can be integrated into the prevention and rehabilitation of a number of medical and psychological conditions such as comorbid diabetes and depression [11].

Pharmacological Therapy

Selective serotonin reuptake inhibitors (SSRI) are the preferred antidepressants in older people with comorbid depression and diabetes, because of their efficacy in ameliorating depressive symptoms without worsening glycaemic control [12]. One antidepressant should normally be tried first for at least four weeks before switching to another SSRI or another antidepressant from a different class, such as mirtazapine or venlafaxine. Treatment should be continued for at least six months or longer until complete remission of depression, and then stopped gradually. Long-term treatment is recommended in patients with recurrent episodes of depression to prevent relapses for at least two years, and lifelong in severe cases. There is no one SSRI antidepressant that is more effective than another and selection should be based on patient tolerability. Citalopram, sertraline and escitalopram may be particularly well tolerated in older people due to their favourable pharmacokinetic profiles with fewer adverse effects. When poor sleep and low appetite are particular issues, mirtazapine can be helpful (although weight gain is an adverse effect, which may be undesirable in some patients). Tricyclic antidepressants are associated with unfavourable anticholinergic effects, confusion, hyperglycaemia, orthostatic hypotension and cardiac arrhythmias, making them less appropriate choice for older people with depression.

Psychotherapy

Several modalities of psychotherapy are effective in reducing depressive symptoms in older people with comorbid diabetes and depression, such as cognitive behavioural therapy (CBT), interpersonal psychotherapy, problem-solving treatment and behavioural activation and pleasant activity scheduling. CBT can be delivered individually by mental health providers or trained nurse case managers and mainly promotes medication adherence and self-care through education and reducing negative attitudes towards patients own health. IPT deals with depressive symptoms through improving interpersonal relationships. Problem-solving treatment is a cognitive–behavioural intervention that focuses on training in adaptive problem-solving attitudes and skills. Behavioural activation is to change patients' behaviour to learn to monitor their mood and daily activities and how to increase the number of pleasant activities and positive interactions with the environment. Other measures such as social interventions through day centres, community groups, befriending services, religious ceremonies and family support may help in reducing the negative impact of social isolation and loneliness on depressive symptoms [13]. Combination of pharmacological and psychological therapy may be more effective than either alone in maintaining remission or reducing the number of recurrent episodes [14].

Collaborative Care

Collaborative care is the strategy of combining the treatment of depression and diabetes. Collaborative care that incorporates brief low-intensity psychological therapy delivered in partnership with practice nurses in primary care can reduce depression and improve self-management in patients with diabetes. In a cluster randomised controlled trial in 387 patients with a record of diabetes, heart disease or both associated with depressive symptoms in 36 general practices in the UK, mean depressive scores were 0.23 points lower in the collaborative care compared with the usual care arm after four months of follow-up. Patients in the intervention arm also reported as being better self-managers, rated their care as more patient centred and were more satisfied with their care at follow-up [15]. In another study in four primary care networks in Canada, collaborative care including case managers working with patients to deliver individualised care resulted in greater 12-month improvements in the Patient Health Questionnaire (PHQ), mean 7.3 (standard deviation [SD] 5.6) compared with a control group 5.2 (SD 5.7), $p = 0.015$. Recovery of depressive symptoms (PHQ reduced by 50%) was greater among intervention patients (61% vs. 44%, $p = 0.03$) [16].

Summary

Depression is common in older people with diabetes and the relationship is bidirectional. Regular screening and early identification and treatment of depression is important to improve outcomes. A combination of lifestyle changes, pharmacological and psychological interventions in a collaborative care setting is the best approach for the management of comorbid depression and diabetes.

Clinical Practice Question

Q1. A 75-year-old man with a history of type 2 diabetes mellitus and depression on oral hypoglycaemic therapy and mirtazapine 15 mg once daily for the past five years presented to his general practitioner reporting that he has a dark feeling over himself, a sense of lowness and a struggle for motivation to get out and about for the past six months. He also reported that his sleep has been very poor over the past two months. He has started drinking two glasses of whisky in the evenings to try to get to sleep. On examination, he was unkempt, had poor eye contact and a low affect. He criticises himself: 'I should be stronger and just snap out of it.' What will be your next steps?

Choose the options that apply.

A. Explore further his feeling, whether it is similar when he was first diagnosed with depression.
B. Explain the nature of wellbeing and low mood.
C. Advise to reduce excess alcohol and explain ideas of social prescribing and talk therapy.
D. Increase mirtazapine to 30 mg once daily.
E. Urgent referral to mental health service.

References

Key references only are listed here. For a full list of references visit: `https://www.wiley.com/go/sinclair/1e`.

1. Pouwer, F., Nefs, G., and Nouwen, A. (2013). Adverse effects of depression on glycemic control and health outcomes in people with diabetes: a review. *Endocrinol. Metab. Clin. North Am.* 42: 529–544.
2. Kan, C., Silva, N., Golden, S.H. et al. (2013). A systematic review and meta-analysis of the association between depression and insulin resistance. *Diabetes Care* 36: 480–489.
3. Sullivan, M.D., Katon, W.J., Lovato, L.C. et al. (2013). Association of depression with accelerated cognitive decline among patients with type 2 diabetes in the ACCORD-MIND trial. *JAMA Psychiatr.* 70: 1041–1047.
4. Schmitz, N., Gariepy, G., Smith, K.J. et al. (2014). Recurrent subthreshold depression in type 2 diabetes: an important risk factor for poor health outcomes. *Diabetes Care* 37: 970–978.
5. Kimbro, L.B., Mangione, C.M., Steers, W.N. et al. (2014). Depression and all-cause mortality in persons with diabetes mellitus: are older adults at higher risk? Results from the translating research into action for diabetes study. *J. Am. Geriatr. Soc.* 62: 1017–1022.
6. American Psychiatric Association (2013). *Diagnostic and Statistical Manual of Mental Disorders*, 5e. Washington, DC: American Psychological Association.

7. Kramer, D., Allgaier, A.K., Fejtkova, S. et al. (2009). Depression in nursing homes: prevalence, recognition, and treatment. *Int. J. Psychiat. Med.* 39: 345–358.
8. Cepoiu, M., McCusker, J., Cole, M.G. et al. (2007). Recognition of depression in older medical inpatients. *J. Gen. Intern. Med.* 22: 559–564.
9. Km, P., Pachana, N.A., and McDermott, B.M. (2014). Health professionals' detection of depression and anxiety in their patients with diabetes: the influence of patient, illness and psychological factors. *J. Health Psychol.* 21: 1566–1575.
10. Look AHEAD Research Group (2014). Impact of intensive lifestyle intervention on depression and health-related quality of life in type 2 diabetes: the look AHEAD trial. *Diabetes Care* 37: 1544–1553.

16f Special Issues in Old Age: Foot Care

Solomon Muzulu

Department of Diabetes and Endocrinology, Rotherham General Hospital, Rotherham, UK

Key Points

- All people with diabetes mellitus should receive footcare advice and regular foot examination.
- Older people with diabetes are at risk of foot disease because of increasing frailty and difficulties with self-care.
- Peripheral neuropathy and peripheral vascular disease are major risk factors for diabetic foot ulcer disease.
- Previous foot ulceration is the strongest predictor of future foot ulceration.
- A new diabetic foot problem should be assessed immediately and managed in the community by the foot protection service or, if severe, by the multidisciplinary diabetic foot team.
- Treatment of diabetic foot ulcer disease involves offloading, debridement, treatment of infection, restoration of circulation and good glycaemic control.
- The majority of amputations can be avoided by prevention and aggressive management of diabetic foot ulcers.

Introduction

A diabetic foot problem is any problem affecting the foot of a person with diabetes that is caused by neuropathy or peripheral vascular disease (PVD) [1]. Any 'minor' foot problem can cause serious morbidity

Care of Older People with Diabetes: A Manual for Healthcare Practice, First Edition.
Edited by Alan J. Sinclair and Ahmed H. Abdelhafiz.

Companion website: www.wiley.com/go/sinclair/1e

in people with diabetes. Callus, corns, blisters and bunions can ulcerate and get infected. Interdigital fungal infections and ingrowing toenails can lead to foot cellulitis. Diabetes-related foot problems cost the United Kingdom (UK) National Health Service over £0.5 million a year [2]. In addition to the economic burden, there are associated huge personal costs. Non-healing foot ulcers and lower-extremity amputations lead to reduced physical function and poor quality of life. Furthermore, a person who develops diabetic foot ulcer (DFU) has 50% five-year mortality, and around 50–70% of those who have a minor or major amputation will die within five years of their amputation [3, 4].

Epidemiology

In the UK, an estimated five million people have diabetes mellitus. Their lifetime risk of developing DFU is 19–34% [4, 5]. DFU is the leading cause of admission to hospital for diabetes-related complications. Recurrence of DFU is common-40% within one year and 65% within five years [4]. Previous foot ulceration is the strongest predictor of future foot ulceration. Diabetes is the leading cause of non-traumatic lower-extremity amputation, with a lifetime risk of 20% [4]. In England, there are over 176 diabetes-related minor and major amputations per week [6]. People aged over 65 years, especially men, are at higher risk of diabetes-related foot disease and lower-extremity amputation [7].

Pathogenesis

Diabetic foot ulcer is a break in the epidermis and at least part of the dermis in a person with diabetes. The most common sites are the weight-bearing areas of the foot. Peripheral sensory neuropathy (PSN) causes loss of protective sensation, while motor neuropathy and Charcot's neuroarthropathy result in foot deformity and abnormal gait. Other structural deformities that increase the risk of pressure-induced foot ulceration include clawed toes, hammer toes and callus. Repetitive minor trauma causes ulceration due to increased pressure, friction and shearing from ill-fitting footwear and abnormal gait in an insensate foot. Peripheral autonomic neuropathy leads to dry cracked skin that can get infected, and neuropathic oedema results in poor wound healing. In addition, people with diabetes have a higher prevalence of PVD, which increases the risk of non-healing ulcers, infection, gangrene and amputation. The underlying aetiology of DFU is peripheral neuropathy

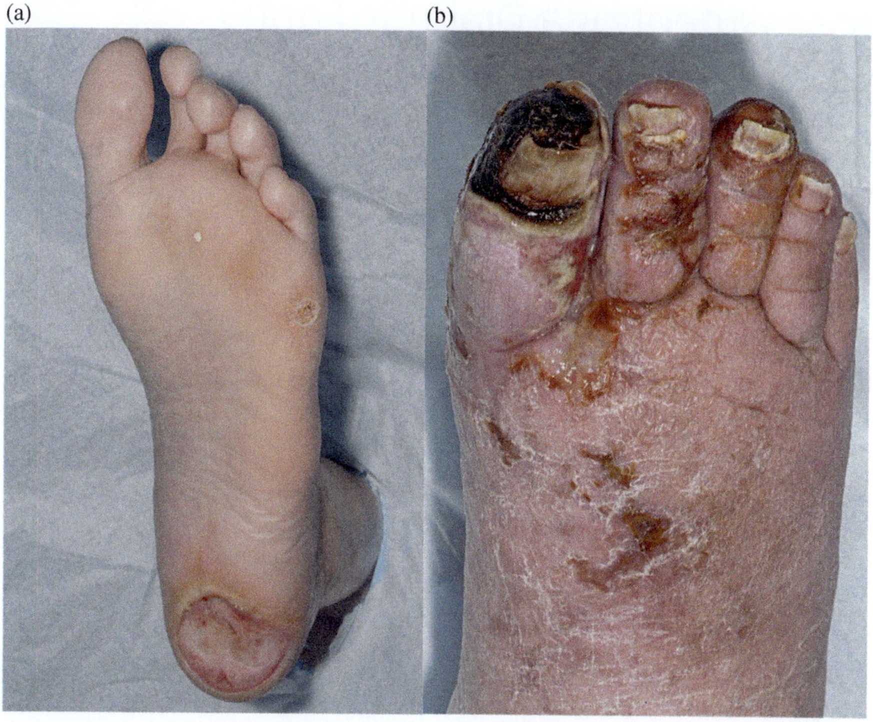

Figure 16f.1: (a) Typical neuropathic ulcer. (b) Ischaemic toe.

and/or ischaemia. DFU is classified as neuropathic (40–60%), ischaemic (12–15%) or neuroischaemic (30–50%) (Figure 16f.1). Closed lesions that do not penetrate to the dermis, such as callus and blisters, are termed pre-ulcerative. These lesions have a high risk of progressing to an ulcer.

Ageing and Diabetic Foot Ulcer Disease

Ageing in diabetes increases the risk of PSN and PVD, partly due to long duration of diabetes and poor glycaemic control. In addition, impaired immune response in older people with diabetes (immunosenescence) predisposes to unopposed tissue inflammation that encourages atherosclerosis [8]. The impaired immune response also permits infection and impairs healing of DFU that can lead to cellulitis and osteomyelitis. Frailty and sarcopenia, which are common in older people with diabetes, increase the risk of DFU, amputations and death after amputation [9, 10].

Assessment of a Diabetic Foot

When assessing a diabetic foot, it is important to remove shoes, socks, bandages and dressings. Examine both feet for neuropathy, ischaemia, ulceration, callus, infection, deformity, gangrene and features of Charcot's neuroarthropathy (Box 16f.1) [1].

Testing for Peripheral Sensory Neuropathy

Three equally reliable tests can be used to test for PSN: (1) 10-g monofilament, (2) 128-Hz tuning fork and (3) the Ipswich touch test (IpTT). It is important to avoid callus, scars, necrotic tissue and the ulcer itself when performing these tests.

Box 16f.1: Assessment of Diabetic Foot Ulcer

- Describe the site, appearance, size and depth
- Probe the ulcer with a blunt sterile probe (only if competent to do so)
- Undermining of ulcer:
  - 'Blow-out' lesions and/or sinuses/tracking
  - Probing to joints and bones (an ulcer that probes to bone suggests the presence of osteomyelitis)
- Assess for presence and severity of infection:
  - Odour (e.g. 'anaerobic smell')
  - Exudate or pus
  - Presence and extent of cellulitis
  - Constitutional symptoms
- Take microbiological samples if there are signs of infection:
  - Swab exudate or pus
  - Swab ulcer base after debridement
  - Bone fragments
- Ascertain aetiology of ulcer–neuropathic, ischaemic or neuroischaemic:
  - Assess for peripheral neuropathy
  - Assess vascular status and request ankle brachial pressure index if ischaemia is suspected

- Request imaging:
  - Plain radiographs (may not show changes of osteomyelitis in acute bone infection–repeat after a week if feasible)
  - Magnetic resonance imaging if clinical suspicion of osteomyelitis is high despite normal plain radiographs and/or if there is clinical suspicion of abscess formation
- Blood tests:
  - Full blood count may show an elevated white cell count
  - C-reactive protein may be elevated, serial measurements will reflect response to therapy
  - Renal function - estimated glomerular filtration rate will aid the choice and dose of antibiotics
  - Haemoglobin A1c will indicate degree of glycaemic control over the preceding three months

10-g Monofilament Test

In the 10-g monofilament test, a 10-g monofilament is held perpendicular to the skin. With the person's eyes closed, enough force is applied for one to two seconds to buckle the monofilament. PSN is present if the pressure is not felt at two or more sites. Ten sites are traditionally tested on each foot, but five sites are just as reliable (Figure 16f.2).

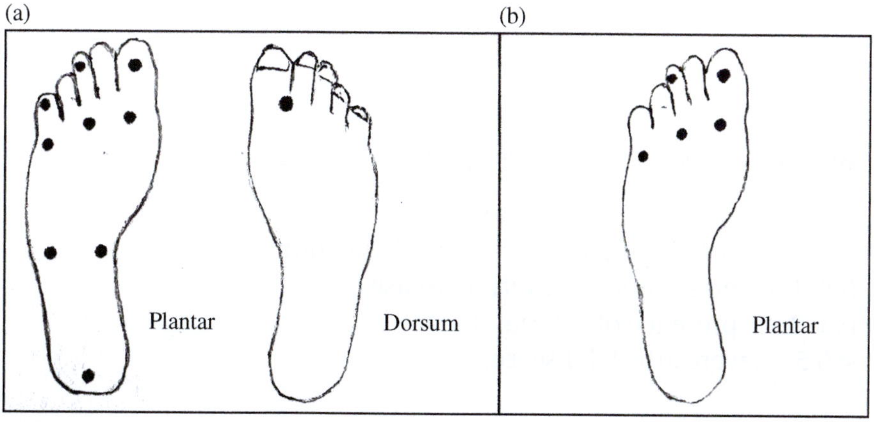

Figure 16f.2: 10 g monofilament test: (a) 10 sites, (b) 5 sites.

128-Hz Tuning Fork

In the 128-tuning fork test, a vibrating tuning fork is placed perpendicular to the distal phalanx of the first (big) toe.

Ipswich Touch Test

The IpTT involves lightly touching by the tip of the index finger for one to two seconds on the tips of the first, third and fifth toes of both feet. PSN is present if two or more of the six sites are insensate [11].

Checking for Peripheral Vascular Disease

Absent posterior tibial and dorsalis pedis pulses with a palpable popliteal pulse is classic of diabetic PVD. Ankle brachial pressure index (ABPI) measurements will reveal the degree of vascular compromise (Box 16f.2).

Management

Assessment and investigations of DFU are summarised in Box 16f.1 and Table 16f.1 [1,12]. After assessment, the patient should be referred to the foot protection service, diabetes podiatrist or multidisciplinary foot team, depending on local arrangements, to be seen within 24 hours of the initial examination. The aim of treatment is to achieve wound

Box 16f.2: Assessment of Peripheral Vascular Disease

Typical ankle brachial pressure index results:
> 1.3 – falsely high due to arterial calcification
0.8–1.3 – no significant arterial disease
0.5–0.8 – presence of arterial disease
< 0.5 – severe arterial disease

Table 16f.1: Interventions based on foot risk stratification in diabetes.

Level	Risk	Intervention
Low	No risk factors except callus (no deformity, no PSN, no PVD and no skin changes)	Give foot care information. Check feet annually
Moderate	Foot deformity, or PSN, or PVD, or skin changes except callus	Refer to foot protection service or podiatrist.[a] Give footcare information. Check feet every 3–6 months with more frequent assessments if cannot check own feet
High	Previous ulceration, or previous amputation, or renal replacement therapy, or PSN with PVD, or PSN with callus and/or deformity, or PVD with callus and/or deformity	Refer to foot protection service or podiatrist. Give footcare information. Check feet 1–2 monthly if no concerns. Check feet 1–2 weekly if concerns. More frequent assessments if cannot check own feet
Active foot disease	Ulceration, cellulitis, spreading infection, suspected acute Charcot neuroarthropathy or unexplained hot and swollen foot with a change in colour with or without pain	Refer to foot protection service or to MDT within 24 hours. Give footcare information
Acute foot attack (active foot disease and systemically unwell)	Ulceration with limb ischaemia. Critical limb ischaemia. Gangrene. Deep seated infection including abscess or osteomyelitis	Acute admission to hospital or to A&E. Must be seen by a member of the foot MDT within 24 hours of admission

A&E, accident and emergency; PSN, peripheral sensory neuropathy; MDT, multidisciplinary team; PVD, peripheral vascular disease.

[a] The foot protection service is a team led by a podiatrist that prevents, treats and manages diabetic foot problems in the community.

healing, restore normal function and improve quality of life. The treatment of DFU involves some or all the following: offloading (rest and pressure relief), wound debridement, wound dressings, control of infection, relief of ischaemia and glycaemic control.

Offloading

Avoiding weight bearing on the affected foot is the most effective method of offloading to heal DFU and suspected acute Charcot's. Non-removable total contact casts are best in the absence of infection. Where no such facilities exist, removable casts or other pressure-relieving footwear such as a modified DH pressure relief shoe can be used.

Debridement

Debridement of DFU, in any setting, must be done by a healthcare professional with the relevant skills and training. Necrotic tissue, fibrous tissue and callus are debrided back to healthy bleeding tissue to aid the healing process.

Dressings

The choice of dressing is guided by a podiatrist or a member of the tissue viability team. Dressings should prevent tissue desiccation, absorb excess fluid and protect the wound from contamination. In an ischaemic ulcer, it is preferable to use simple non-adherent dressings until the vascular supply has been restored.

Infection Control

About 60% of DFUs get infected [4]. The risk of infection increases for non-healing ulcers and ulcers that probe to bone. Infection increases the risk of operative intervention including debridement and amputation. Antibiotics should be commenced as soon as possible for suspected infection in DFU. Microbiological samples should be collected before antibiotic therapy. Where this is not feasible, start empirical antibiotic therapy and collect the microbiological samples as soon as possible thereafter. The most commonly isolated organisms from infected DFUs are *Staphylococcus aureus*, 44%, of which 8% are methicillin-resistant *S. aureus* (MRSA), Streptococci (17%) and Enterococci (15%) [13]. The choice and the route of antibiotic administration depend on the severity of infection (Box 16f.3), previous microbiology results, previous antibiotic use and local antibiotic policy [1, 14]:

Box 16f.3: Assessment of Severity of Diabetic Foot Infection

Mild infection

Localised infection involving only skin and subcutaneous tissue. Erythema is <0.5–2.0 cm around the ulcer (exclude other causes of inflammatory response such as trauma, gout, acute Charcot neuro-arthropathy, fracture, thrombosis or venous stasis).

Moderate infection

Localised infection with erythema >2.0 cm around the ulcer or involving structures deeper than skin and subcutaneous tissues (such as abscess, osteomyelitis, septic arthritis or fasciitis), and no systemic inflammatory response signs.

Severe infection

Local infection with signs of systemic inflammatory response (such as temperature of > 38°C or < 36°C, tachycardia or tachypnoea).

- If there is a previous history of MRSA, teicoplanin, vancomycin or linezolid is used in place of flucloxacillin.
- Deep-seated infections and abscesses require urgent surgical assessment for debridement and/or drainage.
- Duration of antibiotic therapy ranges from seven days for simple infections to six weeks for osteomyelitis (Figure 16f.3).

Ischaemia Relief

If there is critical ischaemia (ABPI <0.5), seek an urgent vascular surgical assessment for vascular imaging and revascularisation. If there is non-critical ischaemia (ABPI 0.5–0.8), seek non-urgent vascular surgical assessment if the ulcers have not healed after four to six weeks of optimal management.

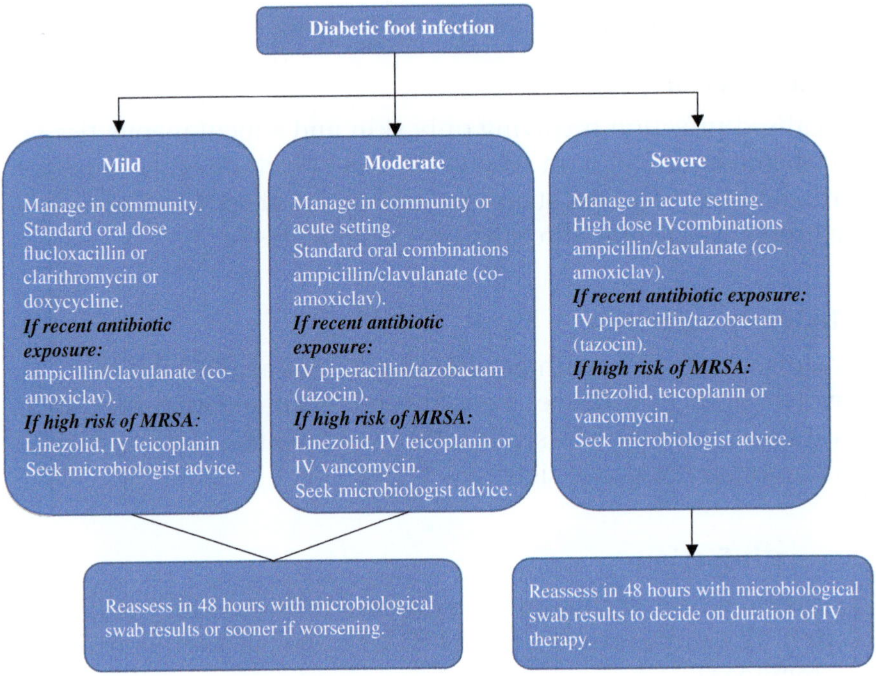

Figure 16f.3: Treatment of diabetic foot infection. IV, intravenous; MRSA, methicillin resistant *Staphylococcus aureus*.

Glycaemic Control

Optimal glycaemic control is essential when treating diabetic foot infection, aiming for capillary blood glucose between 4 and 11 mmol/l. This may require temporary use of insulin therapy if the patient is on oral hypoglycaemic agents. Oral hypoglycaemic agents must be reviewed and altered if necessary (e.g. sodium glucose transporter-2 inhibitors must be stopped temporarily in severe infection because of the risk of diabetic ketoacidosis). Canagliflozin may need to be stopped completely because of its agent-specific slightly increased risk of toe amputations in those 65 years or older with baseline cardiovascular disease [15].

Prevention

Early diagnosis and intervention are key to improved morbidity and reduced mortality from DFU disease. People with diabetes should be given both verbal and written footcare advice at diagnosis to prevent

DFUs. This advice should be reinforced at annual reviews or more frequently if the foot is considered at risk. Footcare advice should include:

- Foot hygiene
- Self-examination of the feet; this can be difficult with increasing age and frailty.
- Footwear should comfortably accommodate the foot.
- Individual risk of DFU, based on risk factors.
- Importance of risk factor reduction.
- Who to contact in an emergency.
- Prompt assessment and treatment of new lesions. People with diabetes must promptly report signs of diabetic foot problems including infection, callus, ulceration and cracked skin. Late presentation of DFU disease is a poor prognostic indicator.
- Regular foot checks-the frequency depends on risk stratification (Table 16f.1).

Summary

Diabetic foot ulcer disease is common in older people with diabetes and the risk increases with increasing age and poor diabetes control. Advice on foot care should be given at diagnosis of diabetes and foot examination should be a fundamental part of diabetes annual reviews. Early detection of diabetic foot disease and timely intervention improve outcomes.

Clinical Practice Question

A 60-year-old woman with insulin-treated type 2 diabetes presents to the emergency department with a painful left foot (see photographs).

She has peripheral neuropathy, ischaemic heart disease and hypertension. Her medications include Humulin® M3 (Eli Lilly, Cambridge, MA) insulin 20 units twice a day, metformin 1 g twice a day, ramipril 5 mg once a day, aspirin 75 mg once a day and bisoprolol 5 mg once a day. On examination, she is apyrexial and haemodynamically stable, with a pulse of 65 bpm and blood pressure 148/72 mmHg. Initial blood tests show white blood cell count 10.7 (reference range 5.0–10.0), C-reactive protein 200 mg/l (reference range < 5 mg/l), creatinine 200 μmol/l

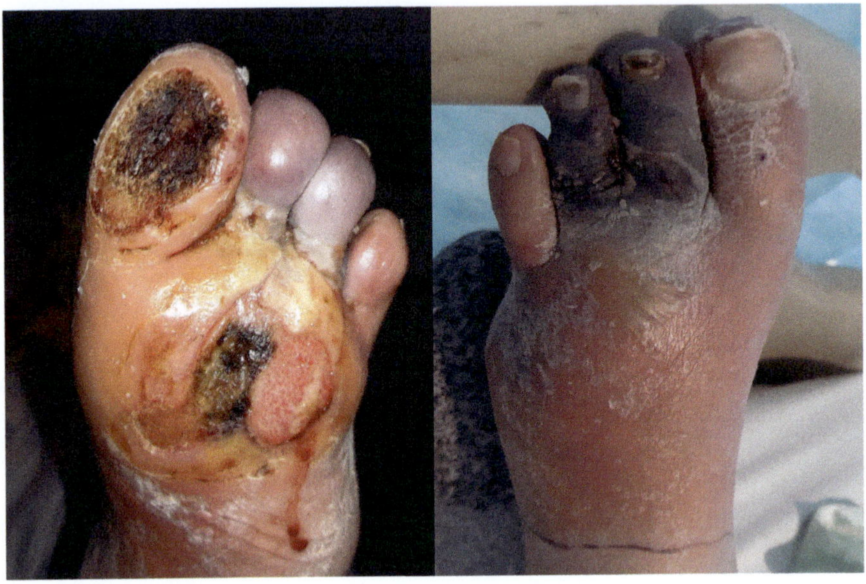

(her baseline creatinine is 78 μmol/l), estimated glomerular filtration rate 25 ml/minute/1.73 m^2, venous plasma glucose 28 mmol/l. Her haemoglobin A1c was 80 mmol/mol a week ago.

Q1. Describe four concerning features about this woman's left foot.
Q2. Is this: (A) neuropathic (B) ischaemic or (C) neuroischaemic foot?
Q3. Outline a management plan.
Q4. Why was this woman's foot at high risk even before this acute presentation?

References

Key references only are listed here. For a full list of references visit: `https://www.wiley.com/go/sinclair/1e`.

1. National Institute for Health and Care Excellence (2019). Diabetic Foot Problems: Prevention and Management. NICE Guideline NG19. London: NICE. `www.nice.org.uk/guidance/ng19` (accessed 2 January 2024).
2. Keer, M., Rayman, G., and Jeffcoate, W.J. (2014). Cost of diabetic foot disease to the National Health Service in England. *Diabet. Med.* 31: 1498–1504.

3. Moulik, P.K., Mtonga, R., and Gill, G.V. (2003). Amputation and mortality in new-onset diabetic foot ulcers stratified by etiology. *Diabetes Care* 26: 491–494.
4. McDermott, K., Fang, M., Boulton, A.J.M. et al. (2023). Etiology, epidemiology and disparities in the burden of diabetic foot ulcers. *Diabetes Care* 46: 209–221.
5. Armstrong, D.G., Boulton, A.J.M., and Bus, S.A. (2017). Diabetic foot ulcers and their prevalence. *N. Engl. J. Med.* 376: 2367–2375.
7. Ahmed, M.U., Tannous, W.K., Agho, K.E. et al. (2022). The burden of diabetes-related foot disease among older adults in Australia. *Int. Wound J.* 19: 1758–1768.
8. Weyand, C.M. and Goronzy, J.J. (2016). Aging of the immune system. Mechanisms and therapeutic targets. *Ann. Am. Thorac. Soc.* 13 (Suppl 5): S422–S428.
9. Morley, J.E. (2012). Sarcopenia in the elderly. *Fam. Pract.* 29 (Suppl 1): i44–i48.
10. Izzo, A., Massimino, E., Riccardi, G. et al. (2021). A narrative review of sarcopenia in type 2 diabetes mellitus: prevalence and associated factors. *Nutrients* 13: 183–201.
14. Schaper, N.C., van Netten, J.J., Apelqvist, J. et al. (2023). Practical guidelines on the prevention and management of diabetes-related foot disease: IWGDF 2023 update. Diabetes Metab. Res. Rev. 40: e3657.

16g Special Issues in Old Age: Skin Care

Grace Keegan and Sarah Mahmoud

Dermatology Department, Rotherham General Hospital, Rotherham, UK

Key Points

- Ageing is associated with dermatological changes that increase the risk of multiple skin pathological conditions.
- Diabetes is associated with significant skin complications, especially in older people.
- Good glycaemic control, education of patients and carers, and regular skin inspection are key to maintaining skin hygiene and preventing diabetes-related skin complications.

Introduction

The prevalence of diabetes is shifting towards old age and is likely to further increase due to increased life expectancy. Skin care is particularly important in older people with diabetes, because of the increased risk of infection and potential complications if untreated, as well as the possible adverse effects of hypoglycaemic medications. In addition, ageing has a large variety of effects on the skin due to loss of collagen and elastin fibres [1]. These degenerative changes in the skin result in a loss of support for the vasculature and lead to increased susceptibility of pressure ulcers and stasis dermatitis [2]. This chapter reviews age-related skin changes, common dermatological conditions in diabetes and their management in old age.

Care of Older People with Diabetes: A Manual for Healthcare Practice, First Edition.
Edited by Alan J. Sinclair and Ahmed H. Abdelhafiz.

Companion website: www.wiley.com/go/sinclair/1e

Age-related Skin Changes

Ageing is associated with skin changes such as thinning of the epidermis, increased dermal vascularity and reduced number of sweat glands. In addition, immune defence characteristics of the skin decline with increasing age. These changes will have significant clinical effects exposing older people to minor trauma, bruising, dehydration and increased risk of skin cancer (Table 16g.1).

Diabetes Mellitus-related Skin Conditions

Several dermatological conditions are common in people with diabetes than in the general population. For example, non-specific conditions such as xerosis, eruptive xanthomas, pruritis, keratosis pilaris

Table 16g.1: Clinical effects of ageing on the skin.

Ageing-related changes	Clinical effects
Thinning of the epidermis with increased vulnerability to trauma	Increased risk of skin tears
Flattening of the dermal papillae and increased risk of blister formation	Increased susceptibility to skin infection
Increased dermal vascularity and susceptibility to vascular damage	Skin more prone to bruising
Reduced thermoregulatory ability of the skin	Increased susceptibility to hypothermia or heat stroke
Decreased inflammatory response and production of cytokines	Impaired immune function and wound healing
Impaired neurological response and reduced sensation	Increased risk of thermal injury
Thinning of the skin and loss of cushioning and support	Increased risk of pressure damage
Atrophy of sweat gland with reduced sweat production and reduced lipids in the stratum corneum	Decreases the ability of the skin to retain water, leading to dry skin
Decreased melanocytes with greater susceptibility to solar radiation	Reduced ability to tan and increased risk of cutaneous neoplasms

and pigmented purpuric dermatoses are commonly associated with diabetes. Diabetes is also strongly associated with specific primary skin conditions, diabetes-related skin infections and diabetes medications-related adverse skin effects.

Primary Skin Conditions

Acanthosis Nigricans

Acanthosis nigricans is a velvety darkening of the skin that often appears in flexural areas such as the axilla, neck creases, under the breasts and in the groin creases. Diabetes and insulin resistance are commonly associated with acanthosis nigricans, but it can also rarely indicate a malignancy. Presentation is often asymptomatic, but the affected skin may be itchy, may have an odour and may develop skin tags. There is no specific treatment available, but good blood glucose control may improve symptoms (Figure 16g.1).

Necrobiosis Lipoidica

Necrobiosis lipoidica is a rare complication of collagen degeneration. It is more common in type 1 diabetes mellitus (T1DM) and presents as a dull red papule or a plaque, often on the shins. It can rarely appear elsewhere on the body, such as on the upper legs, hands, arms, torso, face or scalp. This slowly enlarges into one or more yellowish brown patches with a red rim. It can resolve spontaneously but can be complicated by infection, scarring or ulceration. Treatments include oral, topical or intralesional administration of corticosteroids, antimalarial drugs, ultraviolet radiation, laser therapy and immunotherapy to surgical removal with skin grafting (Figure 16g.2).

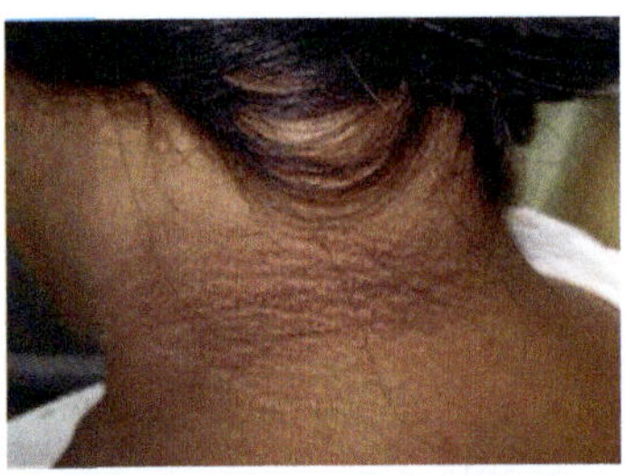

Figure 16g.1: Acanthosis nigricans.

Source: image licence: DermNet (http://dermnetnz.org).

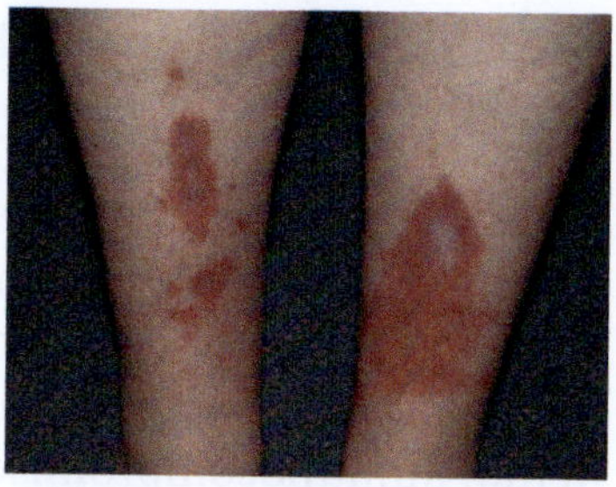

Figure 16g.2: Necrobiosis lipoidica.

Source: image licence: DermNet (http://dermnetnz.org).

Diabetic Dermopathy

Diabetic dermopathy is harmless shin spots, which can affect up to 33% of patients with T1DM and 39% of patients with type 2 diabetes mellitus (T2DM). These lesions present as small and well-demarcated brown atrophic macules or papules on the pretibial area. Lesions heal within one to two years without treatment, leaving atrophic hypopigmented areas [3] (Figure 16g.3).

Bullous Eruption of Diabetes Mellitus

Bullous eruption of diabetes mellitus is also known as bullous diabeticorum. It is recurrent spontaneous blisters developing on the extremities of patients with long-standing diabetes mellitus associated with peripheral neuropathy. The bullae are usually asymptomatic and heal slowly without scar formation in few weeks (Figure 16g.4).

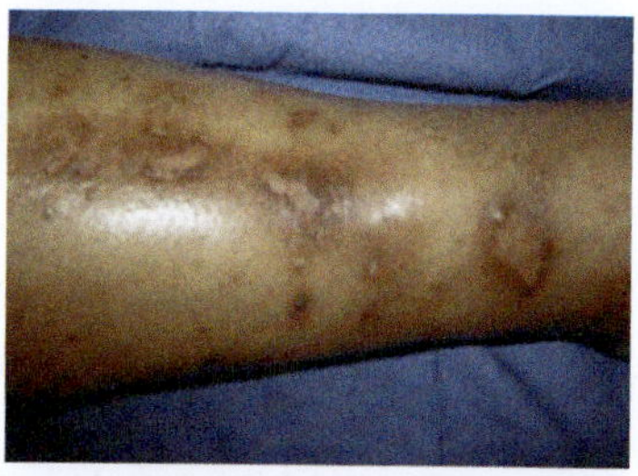

Figure 16g.3: Diabetic dermopathy.

Source: image licence: DermNet (http://dermnetnz.org).

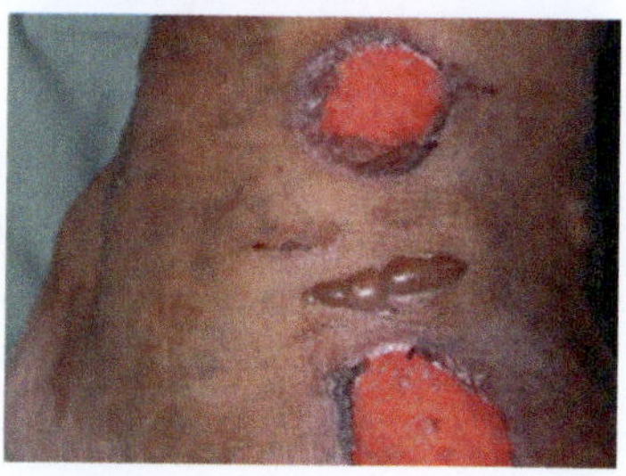

Figure 16g.4: Bullous eruption of diabetes.

Source: image licence: DermNet (http://dermnetnz.org).

Diabetes-related Skin Infections

Bacterial Infections

Bacterial infections in older people with diabetes can sometimes go unnoticed. If there is any concern about skin infection, it is important to seek prompt medical attention, as antibiotics may be urgently needed to avoid spread of infection and the development of sepsis especially in frail immunocompromised individuals (Figure 16g.5). Signs to look for are summarised in Box 16g.1.

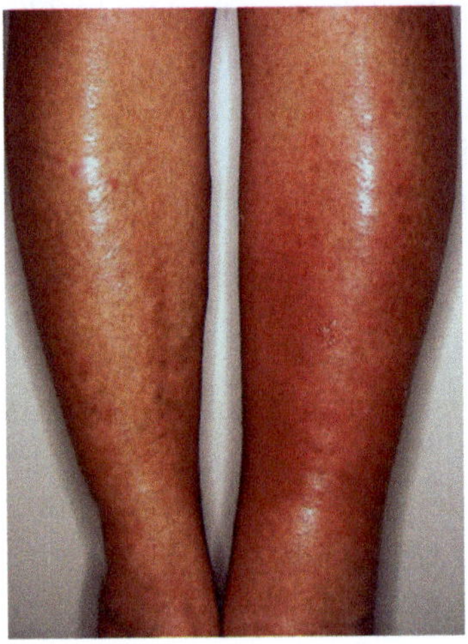

Figure 16g.5: Cellulitis of left leg.

Source: image licence: DermNet (http://dermnetnz.org).

Box 16g.1: Signs to Look for When Assessing a Patient's Skin for Infection

- Redness of the skin.
- The area of skin is hot to touch.
- Pain around the inflamed area. It is important to remember that older people with diabetes may have reduced sensation, so pain may be absent, particularly in the extremities such as feet and lower legs.
- There may be odour or discharge coming from the infected area, particularly if there is a break in the skin.
- Patients who are systemically unwell may also have fever, nausea, vomiting or rigors.
- In severe infections, blisters or bullae may form.

Fungal Infections

The most common cause of fungal infection in older people with diabetes is candida. This type of fungal infection most commonly affects the oral mucosa, skin and genital area. Depending on the area affected, the appearance can differ. To try to prevent fungal infections developing in this at-risk group of patients, it is important to maintain good hygiene practices and make every attempt to avoid moisture damage. If a fungal skin infection is suspected, the patient should seek medical attention. If the patient is systemically unwell because of their infection, they may need hospital admission for further assessment and management. General advice to avoid skin infection is summarised in Box 16g.2.

Box 16g.2: General Advice to Prevent Skin Infection

- Education and awareness: patient and carer education are key in helping to prevent infections developing. Consult patients on the risks of infection and how to identify it and when to seek medical attention.
- Blood glucose control: the patient needs to be involved and well informed about lifestyle and dietary changes and regular monitoring of blood glucose levels. Good blood glucose control is essential to help prevent patients with from developing skin infections.
- Good skin hygiene: it is important to educate patients on the importance of skin hygiene. In patients who are frail and unable to care for themselves, the healthcare team must also be aware of this need. The patient should, preferably, be washed daily and particular attention should be paid to the skin folds, feet and areas prone to the build-up of moisture.
- Moisturising and skin protection: older people with diabetes can often have dry and cracked skin, which is prone to infection. Regular moisturisation can help protect skin from breakdown and therefore infection. It is advisable not to moisturise between the toes as this could lead to fungal infections.

- Oral candida:
  Several mechanisms are linked to higher predisposition of oral candidiasis among older people with diabetes. These include yeast adhesion to epithelial cell surfaces, higher salivary glucose levels, reduced salivary flow, microvascular degeneration and impaired candidacidal activity of neutrophils [4]. Oral candidiasis can present as white or erythematous lesions. White lesions include acute pseudomembranous candidiasis, also known as thrush, which is the most common presentation. Red lesions include angular cheilitis. An antifungal treatment such as nystatin spray may be used. This is sprayed on the affected area in the oral cavity (Figure 16g.6).
- Candidal skin infection:
  Typically presents with soreness and itching. There may also be redness to the skin with small pus-filled lesions (pustules). Scales may accumulate forming a white-yellow curd-like substance on the infected area. If affecting skin folds (candidal intertrigo), infections appear red and moist. Marked skin maceration occurs when fungal infection affects the spaces between the toes. Moreover, multiple studies have reported that *Candida* species are the most common yeast isolated from diabetic foot ulcers [5]. Treatments include topical antifungal creams. If the infection is severe, systemic antifungal therapy may be considered (Figure 16g.7).
- Genital candidiasis:
  Catheters and incontinence, which make the groin, genital and nappy areas prone to moisture, put older people with diabetes at risk. In women, genital candidiasis may present with vulval or vaginal itching and sometimes there may be soreness and irritation. The patient may also complain of a thick white discharge that is different to normal. It is often non-odorous. In men, genital candidiasis can cause balanitis, an inflammation

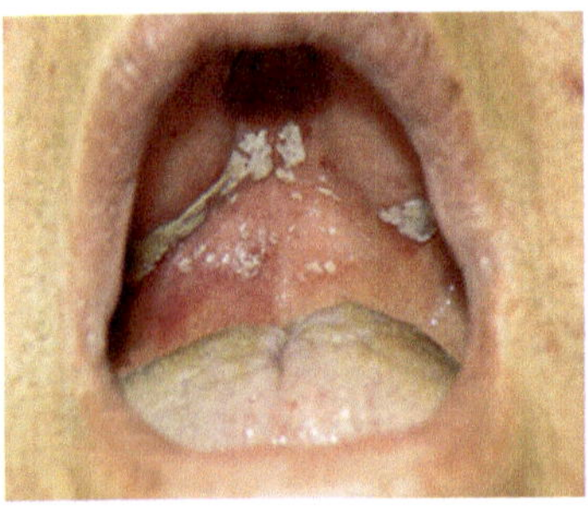

Figure 16g.6: Oral candidiasis.

Source: image licence: DermNet (http://dermnetnz.org).

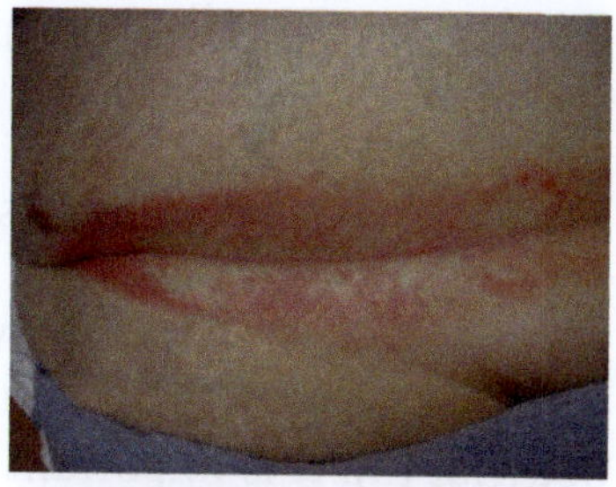

Figure 16g.7: Candida intertrigo.

Source: image licence: DermNet (http://dermnetnz.org).

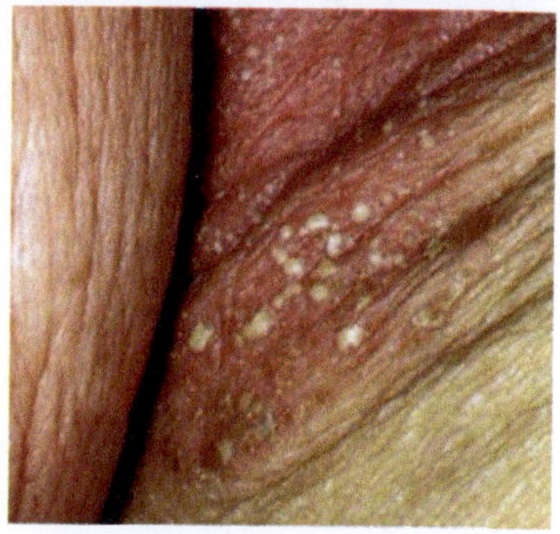

Figure 16g.8: Genital candidiasis.

Source: image licence: DermNet (http://dermnetnz.org).

of the head of the penis. There may be a white, 'cheese-like' discharge. There may also be soreness and itching of the penis or pain and difficulty on passing urine. A range of treatments can be used to treat genital candidiasis, including anti-fungal creams and anti-fungal tablets. In female genital candidiasis, a pessary can be given as an alternative to cream (Figure 16g.8).

- Fungal infection of the nails (onychomycosis):
  Onychomycosis can affect any part of the nail, which may appear discoloured or thickened, with associated pain and discomfort in some individuals. If fungal nail infection is suspected, it is advisable to receive a diagnosis from a medical professional. Management includes antifungal treatment and maintaining good nail hygiene (Figure 16g.9).

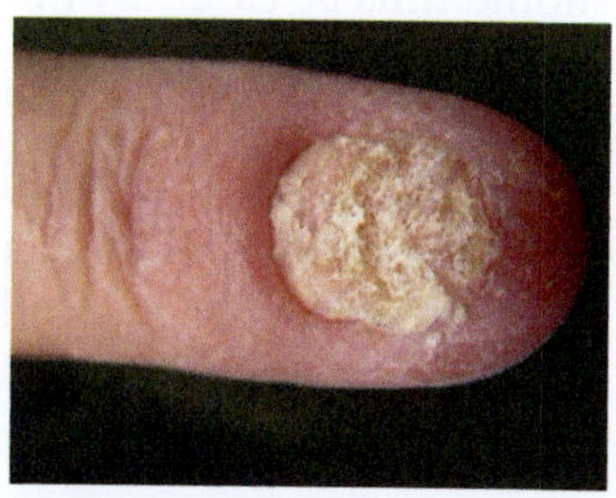

Figure 16g.9: Onychomycosis.

Source: image licence: DermNet (http://dermnetnz.org).

Diabetes Medications-related Skin Adverse Effects

Insulin

Many patients with diabetes may need insulin as part of their medication regimen. It is important to be aware of how insulin may lead to skin changes in some patients. A common adverse effect of subcutaneous insulin injections is lipodystrophy. This is an abnormal distribution of body fat [6]. It is important to recognise lipodystrophy in patients, as repeated injections into affected areas can cause unexplained episodes of hypoglycaemia and therefore inappropriate dosing of insulin. Rotating insulin injection sites and ensuring that the correct injection technique is being used may aid in avoiding the occurrence of lipodystrophy. Rotation from one abdominal quarter to the next on a weekly basis is suggested. There are two types of lipodystrophy: lipohypertrophy and lipoatrophy.

- Lipohypertrophy presents as a soft, fatty lumps under the skin and affects 25–30% of patients with T1DM and less than 5% of patients with T2DM, appearing at the sites where patients commonly inject insulin (e.g. either side of the umbilicus or front of the thigh) [6]. Risk factors include repeated injections at the same site, higher insulin doses, longer duration of insulin therapy and high body mass index [7].
- In contrast to lipohypertrophy, lipoatrophy presents as areas of fat loss. It is more common in T1DM but can be seen in T2DM as well. Lipoatrophy is regarded as an immunological adverse effect of insulin therapy.

Sodium Glucose Transporter-2 Inhibitors

Sodium glucose transporter-2 inhibitors work by reducing the amount of glucose reabsorbed in the kidneys and excreted in the urine, causing glycosuria. The glucose-rich urine can increase the risk of yeast infections, genital and urinary tract infections. Patients taking these medications should thus be carefully monitored for skin and genital complications.

Summary

Diabetes-related skin complications, particularly infections, are common in older people with diabetes. Good glycaemic control, patients and carer education about skin care and regular inspection and hygiene of the susceptible areas for moisture are key to prevent skin infections.

Clinical Practice Question

Q1. David is an 80-year-old man currently residing in a nursing home. He is bedbound and has type 2 diabetes, which is managed with twice-daily insulin injections and metformin 500 mg twice a day. He has developed a new urinary incontinence. His insulin is administered by the staff at the nursing home. David has very erratic blood glucose control, despite receiving the same amount of insulin each day. He has high blood glucose with unpredictable episodes of hypoglycaemia. What might be the cause of his erratic blood glucose control? What are the most appropriate next steps? Choose as many options as apply:

A. Check for lipodystrophy.
B. Check for regular eating pattern.
C. Reduce insulin dose.
D. Exclude urinary tract infection.
E. Increase metformin to 1 g twice a day.

References

1. Waller, J. and Maibach, H. (2005). Age and skin structure and function, a quantitative approach (I): blood flow, pH, thickness, and ultrasound echogenicity. *Skin Res. Technol.* 11: 221–235.
2. Farage, M.A., Miller, K.W., Berardesca, E. et al. (2009). Clinical implications of aging skin. *Am. J. Clin. Dermatol.* 10: 73–86.
3. Duff, M., Demidova, O., Blackburn, S. et al. (2015). Cutaneous manifestations of diabetes mellitus. *Clin. Diabetes* 33: 40–48.
4. Rodrigues, C.F., Rodrigues, M.E., Henriques, M., and Candida sp. (2019). infections in patients with diabetes mellitus. *J. Clin. Med.* 8: 76.
5. Rasoulpoor, S., Shohaimi, S., Salari, N. et al. (2021). Candida albicans skin infection in patients with type 2 diabetes: a systematic review and meta-analysis. *J. Diabetes Metab. Disord.* 20: 665–672.
6. Kadiyala, P., Walton, S., and Sathyapalan, T. (2014). Insulin induced lipodystrophy. *Br. J. Diabetes Vasc. Dis.* 14: 131–133.
7. Ucieklak, D., Mrozinska, S., Wojnarska, A. et al. (2022). Insulin-induced Lipohypertrophy in patients with type 1 diabetes mellitus treated with an insulin pump. *Int. J. Endocrinol.* 2022: 9169296.

16h Special Issues in Old Age: Falls and Bone Health

Nandkishor V. Athavale

Department of Geriatric Medicine, Rotherham General Hospital, Rotherham, UK

Key Points

- Diabetes is a multisystem disorder with significant effects on the musculoskeletal system.
- Falls and fractures are major health issues in older people with diabetes.
- There are many pathophysiological processes leading to increased risk of falls and fractures in older people with diabetes.
- A thorough risk assessment should be carried out using approved risk assessment tools such as the Fracture Risk Assessment Tool.
- Effective evidence-based interventions are available to reduce the risk of fractures and falls in this population.

Introduction

Diabetes is primarily a condition causing hyperglycaemia and is associated with micro- and macrovascular complications. In addition, it has wider effects on other systems such as the musculoskeletal system. For example, diabetes is associated with increased risk of frailty and sarcopenia [1]. These diabetes-related complications increase the risk of falls and fractures, which is now increasingly recognised. These increased diabetes-associated falls and fractures will have a profound effect on morbidity, quality of life and mortality. It is therefore essential

Care of Older People with Diabetes: A Manual for Healthcare Practice, First Edition.
Edited by Alan J. Sinclair and Ahmed H. Abdelhafiz.

Companion website: www.wiley.com/go/sinclair/1e

to risk assess older people with diabetes for falls and fractures, as there are effective interventions available to reduce this risk. This chapter reviews epidemiology, pathogenesis, risk assessment and management of falls and bone health in older people with diabetes.

Epidemiology

Globally, falls are a major public health issue. It is estimated that 30% of adults above the age of 60 years fall every year, with the incidence increasing with increasing age [2]. There is growing evidence from epidemiological studies to suggest that diabetes increases the risk of falls. For example, in the Women's Health and Ageing Study, older women with diabetes had higher risk of any fall (odds ratio [OR] 1.38, 95% confidence interval [CI] 1.04–1.81) and of falling two or more times during the follow-up period (OR 1.69, CI 1.18–2.43) [3]. Another population-based study showed the incidence of falls to be 39% in older people (> 65 years of age) with diabetes, occurring more frequently in those with poor diabetes control (risk ratio [RR] 7.83) [4]. A meta-analysis of 14 685 participants also showed an increased risk of falls with diabetes (RR 1.64, 95% CI 1.27–2.11). The falls were more common in insulin-treated patients [5]. Diabetes also affects multiple aspects of bone metabolism including bone formation, bone resorption and collagen cross-linking, a complication recognised as diabetic osteopathy [6]. The impact of type 1 diabetes (T1DM) on bone health is well known. Although bone mineral density (BMD) is normal or even higher in type 2 diabetes mellitus (T2DM), these patients are also at increased risk of fractures. The risk of hip fracture is estimated to increase sevenfold in T1DM and 1.3-fold in T2DM [7]. The Health, Ageing and Body Composition Study reported increase in fractures of all sites by 64% in people with compared with those without diabetes [8].

Pathophysiology of Fracture Risk in Diabetes

Over past three decades, considerable work has been undertaken to understand the effects of diabetes on bone health. In T1DM, insulin deficiency is recognised as a key factor influencing bone health. Normally, insulin has anabolic effects and works through insulin receptor substrates 1 and 2, stimulating osteoblast proliferation and collagen synthesis. In T1DM, deficiency of insulin and insulin-like growth factor 1 leads to impaired bone formation and mineralisation, leading to increased fragility [6]. In T2DM, BMD can be normal or higher. Therefore, in T2DM, there are other mechanisms independent of BMD affecting bone health. Insulin resistance in T2DM leads to interference with insulin signalling in osteoblasts, which impacts bone quality and bone mass [9]. Prolonged hyperglycaemia has negative effect on osteoblastogenesis by inhibiting the differentiation of mesenchymal stem cells into osteoblasts and by stimulating adipogenesis. It also increases osteoblast apoptosis. The Wnt signalling pathways are a group of signal transducers that begin with proteins that pass signals into the cell through cell surface receptors, which can be negatively affected by hyperglycaemia, thus reducing bone formation. Formation of advanced glycation end-products (AGE) stimulates bone resorption by osteoclasts. AGE cross-links in collagen have a negative impact on bone quality and bone strength by making it more brittle.

The chronic inflammation associated with diabetes promotes osteoclast activity leading to bone resorption. Diabetes-associated vitamin D deficiency affects bone mineralisation and hyperglycaemia causes increased urinary calcium excretion, which may also reduce bone mineralisation. Progressive renal impairment in diabetes may lead to secondary hyperparathyroidism, which affects bone integrity. Finally, certain hypoglycaemic medications, such as thiazolidinediones, may reduce bone density and increase the risk of fractures by stimulation bone resorption [9, 10].

Pathophysiology and Risk Factors for Falls in Diabetes

The presence of diabetic complications partly explains the increased falls risk in diabetes. For example, peripheral neuropathy, which is quite common in diabetes, causes postural instability, reduced mobility and reduced reaction time, leading to increased risk of falls. Diabetes also causes sarcopenia with decreased muscle mass and fibre size predisposing to falls [11]. Other diabetic complications such as retinopathy causing poor vision and reduced renal function, especially patients on dialysis who are frail with multiple morbidities, have been independently associated with risk of falling. Autonomic neuropathy associated with diabetes can cause postural hypotension and also contributes to

Box 16h.1: Pathophysiology and Risk Factors for Fractures and Falls

- Age
- Insulin resistance
- Hypoglycaemia
- Hypoglycaemia unawareness
- Persistent hyperglycaemia
- Formation of advanced glycaemic end products
- Chronic inflammation
- Chronic complications such as neuropathy and retinopathy
- Gait and balance impairment
- Previous falls
- Muscle weakness and sarcopenia
- Orthostatic hypotension
- Impaired calcium and vitamin D metabolism
- Antidiabetic drugs such as thiazolidinediones
- Associated comorbidities like stroke
- Polypharmacy

falls. Higher risk is associated with increased duration of diabetes as incidence of diabetes-related complications such as neuropathy, retinopathy and renal impairment increase with increased duration of diabetes. Hypoglycaemia is another determinant of risk. Tight diabetes control has been shown to increase the risk of falls, especially when treated with insulin [12]. Polypharmacy is common in diabetes where, in addition to glucose-lowering medications, patients may be on medications for associated complications and other comorbidities. Four or more medications are associated with increased risk of falls in patients with diabetes. The falls-related risk factors in diabetes are summarised in Box 16h.1.

Assessment of the Risk of Falls in the Community

The evidence-base for the assessment and management of falls has significantly expanded. The main purposes of the assessment are to understand the mechanism of falling, to address the consequences of falling and to identify potential modifiable risk factors [13]. The first step is assessing patient's risk of falls by risk stratification. This can be

Box 16h.2: Falls Risk Stratification

Three key questions:

1. Have you fallen in the past year?
2. Do you feel unsteady when standing or walking?
3. Do you have worries about falling?

Markers of Falls severity

- Injury
- Two or more falls in the past 12 months
- Inability to get up after falling
- Frailty
- Syncope or loss of consciousness

done by asking three key questions followed by assessing the severity of the fall (Box 16h.2). These procedures will help to determine the most appropriate assessment and intervention (Figure 16h.1). The comprehensive geriatric assessment underpins the falls risk assessment. A detailed history of falling includes circumstances, preceding symptoms, frequency, injuries, detailed past medical history, medication history, followed by environmental and functional history. This should be followed-up with a clinical examination with a focus on cardiovascular, musculoskeletal and neurological examination. The assessment is completed by some basic tests including haemogram, basic biochemistry, vitamin D levels, glycaemic control and electrocardiogram. Those patients with a high risk of falling should be offered a multifactorial falls risk assessment including gait, balance, muscle strength, visual and auditory assessment and medication review [14]. (Box 16h.3) High-risk fallers may need further specialist assessment in secondary care, including cardiac investigations and tilt table testing.

Assessment of Bone Health in Community

Although described separately, assessment of bone health and fracture risk goes hand in hand with falls risk assessment. A thorough history of recent and previous fractures, including mechanism of injury and

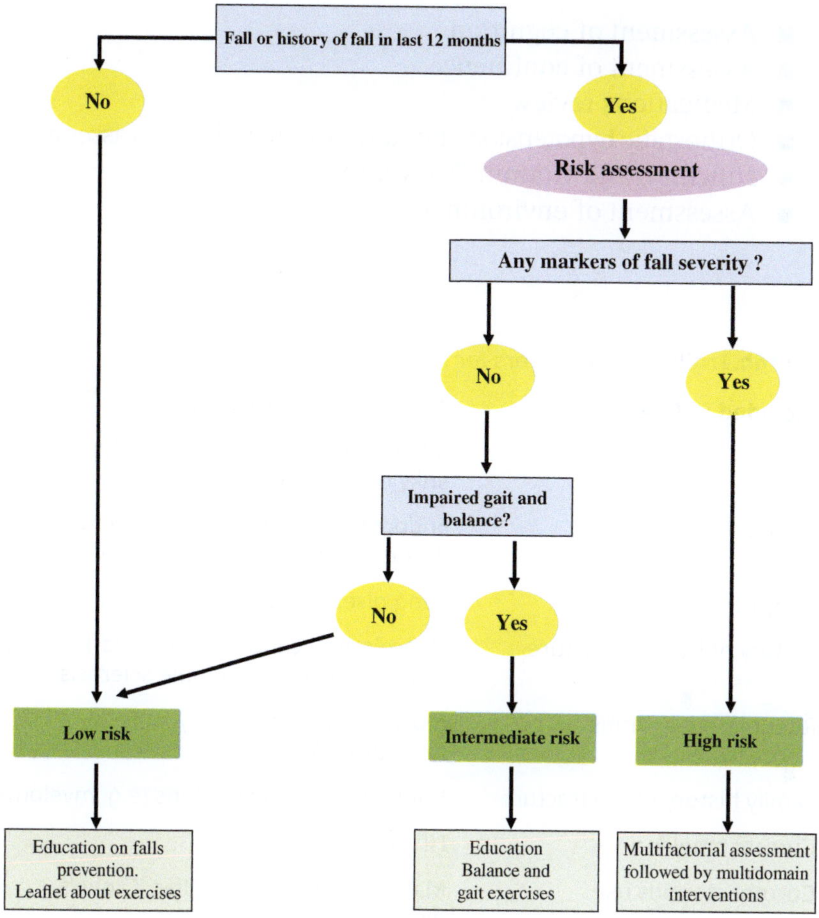

Figure 16h.1: Falls assessment and management algorithm in older people with diabetes-based on world falls guidelines.

Box 16h.3: Components of Multifactorial Falls Assessment

- Thorough history and clinical examination
- Balance assessment (e.g. one-leg stand and tandem stance)
- Gait assessment (e.g. Timed Up and Go)
- Assessment of muscle strength
- Walking aids and footwear assessment
- Vision and hearing assessment
- Assessment of vestibular function
- Assessment of activities of daily living

- Assessment of cognition
- Assessment of continence
- Medications review
- Orthostatic hypotension and cardiovascular diseases assessment
- Nutrition and vitamin D assessment
- Assessment of environment

Table 16h.1: Clinical risk factors for fractures.

Included in FRAX	Additional risk factors
Age	Inflammatory conditions (e.g. lupus or ankylosing spondylitis)
Gender	Endocrine disorders (e.g. Cushing's disease, or hyperparathyroidism)
Body mass index	Lung diseases (e.g. cystic fibrosis or COPD)
History of fragility fracture	Neurological conditions (e.g. Parkinson's disease, stroke or multiple sclerosis)
Rheumatoid arthritis	Muscle diseases (e.g. myositis or myopathies)
Family history of hip fracture	Haematological conditions (e.g. myeloma)
Current smoking	HIV infection
Current steroids use	Malabsorption (e.g. coeliac, Crohn's disease)
Alcohol consumption ≥3 units/day	Falls and frailty
Secondary osteoporosis (e.g. premature menopause and hyperthyroidism)	Medications (e.g. aromatase inhibitors, androgen deprivation therapy and antiepileptics)

COPD, chronic obstructive pulmonary disease; FRAX, Fracture Risk Assessment tool; HIV, human immunodeficiency virus.

history of comorbidities and medications, is essential. It is important to enquire specifically for different risk factors for osteoporosis and fractures as detailed in Table 16h.1. The guidelines recommend risk assessment tools to determine referral to BMD measurement by dual x-ray absorptiometry as well as treatment decision making [15, 16]. Although many tools are available, the Fracture Risk Assessment (FRAX) tool is the most widely used. BMD alone may underestimate the fracture risk in diabetes [6]. The National Osteoporosis Guideline Group has suggested replacing diabetes for rheumatoid arthritis in the FRAX calculations to improve risk stratification [16]. Use of FRAX allows risk stratification to facilitate further investigations and treatment. (Figure 16h.2). A battery of blood tests can be used to look for secondary causes of osteoporosis (Box 16h.4). Very high-risk patients should be referred to specialist centre for further assessment and management. Trabecular bone score can be measured to assess bone quality. It is correlated to trabecular number and disposition. High-resolution peripheral qualitative computed tomography is another tool for bone quality assessment but is not yet widely available in clinical practice.

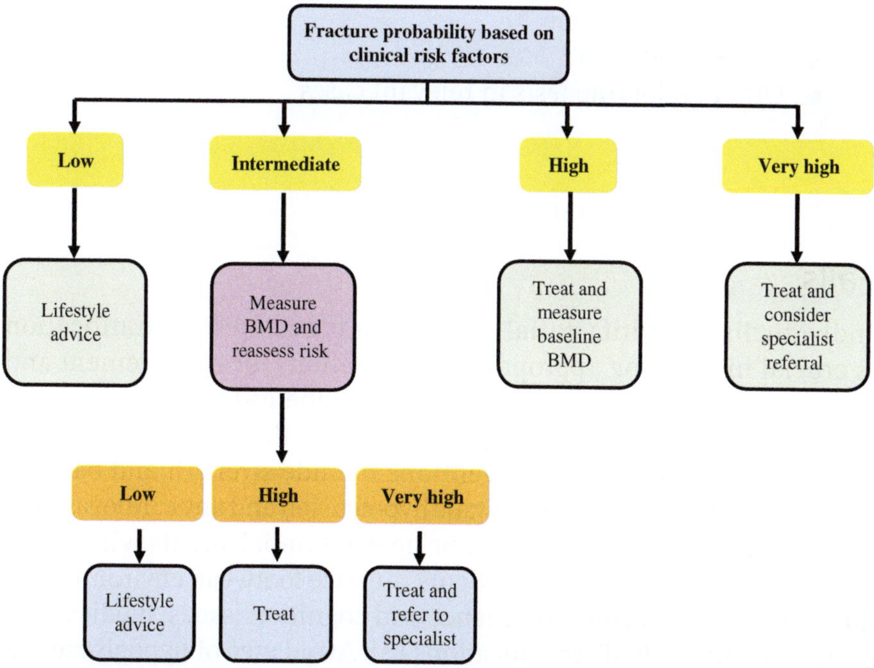

Figure 16h.2: Fracture risk assessment algorithm in older people with diabetes-based on national osteoporosis guideline group. BMD, bone mineral density.

Box 16h.4: Metabolic Screen Blood Tests for Osteoporosis

Baseline tests:

- Full blood count
- Erythrocyte sedimentation rate
- Renal profile
- Liver function tests
- Calcium and bone profile including vitamin D
- Thyroid function tests
- Plasma glucose/haemoglobin A1c

Additional tests:

- Plasma parathyroid levels
- Magnesium
- Coeliac screen
- Myeloma screen
- Serum testosterone
- Urinary calcium
- Other endocrine tests in relevant cases

Management and Prevention

Falls

Individualised multifactorial assessment based on risk stratification is crucial in deciding appropriate interventions for management and prevention of falls in older people with diabetes [13]. Multidomain interventions are designed and targeted to the findings from the multifactor assessment. Interventions include strength and balance exercises, management of orthostatic hypotension and any cardiovascular causes, correction of any visual or hearing impairments, vitamin D supplementation in deficient patients, suitable footwear, environmental adjustments, addressing continence and cognition issues, medications review and individualised education [13]. Avoidance of hypoglycaemia and establishing individualised target for glycaemic control are important. There are a few studies looking into falls prevention in older diabetic people. One review showed that exercise to improve balance, strength and mobility, health education and diabetes self-management is a useful intervention in older people with diabetes [17].

Fractures

Risk assessment including FRAX and BMD measurement allows individualising bone health management for patients. Lifestyle measures are the cornerstone to healthy bones. These include adequate calcium intake, healthy balanced diet, regular weight-bearing exercises, optimum vitamin D intake, reduced alcohol consumption, smoking cessation and falls risk assessment [16]. In high-risk patients, pharmacological interventions can be used. First-line medications are antiresorptive agents such as oral or intravenous bisphosphonates. Alternatives such as raloxifene, denosumab or strontium can be used. In very high-risk patients, anabolic treatments like teriparatide or romosozumab are recommended [16].

Summary

With increasing age, the risk of falls and fractures increases. Diabetes mellitus and the associated complications further increase this risk. Diabetes-related falls are multifactorial and need detailed assessment. Standardised risk assessment tools are available and should be used for every patient presenting with a fall. Intervention and prevention plans, tailored to individual needs, will help reduce the risk of future falls and fractures.

Clinical Practice Question

Q1. A 78-year-old woman with history of type 2 diabetes and dementia, who managed well alone at home, was found on the floor by her son. She had no injuries except a bruise on her left knee. She is on metformin 1 g twice a day, gliclazide 80 mg twice a day, donepezil 5 mg once a day and co-codamol (30/500 mg) two tablets four times a day. She had sustained right wrist fracture two years ago. What would be the best course of action?

Choose one option:

A. Assure her and son and send home, as no injuries were sustained.
B. Admit her to hospital for further assessment.
C. Check blood glucose, lying and standing blood pressure, take history of risk factors, carry out clinical examination and carry out a risk assessment using the Fracture Risk Assessment tool.
D. Prescribe calcium and vitamin D supplements.
E. Start alendronic acid for her recent fracture.

References

Key references only are listed here. For a full list of references visit: https://www.wiley.com/go/sinclair/1e.

2. Ganz, D.A. and Latham, N.K. (2020). Prevention of falls in community dwelling older adults. *N. Engl. J. Med.* 382: 734–743.
5. Yang, Y., Hu, X., Zhang, Q. et al. (2016). Diabetes mellitus and risk of falls in older adults: a systematic review and meta-analysis. *Age Ageing* 45: 761–767.
6. Jackuliak, P. and Payer, J. (2014). Osteoporosis, fractures, and diabetes. *Int. J. Endocrinol.* 2014: 820615.
7. Starup-Linde, J., Frost, M., Vestergaard, P. et al. (2016). Epidemiology of fractures in diabetes. *Calcif. Tissue Int.* 100: 109–121.
8. Strotmeyer, E.S., Cauley, J.A., Schwartz, A.V. et al. (2005). Nontraumatic fracture risk with diabetes mellitus and impaired fasting glucose in older white and black adults: the health, aging, and body composition study. *Arch. Intern. Med.* 165: 1612–1617.
10. Zhu, Z.N., Jiang, Y.F., and Ding, T. (2014). Risk of fractures with thiazolidinediones: an updated meta-analysis of randomised controlled trials. *Bone* 68: 115–123.
13. Montero-Odasso, M., Van der Velde, N., Martin, F.C. et al. (2022). World guidelines for falls prevention and management for older adults: a global initiative. *Age Ageing* 51: afac205.
14. National Institute for Health and Care Excellence (2019). 2019 Surveillance of Falls in Older People: Assessing Risk and Prevention (NICE guideline CG161). London: NICE.
15. National Institute for Health and Care Excellence (2019). 2019 Surveillance of Osteoporosis: Assessing the Risk of Fragility Fracture (NICE guideline CG146). London: NICE.
16. National Osteoporosis Guideline Group. Clinical Guideline for the Prevention and Treatment of Osteoporosis. https://www.nogg.org.uk/full-guideline.

16i Special Issues in Old Age: Avoiding Hospitalisation

Demelza Emmerton and
Ahmed H. Abdelhafiz

Department of Geriatric Medicine, Rotherham General Hospital, Rotherham, UK

Key Points

- Older people with diabetes are at a higher risk of hospitalisation compared with younger people.
- Risk of hospitalisation increases with increasing age, longer duration of diabetes, multiple morbidities and polypharmacy.
- Comprehensive geriatric assessment is a key for a holistic care that may help reduce the risk of hospitalisation.
- Patient and healthcare system-centred interventions are required to avoid hospitalisations.
- Telemedicine and mobile applications are potential future interventions that may help to improve care and avoid hospitalisation of older people with diabetes.

Introduction

Acute decompensation, which leads to hospitalisation, is threefold higher in older (≥ 65 years) compared with younger (< 45 years) people with diabetes [1]. About 30% of hospitalised patients already have a diagnosis of diabetes and an additional 10% are newly diagnosed during the admission [2]. Hospitalised older people with diabetes are less likely to be discharged home, but frequently need transitional care admission for rehabilitation or permanent institutionalisation, which increases the

Care of Older People with Diabetes: A Manual for Healthcare Practice, First Edition.
Edited by Alan J. Sinclair and Ahmed H. Abdelhafiz.

Companion website: www.wiley.com/go/sinclair/1e

burden on healthcare systems [3]. Optimising the care for older people in the community and care-home settings may therefore reduce acute decompensation and hospitalisation. This chapter reviews risk factors for hospitalisation, investigates relevant aspects for optimising care and explores ways of reducing hospitalisation of older people with diabetes.

Risk Factors for Hospitalisation

Multiple morbidities associated with diabetes in older people may lead to avoidable hospital admissions. For example, ambulatory care-sensitive conditions, defined as conditions which could have been treated in outpatient setting, resulted in about 7% of avoidable hospital admissions [4]. Diabetes-associated chronic morbidities and acute infections were responsible for one fifth of potentially preventable hospital admissions that could have been dealt with in a community setting [5]. Acute metabolic decompensation, particularly hypoglycaemia, is a common cause of admission in older (≥ 65 years) compared with younger (< 65 years) people [6]. The very old (≥ 80 years) are more susceptible (3.5 times higher) to hypoglycaemia-related hospitalisations caused by unintentional overdose of insulin or oral hypoglycaemic agents compared with those 65–69 years [7]. Reduced community care, social isolation and deficits in social attachments leading to social vulnerability may increase the risk of acute complications and hospitalisation (Box 16i.1) [8].

Box 16i.1: Risk Factors for Hospitalisations in Older People with Diabetes

- Increasing age
- Long duration of diabetes
- Ambulatory care-sensitive conditions
- Multiple morbidities
- Frailty
- Acute infections
- Hypoglycaemia
- Falls
- Fractures
- Reduced physical function
- Reduced cognitive function
- Depression

- Anxiety
- Poor activities of daily living performance
- Poor self-rated health
- Reduced compliance with medications
- Reduced compliance with self-care tasks
- Poor glycaemic control
- Institutionalisation
- Social vulnerability
- Polypharmacy
- Medication errors
- Poor oral intake
- Erratic eating pattern

Avoiding Hospitalisation

Intervention to avoid hospitalisation could directly target patient care or be directed to improving the operation of the healthcare system (Figure 16i.1).

Patient-Related Interventions

Physical Function

All older people with diabetes should have a comprehensive geriatric assessment when they are first diagnosed and regularly thereafter. Patients with a history of falls should be assessed for their gait and balance. The 'get-up-and-go' test is a simple way to diagnose mobility problems. The patient is asked to stand up and walk for 3 metres then turn round, walk back to the chair and sit down. If they take longer than 30 seconds, impaired mobility is diagnosed and referral to an exercise training programme should be made.

Targeted training exercises that include balance and gait improve joint mobility and gait speed. In addition to exercise, nutrition should be part of regular assessment to help reduce muscle mass loss, delay frailty and prevent disability. The combination of resistance training and protein supplementation has been shown to reduce fat mass and to improve lean muscle mass and strength in frail older people than

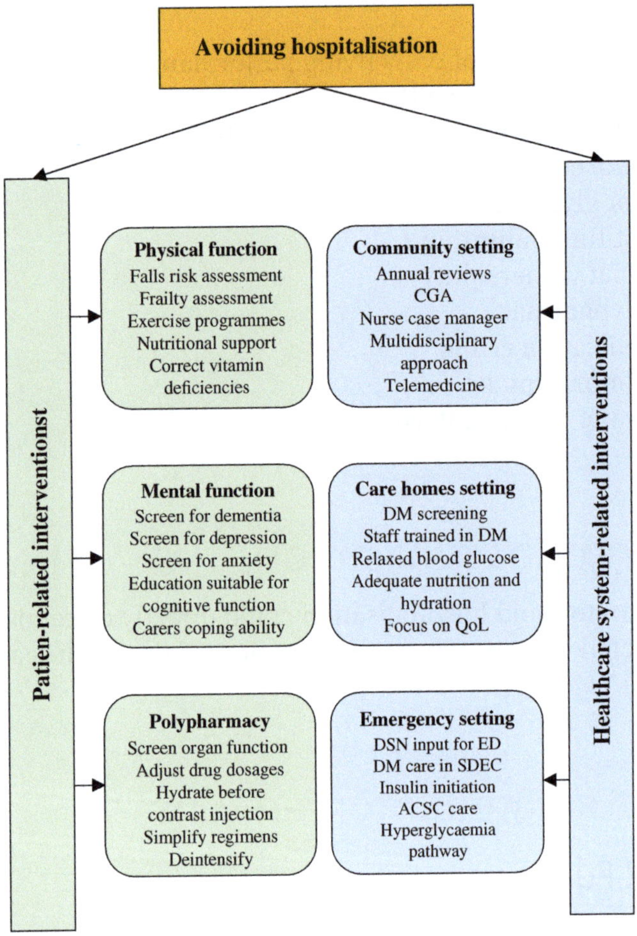

Figure 16i.1: Patient-related and health care system-related interventions to avoid hospitalisation of older people with diabetes. ACSC, ambulatory care-sensitive conditions; CGA, comprehensive geriatric assessment; DM, diabetes mellitus; DSN, diabetes specialist nurse; ED, emergency department; QoL, quality of life; SDEC, same-day emergency care.

exercise alone [9]. In addition, vitamin B_{12} deficiency has been shown in older people with diabetes, especially those taking metformin, which may be associated with neurological disorders, muscle weakness, recurrent falls and increased risk of frailty [10]. Vitamin D supplementation may increase muscle strength and reduce the frequency of falls especially in older people with low vitamin D levels [11].

Mental Function

Cognitive decline may be associated with erratic eating pattern, less compliance with hypoglycaemic medications, which needs close observation by carers to avoid acute glycaemic fluctuations and decompensation. Similarly, the coexistence of depression with diabetes increases healthcare use, costs and adverse outcomes. Depression decreases physical activity leading to, less compliance with self-care tasks, increased risk of functional disability and healthcare service use. The recurrence of unexplained acute glycaemic fluctuations, new difficulties in handling insulin injections, forgetfulness of insulin doses, erratic eating pattern or unexplained non-compliance with self-care should alert physicians to screen for cognitive impairment and depression and plan early interventions.

The FINGER (Finnish Geriatric Intervention Study to Prevent Cognitive Impairment and Disability) study has demonstrated a beneficial effect of exercise and nutrition on cognitive function in older people with diabetes [12]. Similarly, in the Look AHEAD (Action for Health in Diabetes) study, intensive lifestyle interventions significantly reduced the incidence of depressive symptoms (hazard ratio 0.85, 95% confidence interval 0.75–0.97, $p = 0.02$) and preserved better function in the intervention group ($p < 0.01$) [13]. Care plans should be adjusted to reflect the patient's dynamic mental abilities. More regular assessments and regular review of medications are required to avoid unnecessary adverse effects and hospital visits. In addition, carers themselves should be regularly assessed for their ability to care for patient as well as for their own health.

Polypharmacy

Owing to the increased number of diabetes-associated comorbidities and complications, older people are likely to take many medications, with an increased risk of drug interactions and adverse effects that lead to hospital admission. For example, antihypertensive medications may cause postural hypotension, falls and fractures or acute kidney injury. Monitoring of kidney function is thus required. Reduction of blood pressure should be gradual, with close monitoring of both lying and standing blood pressures and regular inquiry about postural symptoms.

With close monitoring of blood pressure, antihypertensive medications can be reduced if blood pressure remains controlled on lower therapy.

Agents associated with increased risk of acute kidney injury, such as nonsteroidal anti-inflammatory drugs, should be used carefully and only for short periods if possible, and contrast agents should only be used only in well-hydrated patients with close monitoring of renal function. With increasing age and development of organ dysfunction, clearance of hypoglycaemic agents will diminish, which may lead to hypoglycaemic episodes, especially in malnourished and frail patients. Therefore, regular review of the need of hypoglycaemic therapy and deintensification or complete withdrawal of these agents in patients with severe weight loss and malnutrition should be considered.

Healthcare System-related Interventions

Community Setting

Development of educational programmes suitable for patients and their carers' abilities and cultural background may help to improve care of diabetes in the community. Annual diabetes reviews that incorporate comprehensive geriatric assessment by general practitioners will help early detection and intervention for a potential cause of diabetes care decompensation. Patients who have already been admitted to hospital will need a discharge summary that includes a problem list and a clear management plan communicated fully to the community care team to prevent hospital readmission. A nurse case manager devoted to diabetes care could ensure efficient general follow-up of patients after hospital discharge. A systematic and a multidisciplinary team approach to care with a focus on providing patients with support to cope with their disease will help to improve outcomes.

Long-term telephone support for disease management and improvement of physical activity and nutrition has been shown to reduce hospitalisations and to improve quality of life of older patients with diabetes living in the community [14]. In addition to conventional community care, future smartphone applications (apps) for diabetes may enhance diabetes self-care in older people. These apps ensure support and close liaison of patients with a trained healthcare professional who is based in an accessible community care setting. Smartphone apps may also provide a management programme that is 'personalised' so that goals of care are intimately linked to clinical needs and functional and comorbid characteristics of the patient.

Care-home Setting

Diabetes is prevalent in at least 25% of care-home residents. Because of the high morbidity burden, especially frailty, cognitive impairment and reduced life expectancy of residents in care homes, less intensive glycaemic control, lower doses of hypoglycaemic agents and simplification of the insulin regimen may reduce treatment errors and risk of hypoglycaemia that could lead to hospitalisation. Owing to the severe frailty and malnutrition prevalent in this population, the choice of long-acting insulin analogues will reduce the risk of hypoglycaemia and so reduce hospitalisation [15]. Patients who have erratic eating patterns and unpredictable caloric intake could be managed with hypoglycaemic medications that have less risk of hypoglycaemia or an insulin regimen where short-acting insulin analogues are administered only after meals, thus preventing insulin-induced hypoglycaemia if a meal is missed or only partly consumed. Maintaining a random blood glucose greater than 5 but less than 15 mmol/l is a reasonable target to avoid extreme blood glucose levels.

Maintenance of exercise and nutrition will help to improve overall function. For these frail patients, aquatic exercise or other exercise modalities such as whole-body electromyostimulation, vibration, yoga and tai chi may have some benefits and can be considered as an alternative to conventional exercise to improve adherence and compliance. In addition to adequate nutrition, hydration should be maintained, due to impaired thirst sensation in this very old population, to avoid risk of volume depletion and hyperglycaemic crises.

Emergency Setting

A dedicated team of healthcare professionals with an interest in diabetes in old age will ensure early specialist input to avoid admission for patients visiting the emergency department, reduce the length of hospital stay and facilitate early discharge of those admitted to hospital [16]. Access to the emergency department for specialist nurse input can avoid the admission of patients presenting with mild acute metabolic decompensation of diabetes and provide early follow up appointments.

The incorporation of same day emergency care and ambulatory care into the emergency department will enable treatment of patients with mild diabetes-related complications and can help to avoid hospitalisation. For example, hyperglycaemia is considered an ambulatory care-sensitive condition, which means that it can potentially be managed by ambulatory emergency care, rather than inpatient care. An ambulatory hyperglycaemia pathway could reduce unnecessary hospital admissions. Multidisciplinary input to these services, which involves, in addition to treatment, education in diabetes self-care, such as preventative foot care and avoiding hypoglycaemia, may reduce future admissions. In addition, these settings can be used for initiation of insulin when required, and education of ways of insulin administration and glucose monitoring instead of hospital admission. Recommendations to reduce hospitalisation are summarised in Box 16i.2.

Box 16i.2: Recommendations for Reducing Hospitalisation of Older People with Diabetes

- Regular patient assessment for risk factors of hospitalisation
- A register of patients at risk with available action plan when required
- Patient-centred care plan
- Clear individualised goals of therapy
- Regular check for susceptibility to infections
- Regularly educational programmes for patients and carers appropriate for cognitive abilities and sensitive to cultural background
- Regular review of patients' ability to administer insulin and monitor glucose levels
- Easy access to community-based diabetes services
- Regular exercise programmes appropriate for patient's physical function
- Regular dietician input, especially for frail people at risk of malnutrition
- Care-home residents should be screened for diabetes on admission and staff trained for diabetes care
- Regular pneumococcal, influenza and herpes zoster vaccination
- Shared care plans between primary and secondary care

- A clear hospital discharge plan with preventative measures well communicated to primary care
- Comprehensive geriatric assessment for all admitted patients with multidisciplinary plans on discharge
- Foot care for all admitted patients and easy access to community podiatry service on discharge
- Screen all admitted patients for frailty with appropriate interventions on discharge

Summary

Many hospitalisations for older people with diabetes are avoidable. Regular addressing of risk factors of hospitalisation with a structured patient and health care system-related interventions will reduce the risk hospitalisation. Future application of telemedicine will further reduce this risk.

Clinical Practice Question

Q1. A 77-year-old woman with type 2 diabetes for 26 years lives alone and is self-caring. She is on Humulin® (Eli Lilly, Basingstoke, UK) insulin I 14 units in the morning and 8 units in the afternoon, together with metformin 1 g twice a day and linagliptin 5 mg once a day. Her diabetes is well controlled: latest haemoglobin A1c 58 mmol/mol. She recently had two visits to the emergency department because of hypoglycaemia and another hospital admission because of hyperglycaemia. Staff noticed that she was not compliant with self-care tasks and made errors in insulin doses and times of administration. What is the most appropriate treatment for her?

Choose one option:

A. Change insulin to long-acting insulin analogue.
B. Screen for cognitive impairment.
C. Organise home help with regular carer visits.
D. Take over insulin administration by district nurse.
E. Reduce insulin dose and add another oral hypoglycaemic agent.

References

Key references only are listed here. For a full list of references visit: https://www.wiley.com/go/sinclair/1e.

1. McDonnell, M.E. and Umpierrez, G.E. (2012). Insulin therapy for the management of hyperglycemia in hospitalized patients. *Endocrinol. Metab. Clin. N. Am.* 41: 175–201.
2. Gosmanov, A.R. (2016). A practical and evidence-based approach to management of inpatient diabetes in non-critically ill patients and special clinical populations. *J. Clin. Transl. Endocrinol.* 5: 1–6.
3. Umpierrez, G.E., Hellman, R., Korytkowski, M.T. et al. (2012). Endocrine Society. Management of hyperglycemia in hospitalized patients in non-critical care setting: an Endocrine Society clinical practice guideline. *J. Clin. Endocrinol. Metab.* 97: 16–38.
4. Niefeld, M.R., Braunstein, J.B., Wu, A.W. et al. (2003). Preventable hospitalization among elderly medicare beneficiaries with type 2 diabetes. *Diabetes Care* 26: 1344–1349.
5. Hongsoo, K., Helmer, D.A., Zhao, Z. et al. (2011). Potentially preventable hospitalizations among older adults with diabetes. *Am. J. Manag. Care* 17: e419–e426.
6. Fu, H., Curtis, B.H., Xie, W. et al. (2014). Frequency and causes of hospitalization in older compared with younger adults with type 2 diabetes in the United States: a retrospective, claims- based analysis. *J. Diabetes Complicat.* 28: 477–481.
7. Budnitz, D.S., Lovegrove, M.C., Shehab, N. et al. (2011). Emergency hospitalizations for adverse drug events in older Americans. *N. Engl. J. Med.* 365: 2002–2012.
8. Gupta, N. and Sheng, Z. (2021). Reduced risk of hospitalization with stronger community belonging among aging Canadians living with diabetes: findings from linked survey and administrative data. *Front. Public Health* 9: 670082.
9. Liao, C.D., Tsauo, J.Y., Wu, Y.T. et al. (2017). Effects of protein supplementation combined with resistance exercise on body composition and physical function in older adults: a systematic review and metaanalysis. *Am. J. Clin. Nutr.* 106: 1078–1091.
10. Pflipsen, M.C., Oh, R.C., Saguil, A. et al. (2009). The prevalence of vitamin B12 deficiencyin patients with type 2 diabetes: a cross-sectional study. *J Am Board Fam Med* 22: 528–534.

16j Special Issues in Old Age: Use of Technology

Anna Kahkoska[1,2,3]*, Aastha Dubal*[1]*, Josh Weinstein*[4] *and Ruth S. Weinstock*[5]

[1] *Division of Endocrinology and Metabolism, University of North Carolina at Chapel Hill, Chapel Hill, NC, USA*
[2] *Department of Nutrition, Gillings School of Global Public Health, University of North Carolina at Chapel Hill, Chapel Hill, NC, USA*
[3] *UNC Center for Aging and Health, University of North Carolina at Chapel Hill, Chapel Hill, NC, USA*
[4] *Department of Health Policy and Management, Gillings School of Global Public Health, University of North Carolina at Chapel Hill, Chapel Hill, NC, USA*
[5] *Division of Endocrinology, Diabetes and Metabolism, Department of Medicine, SUNY Upstate Medical University, Syracuse, NY, USA*

Key Points

- Technological solutions to diabetes management (e.g., insulin pumps, continuous glucose monitoring, automated insulin delivery systems) and more general remote patient monitoring (e.g., vital signs, wearables, smartphone application-based trackers) have the potential to improve quality of diabetes care, inform self-management regimens and increase the safety of older adults.
- Many older adults face unique barriers to technology access and effective use and perceive different technology burdens than younger individuals.
- Continuous glucose monitoring is associated with improved safety, glycaemic, and patient-oriented outcomes among older adults, and

Care of Older People with Diabetes: A Manual for Healthcare Practice, First Edition.
Edited by Alan J. Sinclair and Ahmed H. Abdelhafiz.

Companion website: www.wiley.com/go/sinclair/1e

it is recommended for older adults with type 1 and type 2 diabetes with hypoglycaemia.
- Use of automated insulin delivery systems in older adults with type 1 diabetes can reduce hypoglycaemia. There remain challenges in scaling use of these technologies, spanning patient, provider and healthcare system factors.
- Studies on the use of diabetes technologies in older adults are urgently needed in special populations, such as those with cognitive impairment, and those in nursing homes and long-term care facilities. Solutions to integrate and monitor remote patient data securely are needed.
- Future efforts to implement technology in this population will need to ensure that technologies are accessible and training and support are available to all patients and their caregivers.

Introduction

Older adults with diabetes are a heterogenous and complex group with diverse clinical needs, living situations, functional and cognitive impairments, comorbidities, historical self-management experiences and preferences for care [1–3]. These factors can rapidly change or evolve as individuals grow older. Older adults are at an increased risk for hypoglycaemia related to increasing diabetes duration and comorbidities, cognitive impairment, frailty, variable nutritional status, polypharmacy and hypoglycaemia unawareness [3, 4]. As such, a focus on patient safety, especially avoiding hypoglycaemia, alongside accommodating patient preferences and preserving quality of life, defines the philosophy of diabetes care and management of diabetes in older adults [3, 5–7].

Innovative technologies can improve health outcomes and increase the length and quality of life for older adults with chronic medical conditions [8]. In this chapter, we focus on the use of diabetes technologies and other remote patient monitoring (RPM) technologies. We describe key terms and discuss key issues and management considerations for older adults.

What Is Diabetes Technology?

Diabetes technology is used to describe 'hardware, devices and software' for glucose monitoring and insulin dosing and delivery, which may include continuous glucose monitoring (CGM), continuous

Table 16j.1: Key diabetes technologies.

Technology	Description
Continuous glucose monitoring (CGM)	Involves the use of a small sensor placed under the skin to measure glucose levels in the interstitial fluid every few minutes throughout the day and night. These real-time data are transmitted to a monitoring device (a receiver, smartphone, tablet or watch), allowing individuals, their caregivers and healthcare providers to view glucose levels and trends. Alarms are available to alert the user of hypo- and/or hyperglycaemia
Bluetooth-enabled insulin pens	An insulin pen that wirelessly connects to a mobile application via Bluetooth. It allows for convenient insulin dose tracking and more accurate bolus delivery compared to syringes.
Insulin pumps	Devices that provide continuous subcutaneous infusion of fast-acting insulin, allowing more precise and flexible insulin dosing over the day and night, compared to insulin injections.
Automated insulin delivery and hybrid closed loop systems	Insulin delivery systems that use a controller algorithm alongside insulin pumps to automatically adjust insulin delivery based on real-time CGM readings. The user is often still required to manually dose mealtime insulin or announce meals

subcutaneous insulin infusion (insulin pumps), automated insulin delivery (AID) systems (also called hybrid closed loop or artificial pancreas systems) and smart insulin pens (Table 16j.1) [4]. These systems are rapidly advancing [9]. The American Diabetes Association Standards of Care recommend the individualised use of these technologies in all people with diabetes, including older adults [10].

What Is Remote Patient Monitoring?

Remote patient monitoring allows for patients' health status to be monitored outside clinical settings, such as in their homes or other non-hospital environments. This is facilitated by the use of minimally invasive or non-invasive technological devices and tools that collect and transmit patient data to healthcare providers, systems, and other caregivers [11]. The primary goal of RPM is to enhance the management of chronic diseases, provide timely interventions, and improve overall patient care while minimising the need for in-person visits. RPM typically involves the use of devices that can measure and transmit vital signs, such as heart rate, blood pressure, blood glucose levels, sleep patterns, VO_2 and other relevant health metrics to healthcare providers.

Closely related to RPM is remote activity monitoring (RAM): the use of electronic devices to monitor a person's mobility or activities of daily living [12]. While RPM primarily focuses on monitoring the health and medical parameters of patients, RAM encompasses a broader range of monitoring activities, including physical activity, movement, mobility, medication adherence and general daily behaviours.

In both cases, the collected data are transmitted securely to a healthcare system where they can be reviewed and analysed. Healthcare providers can use this information to track the patient's health status and identify and address potential problems. RPM is particularly beneficial for patients with chronic conditions needing ongoing management and for those who need post-acute care after hospitalisation.

Diabetes Technology and Remote Patient Monitoring in Older Adults

Using technological advancements in diabetes management, such as insulin pumps, CGM and AID, together with broader applications like RPM (e.g. vital signs, wearables, smartphone application-based trackers), hold the promise of enhancing the quality of diabetes care, guiding self-management practices and bolstering patient safety in older adults. These technologies are advancing rapidly, and while the scientific evidence and clinical experience regarding their use in older adults are expanding, they remain relatively limited. Unique challenges in accessing and effectively using technology may exist for individual older adults, and their perceptions of technological burdens may differ from those of younger age groups. An overview of these technologies and their applications to diabetes care in older adults can be found in Figure 16j.1 [13].

Despite potential, there are known barriers to the use of medical technology among older adults, including low technological literacy,

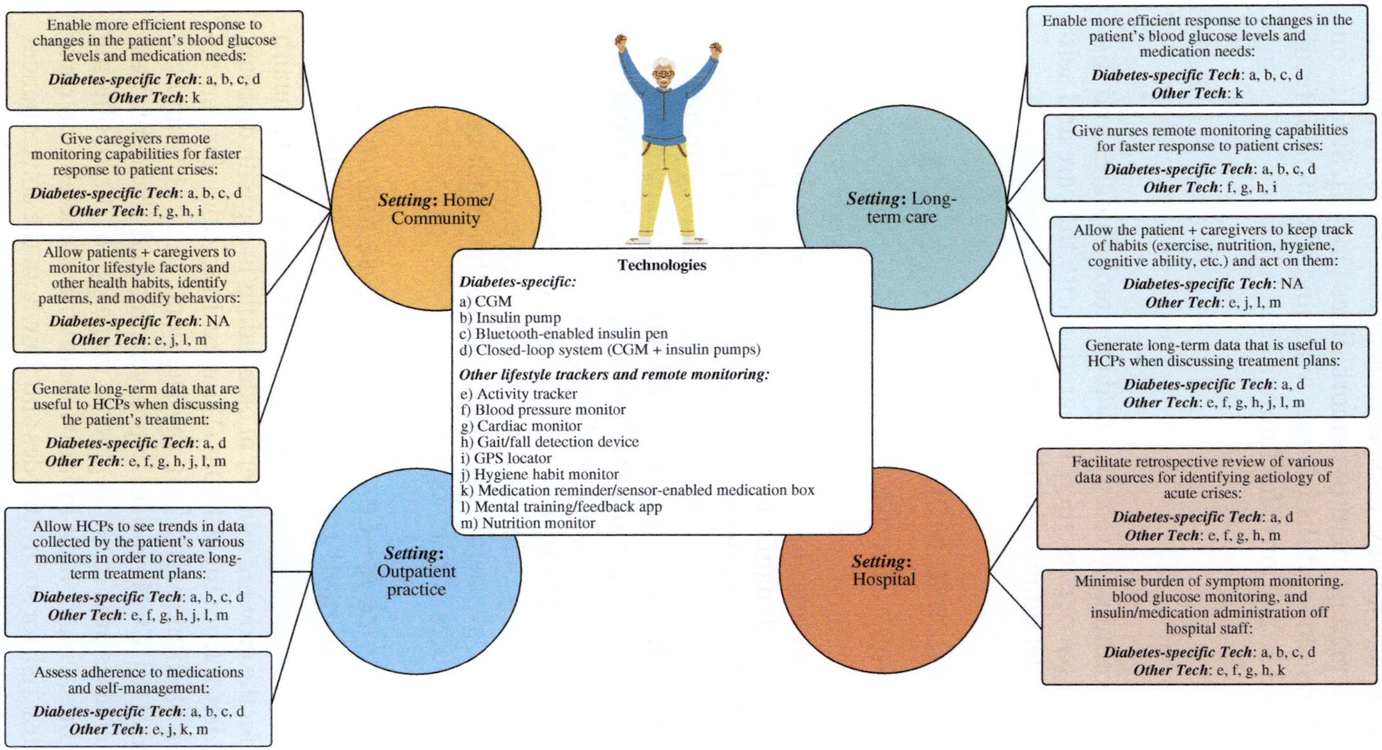

Figure 16j.1: Potential roles of technology in the care of older adults with diabetes across settings. CGM, continuous glucose monitoring; HCPs, healthcare providers; NA, not applicable; Tech, technology.

Source: adapted from Huang et al. [13] American Diabetes Association [The Growing Role of Technology in the Care of Older Adults With Diabetes, American Diabetes Association, 2023]. Copyright and all rights reserved. Material from this publication has been used with the permission of American Diabetes Association.

attitudes towards technology, perspectives of caregivers, functional impairments and management of comorbidities [14, 15]. Studies on the ways in which older adults interact with, and may benefit from, technology should be a priority for future research [1].

Management

We focus on two clinically relevant diabetes technologies and discuss benefits and barriers of their integration into the care and self-management of older adults with diabetes.

Continuous Glucose Monitoring

What Is Continuous Glucose Monitoring?

Continuous glucose monitoring comprises an on-body sensor that transmits glucose readings to a receiver or smart device that provides users with real-time, dynamic information about their glucose levels around the clock [4]. CGM also provides alerts to prevent dangerously high or low glucose levels, leading to better diabetes management and, ultimately, improved health outcomes. CGM is now standard care for all people with diabetes who require insulin therapy [3]. Clinical practice guidelines state that CGM should be offered to people capable of using CGM themselves or with help from a caregiver [10]. Professional CGM use may be used for any older adult to ascertain glycaemic patterns (i.e. hypoglycaemia, glycaemic variability) since this is not captured by laboratory measures of haemoglobin A1c.

What Is the Evidence for Continuous Glucose Monitoring as Part of Management for Older Adults with Diabetes?

Accumulating evidence suggests that CGM can increase safety, health and wellness for the growing number of older adults living with diabetes, including evidence from the WISDM (Wireless Innovation for Seniors with Diabetes Mellitus) study [16], the Diamond study [17], and the MOBILE study [18]. CGM reduces hypoglycaemia and glycaemic variability and increases time in target glucose range [3, 16, 19, 20] offering a potentially lifesaving benefit in individuals with diabetes who carry both the greatest risk for such episodes and for whom the consequences can be devastating. CGM is now recommended as standard care for older adults with T1DM and T2DM requiring insulin [3]. CGM may also facilitate more flexible management and involvement of care partners.

Real-world evidence for the clinical effects of CGM is limited in older adults. However, electronic health record data from the Veterans Affairs Health Care System ($n = 5015$ with T1DM and $n = 15\,706$ with T2DM; 2015–2020) showed that initiation of CGM reduced risk of admission to an emergency room or hospital for hypo- and hyperglycaemia in an older population with diabetes [21]. Among those with T1DM, CGM use was associated with reduced risk of hypoglycaemia, while in those with T2DM, CGM use was associated with a reduce risk of hyperglycaemia [21].

What Are Challenges for Continuous Glucose Monitoring Use in Older Adults?

Despite significant potential benefits, adoption of CGM by older adults remains low: just 27% of adults over 60 years with T1DM and 3% of adults with T2DM are using CGM [22, 23]. This may reflect, at least in part, that older individuals perceive greater burdens with CGM incorporation [15, 24].

There are also age-specific barriers to CGM uptake that probably underly these trends [19]. Learning to use and integrate technology for diabetes management into daily routines can be extremely complex for older adults [14, 15], particularly in the context of unique biopsychosocial needs for successful uptake and sustained use. For example, anecdotal experience from device trials suggests that older adults require more time and support to learn and use CGM compared with younger adult counterparts [15]. Similarly, qualitative studies engaging older adults and their care partners have revealed that for many older adults, learning how to use CGM is a complex learning process fraught with opportunities for failure [25]. Older adults have highly individualised needs for support to reap the clinical and quality of life benefits of CGM [26].

Automated Insulin Delivery Systems

What Is Automated Insulin Delivery?

AID systems use CGM data to adjust insulin delivery from an insulin pump using a controller algorithm. There have been several types of AID systems, each with varying degrees of automation. Predictive low glucose suspend (PLGS) or low glucose suspend (LGS) systems alter insulin dosing based on CGM readings; if a PGLS or LGS system predicts or detects hypoglycaemia, it will reduce or suspend insulin delivery [27]. Hybrid closed loop (AID) systems use glucose levels provided by the CGM to alter insulin dosing, both increasing and decreasing insulin delivery based on current and predicted glucose levels [27]. Each of these systems requires the user to administer prandial insulin doses. Full AID systems that automatically administer insulin, including for meals, without input of the user, are not yet commercially available.

Evidence on Automated Insulin Delivery for Older Adults

Boughton et al. [28] conducted an open-label randomised trial assessing the effectiveness of a AID system compared to the use of CGM and insulin pump without automation in older adults and found that the AID system improved markers of glycaemic management [28]. Multiple other studies that were not primarily focused on older adults have found statistically and clinically significant improvements in glycaemic control among older adults as a subgroup in their studies [29, 30]. Importantly, the evidence does not only indicate improvements in time-in-range measures, but also hypoglycaemia endpoints.

Clinical Guidelines for Automated Insulin Delivery Usage among Older Adults with Type 1 Diabetes

A set of consensus recommendations for the use of AID technology published by the Endocrine Society in 2023 state that AID should be an option for glycaemic management in all populations with T1DM [31]. Older adults (> 65 years) are a subgroup that these consensus recommendations specifically highlight for considering recommending AID [31].

What Are Challenges for Automated Insulin Delivery Use in Older Adults?

Many challenges for CGM use in older adults also apply to AID use (Table 16j.2). Aside from access concerns, Aiello et al. identified key considerations and challenges for the use of AID systems by several subgroups with T1DM [33]. Among older adults, they noted that comfort with technology and cognition played substantial roles in the relationship between older adults and their insulin delivery systems,

Table 16j.2: Challenges for continuous glucose monitoring and automated insulin delivery use in older populations.

Issue	Challenges
Access	Access to providers with high degree of familiarity with CGM; availability in retail pharmacies (CGM) or from distributors (automated insulin delivery)
Financial	High cost; variable US-based insurance coverage policies and reimbursements
Usability	Requisite fine motor skills and both technological and health literacy; lacking accommodation for visual and hearing impairments
Education and support	Access to certified diabetes care and education specialists; availability of adequate training; training for caregivers
Caregiver	Caregiver's level of technological and health literacy; caregiver's fine motor skills
Special populations: hospitalisation, cognitive impairment, nursing homes	Availability of trainers; access to trained staff in acute and chronic care facilities technologies for management; capabilities of nursing homes/long-term care facilities; fine motor skills

CGM, continuous glucose monitoring.

and that cognitive impairments can contribute to difficulties in adhering to their glycaemic management regimen [33]. Qualitative studies have unearthed barriers faced by older adults in their experience with diabetes technology that extend to AID. As these devices become more advanced and easier to use, these barriers should diminish.

Integration of Diabetes Technologies with Remote Patient Monitoring

The COVID-19 pandemic increased the use of RPM technologies, providing proof of principle for how these data sources could be applied in healthcare [8]. It is also recognised, however, that implementation of these technologies must be done with geriatrics principles in mind, including an emphasis on case-by-case evaluation and tailoring their use to an individual's physical, mental and social health, mobility and preferences [8].

There is an intention to integrate data from RPM to bring context to glucose data conferred by CGM; this is termed 'precision monitoring'. For example, care providers may be able to develop more effective and individualised plans for care with additional information on dietary intake, physical activity, sleep patterns and medication adherence [34]. This may have special, geriatric-relevant extensions. Ecological momentary assessment, a tool used to coalesce repeated assessments of behavioural, physiological and psychological processes, allows for novel insight into CGM metrics. Ecological momentary assessments coupled with cognitive assessments to passive interstitial blood glucose levels found that CGM metrics were associated with short-term fluctuations in cognitive function [35]. By leveraging CGM alongside other technologies for RPM, diabetes care may be able to more proactively address health concerns, reduce hospital readmissions and improve overall patient outcomes [34].

What Are the Key Issues?

Key issues for the effective and equitable implementation of technology in older adults are summarised in Figure 16j.2 and discussed below.

- Studies are needed for geriatric populations that are typically excluded from randomised trials, such as those with cognitive impairment, frailty, those in nursing homes and long-term care facilities.
- Strategies are needed to introduce and disseminate evidence-based health technologies to older adults, addressing patient factors including cognitive functioning (memory, learning, executive functioning), functional impairments, hearing and visual impairments, dexterity and mobility, available support from formal and informal caregivers, technological literacy and diabetes management preferences.
- Expanding the use of technology in diabetes management may exacerbate pre-existing structural inequities (i.e. the digital divide). Equitable access to technological devices, reliable Internet connection and technologically aware educators are

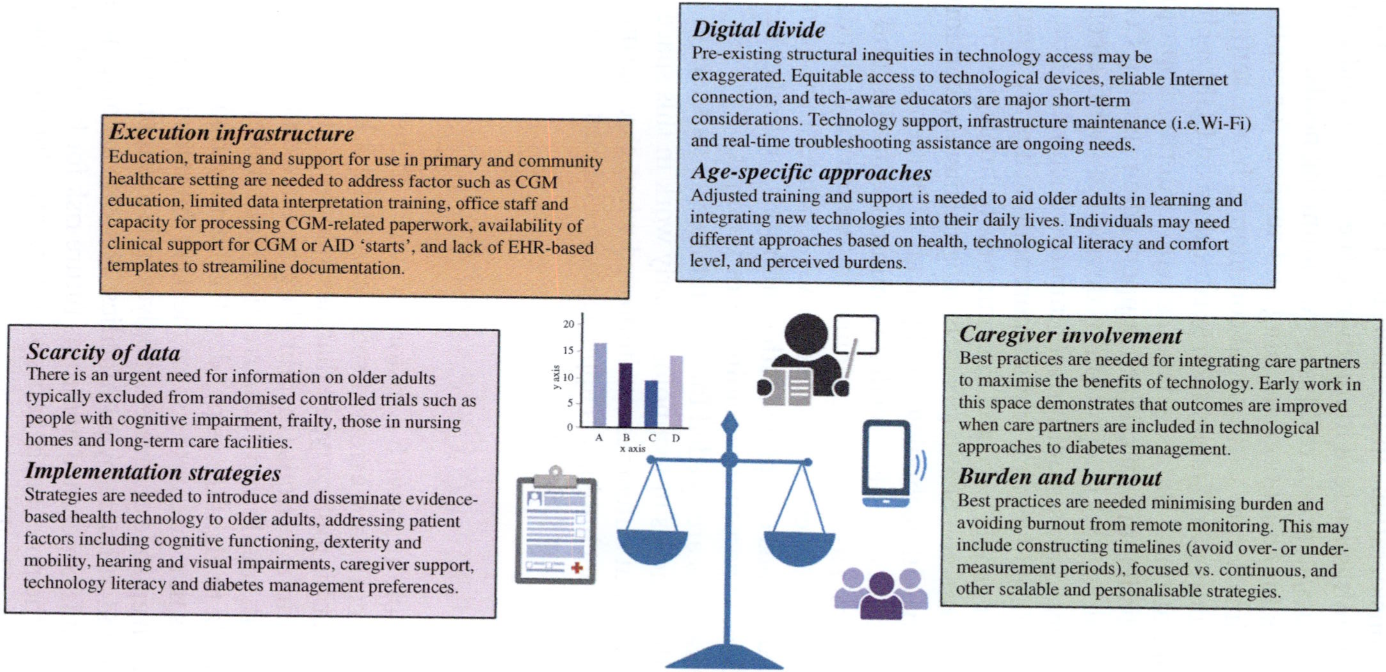

Figure 16j.2: Key issues for the effective and equitable implementation of technology in older adults with diabetes. AID, automated insulin delivery; CGM, continuous glucose monitoring.

major considerations in the short term. Long-term technology support, infrastructure maintenance (i.e. Wi-Fi), and trouble-shooting assistance in real time are continuing needs.

- Strategies for education, training and support for continuing use in primary care settings and community health settings are needed, addressing factors such as education on CGM including interpretation of data, assistance with ordering appropriate devices, availability of clinical support when starting CGM or AID systems, and integration of device data with electronic health records to streamline and improve documentation.
- Individualised training and support approaches are needed to assist older people learn and integrate new technologies into daily routines based on health and technological literacy, comfort and familiarity with technology, and perceived burdens.
- Best practices are also needed to minimise burden and avoid burnout from use of remote monitoring, which may include constructing timelines (avoid waste of over- or under-measurement), focused periods compared with continuous, and other scalable strategies to personalise reminders or prompts.
- Best practices are needed for integrating care partners to maximise the benefits of technology. Early work in this space demonstrates that outcomes are improved when care partners are included in technological approaches to diabetes management and monitoring [36, 37].

Clinical Practice Questions

Q1. A 78-year-old man with a history of type 1 diabetes of 48 years duration, coronary artery disease and stage 3 kidney disease presents for his routine type 1 diabetes follow-up. He uses multiple daily insulin injections (insulin glargine once daily and insulin aspart with meals and for correction) and monitors his blood glucose six to eight times per day. His haemoglobin A1c is 6.9%. He reports that he eats the same meals at the same time each day. He had an episode of severe hypoglycaemia one month ago, which was treated at home by paramedics. His wife accompanies him today and is concerned about his future risk for hypoglycaemia. What are the potential benefits of continuous glucose monitoring for this individual?

Choose the options that are relevant:
A. Increased insights into glycaemic patterns.
B. The opportunity to share his glucose levels with a care partner for support.
C. Data to share with his clinical team to help guide need for changes in insulin regimen.
D. Use of arrows and alarms to help avoid serious hypoglycaemia.

Q2. Selection of diabetes and remote patient monitoring technologies must be individualised to different older adults and their unique needs for care, abilities and preferences.
A. True
B. False

References

Key references only are listed here. For a full list of references visit: `https://www.wiley.com/go/sinclair/1e`.

1. Munshi, M.N., Meneilly, G.S., Rodríguez-Mañas, L. et al. (2020). Diabetes in ageing: pathways for developing the evidence base for clinical guidance. *Lancet Diabetes Endocrinol.* 8 (10): 855–867.
3. ElSayed, N.A., Aleppo, G., Aroda, V.R. et al. (2024). 13. Older adults: standards of care in diabetes 2024. *Diabetes Care* 47 (Suppl 1): S244–S257.
10. ElSayed, N.A., Aleppo, G., Aroda, V.R. et al. (2023). 7. Diabetes technology: standards of care in diabetes 2024. *Diabetes Care* 47 (Suppl 1): S126–S144.
13. Huang, E.S., Sinclair, A., Conlin, P.R. et al. (2023). The growing role of Technology in the Care of older adults with diabetes. *Diabetes Care* 46 (8): 1455–1463.
16. Pratley, R.E., Kanapka, L.G., Rickels, M.R. et al. (2020). Effect of continuous glucose monitoring on hypoglycemia in older adults with type 1 diabetes: a randomized clinical trial. *JAMA* 323 (23): 2397–2406.
17. Beck, R.W., Riddlesworth, T., Ruedy, K. et al. (2017). Effect of continuous glucose monitoring on glycemic control in adults with type 1 diabetes using insulin injections: the DIAMOND randomized clinical trial. *JAMA* 317 (4): 371–378.
19. Munshi, M.N. (2023). Continuous glucose monitoring use in older adults for optimal diabetes management. *Diabetes Technol. Ther.* 25 (Suppl 3): S56–S64.

21. Reaven, P.D., Newell, M., Rivas, S. et al. (2023). Initiation of continuous glucose monitoring is linked to improved glycemic control and fewer clinical events in type 1 and type 2 diabetes in the veterans health administration. *Diabetes Care* 46 (4): 854–863.
25. Kahkoska, A.R., Smith, C., Thambuluru, S. et al. (2022). 'Nothing is linear': characterizing the determinants and dynamics of CGM use in older adults with type 1 diabetes. *Diabetes Res. Clin. Pract.* 196: 110204.
28. Boughton, C.K., Hartnell, S., Thabit, H. et al. (2022). Hybrid closed-loop glucose control compared with sensor augmented pump therapy in older adults with type 1 diabetes: an open-label multicentre, multinational, randomised, crossover study. *Lancet Health Longevity* 3 (3): e135–e142.

16k Special Issues in Old Age: Annual Reviews

Puja Merwaha and Ahmed H. Abdelhafiz

Department of Geriatric Medicine, Rotherham General Hospital, Rotherham, UK

Key Points

- Diabetes in old age is associated with multiple morbidities, frailty and impairment of physical and mental health.
- In addition to diabetes-related care, an annual review should include a comprehensive geriatric assessment at physical, functional and social level.
- A multidisciplinary approach to the annual review with a holistic care may help to enhance diabetes care, reduce acute complications, improve function and maintain quality of life.

Introduction

Diabetes is a chronic and progressive disease, which affects all body systems. It requires close regular monitoring of blood glucose, investigation of the impact of the disease on the body organs and the assessment of wider aspects of patient care. Annual reviews aim to assess glycaemic control, detect complications, plan early interventions and initiate prevention. They also aim to review patients' care plans, self-care and coping. However, in older people with diabetes, ageing-related morbidities add to the burden of diabetes care. Therefore, an annual review of diabetes in this group of patients should also include elements of comprehensive geriatric assessment (CGA) to address other

Care of Older People with Diabetes: A Manual for Healthcare Practice, First Edition.
Edited by Alan J. Sinclair and Ahmed H. Abdelhafiz.

Companion website: www.wiley.com/go/sinclair/1e

age-related complications. This chapter reviews common geriatric morbidities associated with diabetes and suggests an annual review format that ensures a holistic patient care.

Diabetes Phenotype in Older People

With increasing age, diabetes in older people is associated with multiple morbidities and diabetes-related complications, which leads to frailty. In addition, increasing age is associated with geriatric syndromes, which are a group of medical conditions common in this age group. (Box 16k.1)

Multimorbidity

Multimorbidity is more than two diseases occurring in the same person at the same time. The impact of this is termed the morbidity burden, and considers the severity of the conditions. Patient complexity considers severity as well as other cultural, socioeconomic, environmental and behavioural attributes. Diabetes leads to increased atherosclerosis, premature ageing and increased disability. The majority of older people with diabetes have at least one comorbid chronic condition and up to

Box 16k.1: Diabetes Phenotype in Older People with Diabetes

- Multiple morbidities
- Cognitive dysfunction
- Physical dysfunction
- Frailty
- Sarcopenia
- Urinary incontinence
- Depression
- Anxiety
- Falls and fractures
- Polypharmacy and drug errors
- Undernutrition and prone to dehydration
- Anorexia
- Irregular eating pattern
- Vulnerability to hypoglycaemia

40% have three or more morbidities [1]. The morbidity burden is even higher in care-home residents with diabetes. Residents with diabetes have increased incidence of cardiovascular disease, visual problems, pressure sores, limb amputations and kidney failure compared with residents without diabetes [2].

Geriatric Syndromes

Geriatric syndromes consist of physical and cognitive dysfunction, depression, falls and urinary incontinence. These conditions are common in older people with diabetes and may have subtle presentations [3]. When compared with older people without diabetes, those with diabetes have a twofold increased risk of being unable to perform daily physical tasks, such as walking, household chores or climbing stairs, and a 1.6-fold greater risk of difficulties performing basic personal care, such as bathing, using the toilet, dressing and eating. These physical disabilities are attributed to diabetes-related complications, such as neuropathy, pain, poor vision and vascular disease [4]. Additionally, the risk of developing Alzheimer's disease or vascular dementia is twofold and the risk of depression is 1.3-fold higher in older people with diabetes compared with people without diabetes [5, 6].

Frailty

Frailty is a new category of complication in older people with diabetes, in addition to the traditional macro- and microvascular diseases. Diabetes increases the risk of frailty by 1.5-fold [7]. Frailty is a wasting disease characterised by weight loss and loss of muscle mass (sarcopenia) and is linked with undernutrition, especially in people living in care homes. This may be due to reduced muscle protein synthesis because of lower testosterone and insulin-like growth factor I. In addition, diabetes-related chronic inflammation and intramuscular lipid accumulation may lead to increased muscle protein breakdown [8].

Functional Implications

Multimorbidity, geriatric syndromes and frailty appear to have common pathophysiological mechanisms, which increase the risk of each other and eventually lead to disability. The trend of disability in diabetes increases steadily with increasing age from 13.5% for activities of daily living and 8.8% for instrumental activities of daily living among individuals aged 50–59 years to 28.4% and 18.2%, respectively, among those aged ≥ 80 years [6]. Diabetes-associated disability is related to the underlying traditional diabetic complications, the associated comorbidities and frailty. These additional factors need to be addressed during diabetes annual review of older people.

Annual Review Contents

Demographics

Establishing a comprehensive patient's background is a key to diabetes annual review in older people. Information include height, weight, body mass index and waist circumference, and lifestyle factors such as smoking history, alcohol, diet and exercise. Any changes to this information should be noted. Living circumstances, activities of daily living, including self-care and support at living place, should be collected (Figure 16k.1).

History

History taking helps to identify concerns of patients and challenges with the management of their diabetes and general wellbeing. The history will also aim to uncover any acute complaints, which may be biological, psychological or social. It gains insight into their current understanding of diabetes, their management plan, compliance and any barriers to this. History includes notes of patients' diabetes type, duration, haemoglobin A1c (HbA1c), past medical history, medications list and any changes and current diabetes-related complications. A review of how a patient is monitoring his blood glucose, glucose diary, target HbA1c and blood glucose ranges should be reviewed tailored to each patient' plan.

Physical Examination

The purpose of a physical examination is to help identify, prevent and manage common diabetes-related or other morbidity-related complications. The examination should focus on both pathology and

Patient details
Name:
DOB:
Gender:
Patient identifier:

Demographics
Height:
Weight:
BMI:
Waist circumference:

Lifestyle
Smoking:
Alcohol:
Exercise:
Diet:
Appetite:
Home and household:
Sensory aids:

Activities of Daily Living
Washing and dressing:
Feeding:
Continence:
Toilet use:
Shopping and finance:
Driving:
Bartell Index:
Independent (I), Aid (A), Dependent (D)

Past medical history
Diabetes type:
Duration:
Comorbidities:

Medication
Hypoglycaemic agents:
Others:
Allergies:
Medication review:

Frailty and function
Clinical frailty scale:
Formal functional assessment:
FRAX score:
Falls risk:
Bone health:
Gait:
Pain:
Mobility aids:

Sexual function
Via direct enquiry

Initial assessment
Acute complaints:
Blood glucose diary:
HBA1c

Macrovascular Complications
Ischaemic heart disease
Cerebrovascular disease
Peripheral arterial disease
Other:
Check
BP and diary:
Peripheral pulses:
Lipids:
Cardiovascular assessment:

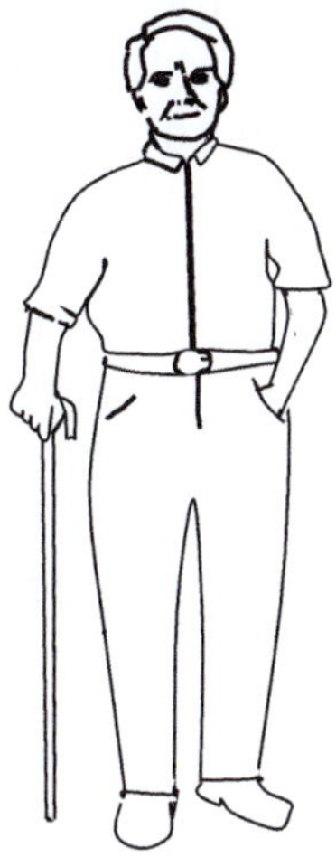

Diet and nutrition
MUST score:
Diet:
Oral hygiene:
Hydration:
Challenges:

Cognition and Mood
Standardised cognitive assessment:
Mood:
Self-care:

Microvascular Complications
Retinopathy
Nephropathy
Neuropathy
Diabetic foot
Other:
Check
Annual retinopathy screening
Renal function and urine ACR
Foot care and neuropathy
Regular dental checks and oral hygiene

Foot care
Peripheral pulses:
Neurology:
Nails:
Footwear:
Ulcers:
Skin condition:
Infection:
Education:

Infection prevention:
Review sick day rules
Vaccinations

Education to patient and carers
Acute illness
Emergency management
Diet and lifestyle
Compliance
Monitoring
Self-care
Screening
Support

Future Planning
Hospital avoidance
Advanced care planning
End-of-life considerations

Key Concerns
Metabolic targets:
Functional:
Coping:
Social:
Medication burden:
Frequency of follow up:

Figure 16k.1: Contents of a comprehensive annual review in older people with diabetes. ACR, albumin to creatinine ratio; BMI, body mass index; DOB, date of birth; FRAX, Fracture Risk Assessment Tool; HbA1c, haemoglobin A1c; MUST, Malnutrition Universal Screening Tool.

function. This covers a top-to-toe examination. It involves but is not limited to an examination of the eyes, oral hygiene, cardiovascular system, skin, peripheral pulses, neuropathy and a thorough foot examination. Note any weakness in the limbs, joint pain and mobility limitations. Note any other issues such as the need for hearing or mobility aids.

Vascular Complications

Macrovascular complications should cover cerebral, cardiac and peripheral vascular diseases. Enquire about exertional chest pain or intermittent claudication or erectile dysfunction, which may suggest underlying macrovascular disease. Enquire about history of vascular disease-related recent hospital admission. Microvascular complications typically affect the eyes, kidneys and nerves, in the form of retinopathy, kidney disease and neuropathies. They can be monitored with annual screening for retinopathy, urinary albumin tests, regular blood pressure checking, blood tests for renal function, lipids, HbA1c and examinations of the feet and peripheral nerves. Recognition and monitoring of chronic kidney disease and timely medication adjustment for acute kidney injury during illness are key in the prevention of diabetic kidney disease.

Sexual Function

Sexual dysfunction affects both men and women and is more common in both older age and in diabetes. This can affect a patient's quality of life. This is multifactorial and influenced by neuropathies, vascular changes, hormones and psychological factors. Sexual function is often forgotten and should be enquired about directly as patients may not voluntarily complain about it.

Cognition and Mood

Cognitive screening should be carried out at the outset to establish a baseline and then regular screening for signs or symptoms of cognitive decline. A standardised test can be used such as a Montreal Cognitive Assessment. The same applies to mood assessment including anxiety and depression. Tools such as Hamilton Rating Scale for Anxiety or the Geriatric Depression Scale may be used.

Physical Function and Frailty

A patient's ability to perform activities of daily living can be assessed using tools such as the Barthel index. Timed Get Up and Go is a good assessment of mobility, and tools such as the clinical frailty scale are easy and simple to screen for frailty. The Fracture Risk Assessment tool is useful for calculating fracture risk and bone health and is also a guide to whether further assessment by dual energy x-ray absorptiometry is required. Falls risk assessment, while considering disability, postural instability and current aids, help to tailor preventative management and aims to improve balance and mobility. Pain should also be assessed as it reduces physical activity by limiting mobility, functional ability, and emotional wellbeing.

Foot Care

A comprehensive foot and neurological examination are needed to detect any current and potential complications. Pulses and sensory changes should be recorded. Examination of the foot nails and skin for infections, wounds and deformities is needed. Education on foot care, footwear, aids and when to seek additional help should be highlighted and provided.

Diet and Nutrition

Nutritional deficiencies and risk of malnutrition should be assessed by reviewing patient's calorie intake, dietary habits, deficiencies, self-reported weight loss, appetite changes and new difficulties with usual activities of daily living such as preparing meals. The Malnutrition Universal Screening Tool can be used here. Conditions such as dementia can lead to reduced food and fluid intake, which can increase the likelihood of adverse events such as hypoglycaemia, acute kidney injury or hyperglycaemic crisis. Thus, assessment of hydration status, both clinically and biochemically is required. Advice should consider patient preferences and be culturally sensitive. It is also beneficial to provide advice surrounding regular oral hygiene and dental checks.

Medication Review

Polypharmacy is a significant problem in older people who often need to take multiple medications for multiple comorbidities. This increases the chances of interactions and adverse reactions. Medication reviews are key to optimising diabetes regimens, stopping unnecessary medications and reducing the risk of drug errors and hospitalisation. Medication reviews also allow education and encourages compliance.

Infection Prevention

Older people with diabetes are prone to infections. Illnesses can also affect blood glucose control, increase the risk of acute diabetic complications and influence an individual's management of their diabetes. Vaccinations for pneumococcal pneumonia, flu and COVID-19 should be offered and discussed. Sick day rules should be revisited with plans for increased monitoring and education on the recognition and management of acute decompensations. A suggested template for a comprehensive annual review of older people with diabetes that can be used in clinical practice is provided in Figure 16k.2.

Summary

In addition to regular diabetes care, older people need a comprehensive geriatric assessment at physical, mental and social levels. A holistic annual review may help control diabetes, prevent acute decompensation, improve function and maintain quality of life.

Clinical Practice Question

Q1. A 77-year-old man with type 2 diabetes for 23 years on oral hypoglycaemic medications has recently started insulin therapy. He has a past medical history of hypertension, ischaemic heart disease, chronic kidney disease and cardiovascular accident. He lives with his wife, is mobile with a stick and has no carers. On annual review, his blood glucose ranges between 5 and 22 mmol/l. What items in his annual review are important to address his fluctuating blood glucose levels?

Choose the most appropriate options:

A. Medication review.
B. Cognitive and mental functions.
C. Education and training.
D. Diet and nutrition.
E. Haemoglobin A1c.

Details

Clinic name and date:
Patient identifier:
Full name:
Date of birth:
Sex: M/F Other:

Past medical history

Diabetes type: [ ] Type 1 [ ] Type 2 [ ] Other:
Co-morbidities:
Active issues:
Hypoglycaemia: [ ] Yes [ ] No
Warning Signs [ ] Y [ ] N

Examination

Height:
Weight:
BMI:
Waist circumference:
BP and heart rate:
Injection sites: [ ] Clean [ ] Infected [ ] Lipodystrophy

Patient lifestyle

Smoking: Smoker – Cigarettes/week:
Ex smoker – Pack years:
Non smoker
Alcohol: Units/week:
Exercise Minutes/week:
Diet and appetite:
Home: [ ] Home [ ] Carers [ ] Care home
Sensory aids: [ ] Glasses [ ] Hearing [ ] Other

Medication

Current diabetes treatment:
[ ] Diet
[ ] Oral hypoglacaemics (Agent, dose):
[ ] Insulin (Agent, dose):
Other Medications
Allergies [ ] Yes list [ ] No

Functional assessment

Physical function and ADL e.g Bartell index
Cognitive function e.g MoCA
Mood e.g GDS, GAD

Sexual function

Current issues:
Inverventions:

Frailty, falls and bone health

Clinical Frailty Scale:
FRAX score: Osteopenia [ ] Y [ ] N
Osteoporisosis [ ] Y [ ] N
Falls risk assessment: Postural instability:
Gait: Balance:
Pain: Arthritis:

Macrovascular complications

Ischaemic heart disease [ ] Yes [ ] No
Cerebrovascular disease [ ] Yes [ ] No
Peripheral vascular disease [ ] Yes [ ] No
Heart failure [ ] Yes [ ] No
New cardiac symptoms [ ] Yes [ ] No

Microvascular complications

Renal function:
CKD stage:
Retinopathy screening [ ] Yes [ ] No
Retinopathy type:
Blindness [ ] Yes [ ] No
Peripheral neuropathy [ ] Yes [ ] No

Labs

Urea and electrolytes:
Liver function tests:
Lipid profile:
Bone profile:
Thyroid function test:
Urine ACR:
Macroalbuminuria:

Mouth care

Regular dental check [ ] Y [ ] N
Oral hygiene [ ] Good [ ] Bad
Dentures [ ] Y [ ] N Caries [ ] Y [ ] N
Gum Disease [ ] Y [ ] Infection [ ] Y [ ] N

Foot examination

Pulses Present	**Right**	**Left**
Dorsalis pedis	[ ] Y [ ] N	[ ] Y [ ] N
Posterior tibial	[ ] Y [ ] N	[ ] Y [ ] N
Peripheral sensation	[ ] Present	[ ] Present
	[ ] Reduced	[ ] Reduced
	[ ] Absent	[ ] Absent

Ulceration:
(Condition, location, infection)
Deformities:
Amputation:

Educational Needs:

[ ] Acute illness
[ ] Emergency management
[ ] Diet
[ ] Compliance
[ ] Monitoring
[ ] Self Care/neglect
[ ] Attend Screening
[ ] Patient/carer support

Advanced care planning:

Additional concerns:

Follow Up:

Key considerations with Goals and treatment changes:

Cardiovascular:
Renal:
Eyes:
Feet:
Sexual function:
Glycaemic control:
Functional needs:
Medications:
Infection prevention
Vaccinations

Specialist team involvement

[ ] Specialist diabetes team
[ ] Diabetic specialist nurses
[ ] Memory services
[ ] Podiatry
[ ] Dietician
[ ] Social prescribing
[ ] Physiotherapy
[ ] Occupational therapy
[ ] Opthalmology
[ ] Mental health teams
[ ] Smoking cessation
[ ] Diabetes education for patients and carers

Figure 16k.2: A template for annual review for older people with diabetes. ACR, albumin to creatinine ratio; ADL, activities of daily living; BMI, body mass index; BP, blood pressure; CKD, chronic kidney disease; GAD, glutamate decarboxylase; GDS, Geriatric Depression Scale; MoCA, Montreal Cognitive Assessment.

References

1. Maddigan, S.L., Feeny, D.H., and Johnson, J.A. (2005). Health-related quality of life deficits associated with diabetes and comorbidities in a Canadian National Population Health Survey. *Qual. Life Res.* 14: 1311–1320.
2. Duffy, R.E., Mattson, B.J., and Zack, M. (2005). Comorbidities among Ohio's nursing home residents with diabetes. *J. Am. Med. Dir. Assoc.* 6: 383–389.
3. Munshi, M., Grande, L., Hayes, M. et al. (2006). Cognitive dysfunction is associated with poor diabetes control in older adults. *Diabetes Care* 29: 1794–1799.
4. Volpato, S., Blaum, C., Resnick, H. et al. (2002). Comorbidities and impairments explaining the association between diabetes and lower extremities disabilities. *Diabetes Care* 25: 678–683.
5. Lu, F.P., Lin, K.P., and Kuo, H.K. (2009). Diabetes and the risk of multi-system aging phenotypes: a systematic review and meta-analysis. *PLoS One* 4: e4144.
6. Maraldi, C., Volpato, S., Penninx, B.W. et al. (2007). Diabetes mellitus, glycemic control, and incident depressive symptoms among 70- to 79-year-old persons: the health, aging, and body composition study. *Arch. Intern. Med.* 67: 1137–1144.
7. Howrey, B.T., Al Snih, S., and Markides, K.S. (2018). Frailty and diabetes among Mexican American older adults. *Ann. Epidemiol.* 28: 421–426.
8. Lee, J.S.W., Auyeung, T.W., Leung, J. et al. (2010). The effect of diabetes mellitus on age-associated lean mass loss in 3153 older adults. *Diabet. Med.* 27: 1366–1371.

16I Special Issues in Old Age: Mouth Care

Nali Ahmed and Ahmed H. Abdelhafiz

Department of Geriatric Medicine, Rotherham General Hospital, Rotherham, UK

Key Points

- Oral health is vital for older people, impacting overall wellbeing.
- Ageing is associated with oral changes that increase the prevalence of oral problems in older people.
- Diabetes-related oral complications are likely due to persistent hyperglycaemia and increased risk of infections.
- Education, rigorous mouth hygiene, good glycaemic control and regular preventative dental care are fundamental part of good mouth care.
- Healthcare providers should raise awareness and promote oral health in this population.

Introduction

Oral health is vital for several essential functions in human physiology. Any disturbance of its functions can drastically affect an older person's quality of life. The stomatognathic system, which consists of teeth and its supporting structures and the associated musculoskeletal components, including the mandible and the maxilla, the temporomandibular joints and the muscles of mastication, is responsible for biting, mastication and initial digestion of food. The oral cavity is a host for many infectious agents and is prone to a wide array of illness when exposed

Care of Older People with Diabetes: A Manual for Healthcare Practice, First Edition.
Edited by Alan J. Sinclair and Ahmed H. Abdelhafiz.

Companion website: www.wiley.com/go/sinclair/1e

to insults or when its protective mechanisms are disrupted. Dental diseases are the most common chronic disorders affecting humans. For example, gingivitis occurs across all age groups and periodontitis prevalence increases with increasing age. Cumulative oral problems increases with increasing age. In addition, older people with diabetes and persistent hyperglycaemia may have a higher risk of tooth problems and gum disease than people without diabetes, due to their lower immunity. This chapter reviews age and diabetes-related oral changes and addresses common oral problems and mouth care in older people with diabetes.

Age-related Oral Changes

With increasing age, there is wearing of the enamel, chipping and fractures of teeth with staining of the fracture lines and chipped areas. This leads to exposure of the dentin, which wears more quickly than the enamel. As a result, ageing teeth appear darker in colour due to dentin exposure and increased surface staining. The risk factors for tooth wear include increasing age, increased teeth use, such as night time bruxism, as well as food characteristics such hard or acidic food [1]. Ageing is associated with a modest reduction in periodontal support, which can be considered physiological if the tooth is functional and not painful or loose. Ageing is also associated with loss of elastic fibres, thick and disorganised collagen bundles in the connective tissue and a reduction of the microvasculature, which lead to less resilient buccal mucosa and impaired its ability of wound healing [2]. Mastication may be reduced with increasing age likely due to reduced muscle mass or sarcopenia affecting the muscles of mastication (Box 16l.1) [3].

Diabetes-related Oral Changes

Diabetes mellitus is associated with several soft-tissue abnormalities in the oral cavity. These abnormalities include periodontal diseases (periodontitis and gingivitis) and salivary glands dysfunction, which lead a reduction in the salivary flow, changes in saliva composition and taste dysfunction. Periodontal diseases are considered the sixth most prevalent complication of diabetes mellitus [4]. Oral bacterial

Box 16I.1: Age-related Oral Changes

- Wearing of enamel
- Teeth chipping and fracture
- Staining of chipped areas and fracture lines
- Exposure of dentin
- Darker teeth
- Reduced periodontal support
- Recession of gum lines
- Reduced elastic tissues in buccal mucosa
- Thickened and disorganised collagen tissue in buccal mucosa
- Reduction of microvasculature of buccal mucosa
- Reduced resilience and wound healing of buccal mucosa
- Reduced masticatory function of muscles of mastication

Box 16I.2: Diabetes-related Oral Changes

- Periodontitis and gingivitis
- Reduced salivary flow
- Taste dysfunction
- Increased bacterial and fungal infections
- Stomatitis
- Geographic, fissured tongue and migratory glossitis
- Traumatic ulcers
- Lichen planus and lichenoid reaction
- Angular cheilitis
- Mucosal neurosensory dysfunction
- Dental caries
- Teeth loss

and fungal infections increases with uncontrolled diabetes. Other diabetes-related oral conditions include stomatitis, geographic tongue, fissured tongue, benign migratory glossitis, traumatic ulcer, lichen planus, lichenoid reaction and angular cheilitis. Delayed mucosal wound healing, mucosal neurosensory disorders, dental caries and tooth loss are also associated with diabetes. These conditions are higher in patients with diabetes compared with healthy controls (Box 16I.2) [5].

Common Oral Conditions in Older People with Diabetes

The persistent metabolic and haemodynamic disturbances of diabetes can lead to widespread systemic complications, including oral cavity. Several oral complications are common in older people with diabetes.

Periodontal Disease

Periodontal disease includes gingivitis, which is gum inflammation without loss of tooth support and periodontitis that extends to include the tissues and the surrounding structures around the teeth and can lead to difficulty in chewing and even tooth loss. Diabetes mellitus is a major risk factor for the development, progression and severity of periodontitis. The prevalence increases with increasing age. The incidence of periodontitis is also linked to diabetes control, which is twice as high in patients with poorly controlled diabetes compared with those with well-controlled or no diabetes [6]. The risk of alveolar bone loss and the severity of disease progression is also higher in poorly controlled diabetes [7]. Therefore, uncontrolled diabetes seems to be particularly important for the development and severity of periodontal disease and glycaemic control appears to be vital in reducing the incidence and the complications of periodontal disease. Other factors such as disruption of the oral cavity flora, change in vascularity or decreased function and white blood cell count may increases the susceptibility to periodontal disease. Key recommendations to address periodontal disease are summarised in Box 16l.3.

Dental Caries

Dental caries or dental cavities are the localised destruction of the susceptible hard dental tissue by the acidic byproducts resulting from bacterial fermentation of dietary carbohydrates. Dental caries increase with increasing age. Poor oral hygiene and regular intake of sucrose-rich food increase the risk of dental caries. Dental caries are more common in patients with diabetes mellitus and may be associated with poor glycaemic control. Compliance with a healthy diet, especially

Box 16l.3: Key Recommendations to Address Periodontal Disease

- Regular dental cleaning every six months by a licensed dental care provider
- Routine oral self-care, brushing morning and night and daily flossing; toothbrushes should be replaced every three to four months
- An antideptic mouthwash and chlorhexidine can reduce bacterial load and prevent periodontal disease
- Acute episodes of oral infection should be addressed immediately
- Amoxicillin 250 mg three times a day for seven days or clindamycin 300 mg four times a day for seven days should be prescribed

one that is low in fermentable carbohydrates, may reduce the risk of dental caries. In older people, the increased prevalence of periodontal disease and the reduced salivary flow and composition, which normally buffers the acidity arising from carbohydrate fermentation, may also increase the risk of dental caries. Pain, halitosis and infections can be the presentation. Strategies to prevent dental caries include fluoride, daily effective oral hygiene and regular visits to dental services.

Dry Mouth

Dry mouth includes xerostomia and hyposalivation. Xerostomia is the subjective sensation of dry mouth. Hyposalivation is objective dry mouth, which can be measured by reduced salivary flow due to salivary gland hypofunction. The prevalence of both xerostomia and hyposalivation increases with increasing age [8]. Dry mouth is one of the manifestations of diabetes due to persistent hyperglycaemia and also may be related to the anticholinergic or xerogenic effects of medications commonly used in older people with diabetes and associated multiple morbidities. Dry mouth in diabetes can also be due to autonomic neuropathy or salivary glands atrophy, which may lead to reduced salivary secretion. Older age, reduced fluid intake, poor glycaemic control and polypharmacy are contributing factors to dry mouth in older people with diabetes. Recommendations to reduces xerostomia are summarised in Box 16l.4.

Box 16l.4: Recommendations to Reduce Xerostomia

- Frequent use of sugar-free beverages, topical fluoride and regular oral hygiene after meals
- Removable prostheses must be kept clean and out of the mouth during sleeping hours
- Frequent lubrication of the lips helps prevent lip cracking and infections
- To enhance salivary production, gustatory (sugar-free mints or candies), masticatory (sugar-free gums) and pharmacological (pilocarpine 5 mg three times a day) means can be used in patients with remaining salivary function
- Salivary substitutes, rinses and moisturising gels can assist patients who have little or no remaining salivary function

Candida

Candida is a type of yeast that exists in healthy individuals as a commensal organism. *Candida albicans* is the most common *Candida* species that causes opportunistic infections of the oral mucosa in immunocompromised and susceptible patients such as those with uncontrolled diabetes. Candidiasis can affect the tongue (glossitis), corners of the mouth (angular cheilitis) and beneath dentures (denture stomatitis). Overall fungal infections, including candidiasis, increase in patients diabetes compared with healthy individuals. For example, one study found that a prevalence of 15% of *Candida*-related lesions in patients with diabetes compared with only 3% in patients without diabetes [9].

Other risks of *Candida* infection include smoking, wearing dentures and the use of steroids or antibiotics. Addressing polypharmacy, maintaining oral hygiene and antifungals such as nystatin or fluconazole can be used for treatment.

Oral Cancer

Diabetes mellitus increases the risk of oral cancer [10]. In addition to the increased prevalence of oral cancer in people with diabetes compared with control, precancerous lesions such as actinic cheilitis, leukoplakia, nicotinic stomatitis and lichen planus are more common in people with diabetes [10]. Diabetes is also associated with increased mortality from oral cancer and decreased recurrence-free survival. The pathogenesis of diabetes-related oral cancer risk remains not very clear.

Taste Impairment

Diabetes is associated with reduced taste sensation, which may have negative consequences such as consuming beverages with high sugar contents with high intense sweet taste and high calories leading to obesity and uncontrolled diabetes. Taste impairment may be due to diabetes-related xerostomia and hyposalivation.

Mouth Care

Rigorous oral hygiene is required for the prevention of oral infections, gum diseases and dental caries in older people with diabetes. Regular teeth brushing, at least twice a day, and cleaning interdental spaces may be compromised in old age due to associated reduced ability for self-care tasks. In addition, for the same reason, regular annual teeth checks and contact with healthcare professional may not be optimal. Therefore, education about mouth care, good glycaemic control and preventative measures are required to reduce the risk of diabetes-related oral complications. Suggested oral health inquiry is summarised in Box 16I.5.

Education

Patients and carers should be educated about the potential oral complications of diabetes mellitus and the importance of regular oral checkups with dental health services. Particular attention should be paid to patients from the lower socioeconomic status, as they are likely to suffer more from unhealthy habits, lack of appropriate information, negative attitude towards oral health and less use of dental services. Adequate education and information about oral health is positively associated with frequent toothbrushing, good periodontal health and compliance with dental visits [11]. In addition to education, information about the importance of looking after their own oral health and how to do it, should be provided on a regular basis whenever patients contact healthcare services.

Box 16l.5: Suggested Enquiries About Oral Health

- Regular check whether patients have noticed any signs of infection, bad breath or taste impairment
- All patients should be registered with a dentist
- Regular check on compliance with dental service attendance
- Regular dental checks every six months, or more often if required
- Recommend urgent dental check when symptoms of infection arise such as painful, swollen or bleeding gums
- Regular and thorough oral examination
- Recommend regular toothbrushing, preferably using an electric toothbrush
- Recommend regular use of antiseptic mouthwash
- Recommend smoking cessation
- Maintain good glycaemic control

Glycaemic Control

Hyperglycaemia will lead to increased glucose content of the saliva increasing the risk of oral infections and dental caries. Increased production of advanced glycation end-products leads to increased risk of periodontal disease, so adequate glycaemic control is crucial for maintenance of oral health. In addition to long-term glycaemic control, short-term blood glucose levels should be kept under control, especially in acute illness such as infections when blood glucose tends to spike. Diet with carbohydrates with a low glycaemic index may help reduce postprandial surges in blood glucose levels.

Preventative Measures

Routine preventive dental care visits are needed for older people with diabetes for prevention and early detection of diabetes-related complications. In a study to investigate the use of preventative dental care older people (≥ 65 years) with diabetes, participants with diabetes were statistically less likely to have preventive dental care than participants without diabetes [12]. Annual diabetes reviews should include an enquiry about oral health, screening for oral disease and referral to

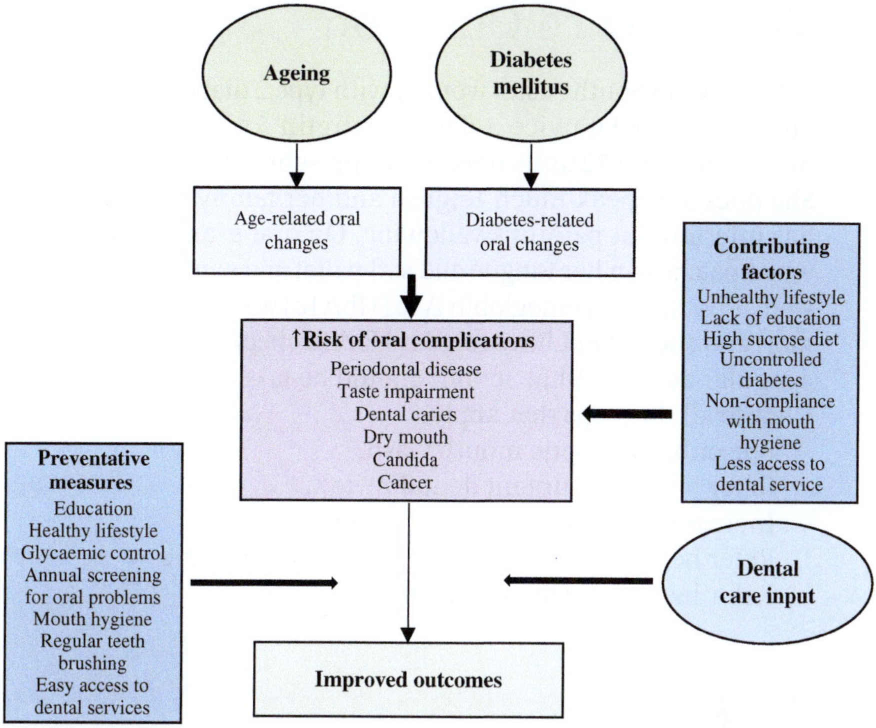

Figure 16l.1: Factors leading to oral complications in diabetes and preventative measures to improve outcomes.

dental services on a regular basis, as well as when required. In addition, specific professional guidelines for criteria for dental referral may be required (Figure 16l.1).

Summary

Ageing is associated with cumulative oral conditions due to age-related oral changes that predispose older people to oral problems. In addition, diabetes-related oral complications is common in older people, probably due to persistent hyperglycaemia, reduced immunity and increased risk of infections. Therefore, mouth care should be an integral part of diabetes care in older people with diabetes, which includes education about oral health, rigorous mouth hygiene, good glycaemic control and regular preventative dental care.

Clinical Practice Question

Q1. A 76-year-old South Asian woman with type 2 diabetes for 27 years on metformin 1 g twice a day, linagliptin 5 mg once a day and insulin glargine 12 units once a day, presented for annual review. She does not speak much English and her family report that she has intermittent painful swallowing. On oral examination, some white patches on her tongue and soft pallet and some missing teeth were found. Her haemoglobin A1c (HbA1c) was 8.6% (70.50 mmol/mol) and she did not have regular HbA1c checks. She does not see a regular dentist. What actions should be taken?
Choose all the steps that apply.
A. Prescribe antiseptic mouth wash.
B. Refer her for an urgent dental review.
C. Increase her hypoglycaemic therapy.
D. Refer her for dental care educational programme.
E. Refer her to speech and language therapy.

References

Key references only are listed here. For a full list of references visit: `https://www.wiley.com/go/sinclair/1e`.

1. Liu, B., Zhang, M., Chen, Y. et al. (2014). Tooth wear in aging people: an investigation of the prevalence and the influential factors of incisal/occlusal tooth wear in Northwest China. *BMC Oral Health* 14: 65.
2. Klein, D.R. (1980). Oral soft tissue changes in geriatric patients. *Bull. N Y. Acad. Med.* 56: 721–727.
3. Goodpaster, B.H., Park, S.W., Harris, T.B. et al. (2006). The loss of skeletal muscle strength, mass, and quality in older adults: the health, aging and body com-position study. *J. Gerontol. A Biol. Sci. Med. Sci.* 61: 1059–1064.
4. Löe, H. (1993). Periodontal disease: the sixth complication of diabetes mellitus. *Diabetes Care* 16: 329–334.
5. Saini, R., Al-Maweri, S.A., Saini, D. et al. (2010). Oral mucosal lesions in non oral habit diabetic patients and association of diabetes mellitus with oral precancerous lesions. *Diabetes Res. Clin. Pract.* 89: 320–326.
6. Nelson, R.G., Shlossman, M., Budding, L.M. et al. (1990). Periodontal disease and NIDDM in Pima Indians. *Diabetes Care* 13: 836–840.

7. Taylor, G.W., Burt, B.A., Becker, M.P. et al. (1998). Glycemic control and alveolar bone loss progression in type 2 diabetes. *Ann. Periodontol.* 3: 30–39.
8. Orellana, M., Lagravere, M., Boychuk, D. et al. (2006). Prevalence of xerostomia in population-based samples: a systematic review. *J. Public Heath Dent.* 66: 152–158.
9. Guggenheimer, J., Moore, P.A., Rossie, K. et al. (2000). Insulin-dependent diabetes mellitus and oral soft tissue pathologies. II. Prevalence and characteristics of candida and candida lesions. *Oral Surg. Med. Oral Pathol. Oral Radiol. Endod.* 89: 570–576.
10. Gong, Y., Wei, B., Yu, L. et al. (2015). Type 2 diabetes mellitus and risk of oral cancer and precancerous lesions: a meta-analysis of observational studies. *Oral Oncol.* 51: 332–340.

16m Special Issues in Old Age: Pain Management

Pann Ei Hnynn Si[1] *and Ahmed H. Abdelhafiz*[2]

[1] *Sheffield Kidney Institute, Sheffield Teaching Hospitals, Sheffield, UK*
[2] *Department of Geriatric Medicine, Rotherham General Hospital, Rotherham, UK*

Key Points

- Chronic pain is common in older people with diabetes compared with those without diabetes and is associated with adverse outcomes.
- Older people tend to under-report pain and perceive it as routine part of ageing, which may lead to the pain being underdiagnosed, undertreated and negative consequences.
- Pain assessment tools should be used appropriately for patient's cognitive ability and cultural background.
- Pharmacological intervention should be started with a low dose and titrated up at slow pace to avoid adverse effects and to improve tolerance.
- A multidisciplinary approach with a comprehensive geriatric assessment is the best policy for pain management to reduce symptom severity and improve health-related quality of life.

Introduction

Pain is an unpleasant, subjective sensory and emotional experience of noxious stimuli and is more common in older compared with younger people. Physiological changes with ageing, such as reduced proprioception and altered peripheral nerves conductivity, increase the risks

Care of Older People with Diabetes: A Manual for Healthcare Practice, First Edition.
Edited by Alan J. Sinclair and Ahmed H. Abdelhafiz.

Companion website: www.wiley.com/go/sinclair/1e

of injuries and development of pain. In addition, pathological changes due to multimorbidity in old age increase and alter sensation of pain. Many older people attribute pain to increasing age or deny pain to avoid hospitalisation. Older people with diabetes are at higher risk of all types of pain, including acute, chronic or intermittent pain, which may lead to increased risk of hospital visits, disability and institutionalisation. Chronic pain is associated with reduced physical function, falls and injuries, which further exacerbates the chronic pain setting up a vicious circle that reduce quality of life. Pain can also be mixed, psychological or unspecified. This chapter reviews assessment and management of pain in older people with diabetes.

Aetiology

Chronic pain is very common and a comorbid condition in older people with diabetes due to disease related factors such as painful peripheral neuropathy, affecting up to one third people with diabetes as reported in one UK study [1]. A cross-sectional US study reported that moderate to extreme general pain was present in 58% of 11 689 participants with diabetes aged 47–73 years [2]. Older people with diabetes have increased risk of rheumatic conditions such as tenosynovitis, capsulitis, periarthritis, carpal tunnel syndrome and osteoarthritis causing increased musculoskeletal pain, which is associated with physical inactivity and reduced quality of life. The other mechanisms of chronic pain in this population include vascular insufficiencies, vitamin D deficiency, decreased insulin-like growth factors, sedentary lifestyle, reduced dietary intake and obesity [3]. Pain can be classified as nociceptive pain, which is associated with normal processing of stimuli that damages normal tissues, and neuropathic pain, which is associated with abnormal processing of sensory stimuli from the peripheral or central nervous system (Table 16m.1).

Assessment

Pain management based on medical assessment alone is usually insufficient and collaborative multidisciplinary comprehensive assessment is crucial to optimal pain management. Associated multimorbidity in older people can affect the accurate assessment of the pain, as well as the response to treatment. Self-reported pain is the gold standard for

Table 16m.1: Types of pain.

Nociceptive	Neuropathic
A. Somatic: originates from skin or musculoskeletal tissues such as joints, bones, muscle or connective tissue. Feels like ache or throbbing and is well localised	A. Centrally generated: originates from injury to central, peripheral nervous system or dysregulation of autonomic nervous system. Examples are phantom pain or stroke associated pain
B. Visceral: originates from visceral organs such as cancer stretching organ capsule, which feels like ache and well localised or obstruction of a viscus, which feels like intermittent cramps and is poorly localised	B. Peripherally generated: originates from peripheral nerves affected by diabetes (diabetic neuropathy) or pain related to an isolated peripheral nerve injury

diagnosis of pain but there are several barriers for pain assessment in people who do not express their pain (Box 16m.1). Older people vary in their expression of pain and healthcare professionals should have skills in observation, active listening, questioning technique, measurement and interpretation. In addition, understanding the impact of pain on the physical, psychological, social and cultural perspectives of the individual is important to develop an effective, patient-centred and holistic management plan.

Box 16m.1: Barriers to Pain Assessment

- Under-reporting
- Perceived as part of ageing
- Inability to access medical care
- Cultural barriers
- Cognitive impairment
- Self-isolation
- Communication problems
- Swallowing problems
- Anxiety about polypharmacy
- Fear of losing independence
- Fear of addiction to pain killers
- Lack of carers support

Visual inspection, including observation of body language, facial expressions and general behaviour is an important first step. Patients in pain may be very quiet and withdrawn or very irritable and agitated. The use of pain assessment tools will aid to obtain objective measurement of the severity of pain, its effects on general wellbeing and quality of life. In addition, it is useful in measuring response to treatment. There are several specifically designed tools for assessing pain severity. Some simple and easy to use unidimensional tools include the numerical rating scale, verbal rating scale and visual analogue scale. Other unidimensional tool such as the Wong–Baker FACES tool can be used for patients with language or communication difficulties as well as cognitive impairment. Multidimensional pain tools provide more information and measurement of pain. The McGill Pain Questionnaire is one example for chronic pain assessment. The Abbey pain scale is useful in people with poor communication or cognitive impairment. The pain assessment in advanced dementia scale is an easy and simple tool, which does not need patient communication but depends on observing a patient's behaviour (e.g. breathing, facial expression, negative vocalisation, consolability and body language). Mnemonic aids can be useful and require no equipment (Box 16m.2). Pain assessment should take into consideration

Box 16m.2: Pain Assessment

Assessment of pain:

- location
- radiation
- severity
- quality
- effects on function
- effects on activities of daily living
- level at rest and activity
- provoking factors
- relieving factors
- related symptoms
- timing
- Pain-relieving medications

Assessment tools:

- Numerical rating scale
- Verbal rating scale
- Visual analogue scale
- Wong–Baker FACES
- McGill Pain Questionnaire
- Abbey pain scale
- Pain assessment in advanced dementia scale

Mnemonics:

- OPQRST (onset, provokes, quality, radiates, severity, time)
- SOCRATES (site, onset, character, radiates, associations, timing, exacerbations, severity)
- PAINED (place, amount, intensifiers, nullifiers, effects, description)

diabetes-related factors contributing to pain, such as peripheral neuropathy, falls or periodontal infections.

Pain in Care-home Residents

The prevalence of diabetes in care homes is high, affecting up to one third of residents [4]. People with diabetes living in care homes are likely to be very old, have multiple morbidities including dementia, frailty, disability, and high prevalence of chronic pain. Residents may perceive pain as a normal part of getting old with no potential to improve. Frail patients may find it harder to regain function after an acute stressful event such as pain. Pain management in these setting is challenging.

Barriers to pain management include communication difficulties due to cognitive impairment and medication intolerance due to multiple morbidities. Suboptimal use of analgesic medications, particularly in patients with dementia, has been reported [5]. There is an unmet need for staff education about pain identification in residents with dementia, regular screening for pain, and the development of simple and easy to use pain assessment tools in this population. In addition, access to specialist pain service is required.

Management

Pain management is an important part of the holistic care plans for older people with diabetes. Pain relief will help reduce the risk of adverse events such as falls, behavioural changes, sleep disturbance, depression, agitation and minimise the need for antipsychotic medications. Given the complexities of managing chronic pain in older people, a multidisciplinary approach that includes several healthcare professionals is required. Management includes non-pharmacological and pharmacological interventions (Figure 16m.1).

Non-pharmacological Therapy

Non-pharmacological measures are particularly suitable in older people because of their low incidence of adverse effects compared with pharmacological therapy. These measures can be adjuvant to pharmacological therapy or used on their own to control pain. Cognitive behavioural therapy can be used to influence patient's beliefs, attitude and emotions to help control and adapt to pain. Psychologists and

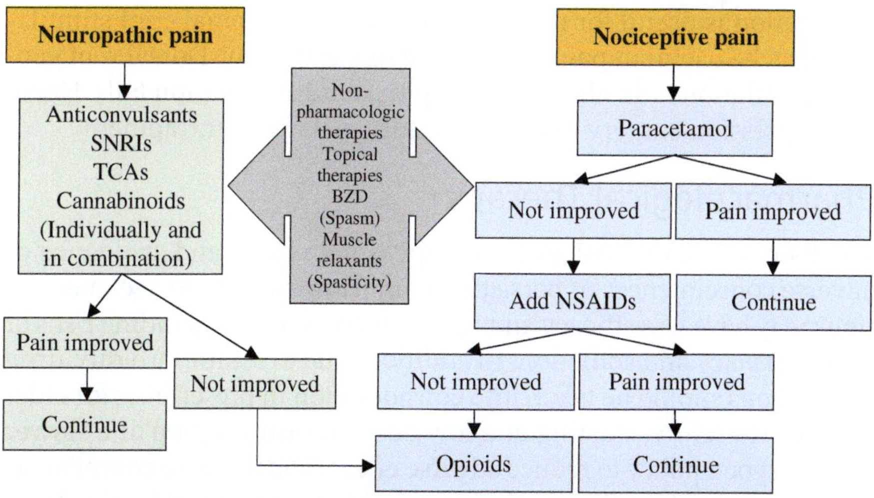

Figure 16m.1: Algorithm of therapeutic options for pain control in older people with diabetes mellitus. Medications for neuropathic and nociceptive pain can be combined in mixed types of pain. BZD, benzodiazepines; NSAIDs, non-steroidal anti-inflammatory drugs; SNRIs, serotonin–norepinephrine reuptake inhibitors; TCA, tricyclic antidepressants.

non-psychologists with training can deliver this mode of therapy. In addition, self-management practice by older people has been shown to improve pain-related distress and disability in primary care [6]. Education about pain, the associated risks of adverse events and ways of relaxation and communication will help to empower patients to control pain. Self-management programmes use a combination of physical, psychological and social perspectives in an educational approach to teach patients specific coping techniques by changing their cognitive, emotional and behavioural responses to manage their pain. Physiotherapy, together with an exercise programme, is an important component of non-pharmacological intervention. Balance training, flexibility, muscle strengthening and endurance may help pain control, improve function and reduce adverse events such as falls [7]. Interventions such as acupuncture and chiropractic care may ease certain rheumatic pains [8,9]. Myofascial release techniques involves applying force on myofascial trigger points or sensitive areas, which improves pain, anxiety, depression, sleep and quality of life [10]. Hypnosis, an altered state of consciousness leading to increased responsiveness to suggestion, may reduce pain intensity, duration and frequency [11]. Mindfulness and meditation are other psychology-based therapeutic modalities, which may reduce pain-related stress [12]. Transcutaneous electrical nerve stimulation is useful for neuropathic pain relief. Spinal cord stimulation may be useful in pain localised in one extremity. Dorsal root ganglia stimulation is an alternative if spinal cord stimulation fails. Nerve decompression surgery may be used for focal nerve entrapment.

Pharmacological Therapy

The focus of pharmacological therapy is pain relief and avoidance of adverse consequences of persistent pain. However, in old age, medications may have less efficacy and more adverse effects, including risks of polypharmacy and addiction. In addition, due to multimorbidity, drug interactions should be taken into consideration in prescribing for older people. Therefore, starting at a low dose and titrating up at a slower pace is a good policy to reduce adverse effects and increase compliance. Paracetamol is first-line analgesic suitable for most mild pain. Non-steroidal anti-inflammatory drugs (NSAIDs) can be used if paracetamol fails to control pain. These drugs are superior to paracetamol in chronic inflammatory pain. Cyclooxygenase-2 inhibitor NSAIDs may have fewer gastrointestinal adverse effects. Opioid analgesics are indicated for severe pain not controlled by other agents. Respiratory depression can occur if dose is increased quickly. Tolerance is another adverse effect. Patients with hepatic and renal impairment are at risk, so close monitoring and dose adjustment is required. Anticonvulsants, serotonin–norepinephrine reuptake inhibitors and tricyclic antidepressants are useful in neuropathic pain relief and may improve pain-related sleep disturbance, depressive symptoms and social functioning. The usefulness of benzodiazepines is limited by their adverse effects of increasing risk of falls, but they can be useful when pain is associated with anxiety or muscle spasm. Muscle relaxants are good for pain associated with spasticity. Specific agents such as calcitonin and bisphosphonates are useful in osteoporosis or cancer-related pain. Cannabinoids are a more recently introduced therapy for neuropathic pain. Micronised NSAIDs are better absorbed with fewer adverse effects than conventional NSAIDs. Several topical agents, such as capsaicin and lidocaine, are useful when oral route is compromised by poor swallowing and can be combined with oral agents for additive effect (Table 16m.2). Newer opioids with a less-sedating effect and less respiratory depression are under development [13].

Table 16m.2: Pharmacological agents for pain control in older people with diabetes mellitus.

Drug	Indication	Remarks
Paracetamol	Mild to moderate pain, dose up to 4 g/day, adjusted in liver dysfunction	Effective in MSK but less effective in inflammatory pain
NSAIDs	Mild to moderate pain, when pain not controlled by paracetamol	Effective in chronic inflammatory pain, caution for GI, renal and CV adverse effects
Opioids	Moderate to severe pain not responding to other therapies	Caution with sedation, cognitive impairment, constipation and drug interactions
Anticonvulsants	Effective in neuropathic pain; may improve sleep deprivation	Dose adjustment in renal impairment

(*Continued*)

Table 16m.2: Continued

Drug	Indication	Remarks
Serotonin-norepinephrine reuptake inhibitors	Effective in neuropathic pain; may improve depressive symptoms	Caution with hypertensive episodes, slow dose titration as adverse effects are dose related
Tricyclic antidepressants	Effective in neuropathic pain; may improve depressive symptoms	Caution with anticholinergic and noradrenergic adverse effects and prolongation of QT interval
Benzodiazepines	Limited for pain associated with muscle spasm or anxiety	Caution with increased risk of falls and cognitive decline
Muscle relaxants	Suitable for pain associated with spasticity	Caution with GI adverse effects, dizziness and somnolence; slow tapering due to risk of delirium and seizures
Calcitonin	Suitable in pain due to osteoporotic fractures or bone metastases	Caution with hypersensitivity reactions; requires monitoring of calcium and phosphate
Bisphosphonates	Suitable in pain due to osteoporotic fractures or bone metastases	Caution with esophagitis and hypocalcaemia; monitor renal function
Cannabinoids	Suitable in neuropathic pain	Caution with CV adverse effects, euphoria, anxiety, psychosis, sedation and dizziness
Micronised NSAIDs	Nanotechnology-developed to increase surface area and absorption	Achieve efficacy at a lower dose to conventional NSAIDs with fewer adverse effects
Topical agents: Topical NSAIDs Capsaicin Lidocaine Opioids Amitriptyline cream, clonidine gel, ketamine cream, medicinal plants extract oils	Alternative to oral NSAIDs with fewer systemic adverse effects; adjuvant analgesic for neuropathic and MSK pain; suitable for localised pain; convenient and long-acting; suitable in patients with poor oral intake	Effective for relief of localised pain e g knee or hand OA pain; caution with burning sensation, especially in patients with skin conditions; caution with skin irritation; good pain relief, less constipation; can reach higher doses with fewer drug interactions and adverse effects

CV, Cardiovascular; GI, gastrointestinal; MSK, musculoskeletal; NSAIDs, non-steroidal anti-inflammatory drugs; OA, osteoarthritis.

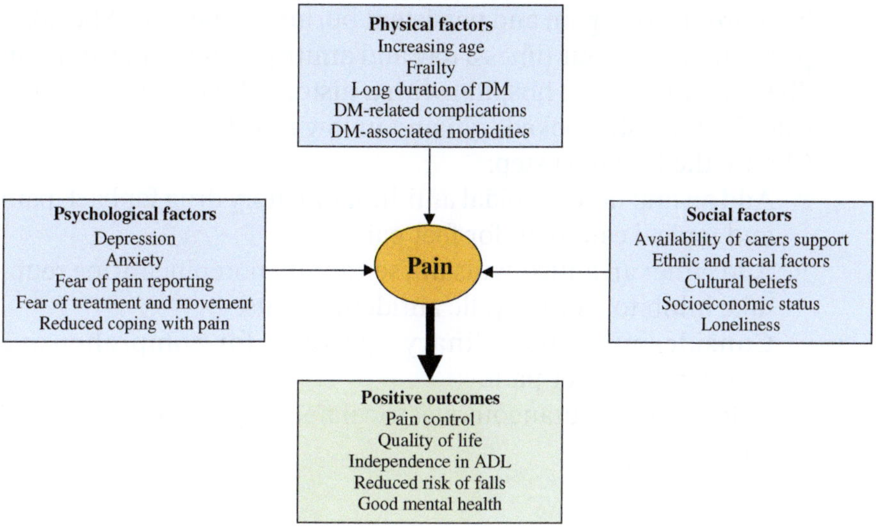

Figure 16m.2: Multidimensional approach for prevention of chronic pain in older people with diabetes, addressing physical, psychological and social aspects of care. ADL, activities of daily living; DM, diabetes mellitus.

Prevention

In addition to non-pharmacological and pharmacological interventions, prevention of chronic pain in older people with diabetes should be holistic, which involves addressing physical, psychological and social aspects. For example, pain is more common in older people with diabetes and associated comorbidities, especially depression [14]. Good glycaemic control, cardiovascular risk prevention, annual screening for depression and adequate social support may reduce the incidence of chronic pain and improve overall outcomes. Therefore, comprehensive approach should aim, in addition to pain control, to prevent deconditioning, maintain both physical and mental function with a focus on quality of life (Figure 16m.2).

Clinical Practice Question

Q1. An 83-year-old woman living alone in the community, known to have type 2 diabetes mellitus for 20 years, with diabetic neuropathy, chronic kidney disease and osteoarthritis of the spine. She has chronic back pain and persistent burning of her feet. She takes paracetamol 1 g four times a day and amitriptyline 50 mg at night. She was admitted to hospital with a history of recurrent falls. On examination, she looked frail and in low mood.

Choose the best next step:

A. Add an oral non-steroidal anti-inflammatory drug for back pain and topical capsaicin for feet pain.

B. Add either an anticonvulsant, serotonin–norepinephrine reuptake inhibitors or tricyclic antidepressants.

C. Consider multidisciplinary approach for comprehensive assessment of her pain.

D. Refer for transcutaneous electrical nerve stimulation or spinal cord stimulation.

References

Key references only are listed here. For a full list of references visit: `https://www.wiley.com/go/sinclair/1e`.

1. Abbott, C., Malik, R., van Ross, E. et al. (2011). Prevalence and characteristics of painful diabetic neuropathy in a large community-based diabetic population in the UK. *Diabetes Care* 24: 2220–2224.
2. Bair, M.J., Brizendine, E.J., Ackerman, R.T. et al. (2010). Prevalence of pain and association with quality of life, depression and glycemic control in patients with diabetes. *Diabetes Med.* 27: 578–584.
3. Sözen, T., Başaran, N.Ç., Tınazlı, M. et al. (2018). Musculoskeletal problems in diabetes mellitus. *Eur. J. Rheumatol.* 5: 258–265.
4. Idrees, T., Castro-Revoredo, I.A., Migdal, A.L. et al. (2022). Update on the management of diabetes in long-term care facilities. *BMJ Open Diabetes Res. Care* 10: e002705.
5. Takai, Y., Yamamoto-Mitani, N., Okamoto, Y. et al. (2010). Literature review of pain prevalence among older residents of nursing homes. *Pain Manag. Nurs.* 11: 209–223.
6. Nicholas, M.K., Asghari, A., Blyth, F.M. et al. (2013). Self-management intervention for chronic pain in older adults: a randomized controlled trial. *Pain* 154: 824–835.
7. Levy, S.S., Macera, C.A., Hootman, J.M. et al. (2012). Evaluation of a multicomponent group exercise program for adults with arthritis: fitness and exercise for people with arthritis (FEPA). *Disability Health J.* 5: 305–311.

8. National Center for Complementary and Integrative Health (2022). Acupuncture: what you need to know. https://nccih.nih.gov/health/acupuncture/introduction#hed1 (accessed 15 June 2023).
9. Meade, T.W., Dyer, S., Browne, W. et al. (1990). Low back pain of mechanical origin: randomized comparison of chiropractic and hospital outpatient treatment. *BMJ* 300: 1431–1437.
10. Castro-Sánchez, A.M., Matarán-Peñarrocha, G.A., Granero-Molina, J. et al. (2011). Benefits of massage-myofascial release therapy on pain, anxiety, quality of sleep, depression, and quality of life in patients with fibromyalgia. *Evid. Based Complement. Alternat. Med.* 2011: 561753.

17 Deintensification of Therapy

Antoine Christiaens[1,2]

[1] *Clinical Pharmacy and Pharmacoepidemiology research group, Louvain Drug Research Institute, Université catholique de Louvain, Brussels, Belgium*

[2] *Fund for Scientific Research, Brussels, Belgium*

Key Points

- Deintensifying treatment is suggested when glucose-lowering treatment places patient at risk of adverse events or when the benefit that can be expected from it is negligible.
- A few studies have shown that reducing the intensity of treatment can be carried out without risk, but no benefits have yet been demonstrated.
- Deintensification of diabetes treatment is currently limited to glucose-lowering treatments.
- Algorithms exist for the practical management of glucose-lowering treatment deintensification.
- Treatments with a high risk of hypoglycaemia (such as sulfonylureas) should be stopped as a priority in patients for whom deintensification is suggested.
- The use of adequate resources to educate patients and healthcare professionals should be promoted, to enable these recommendations to be properly implemented.

Introduction

The treatment of type 2 diabetes (T2DM) must achieve the treatment objective that has been set according to the patient's state of health. For patients with T2DM, it is important to ensure an optimal balance,

Care of Older People with Diabetes: A Manual for Healthcare Practice, First Edition.
Edited by Alan J. Sinclair and Ahmed H. Abdelhafiz.

Companion website: www.wiley.com/go/sinclair/1e

to avoid both under- and overtreatment. Although this principle is probably applicable to all treatment axes used in diabetes (glycaemic control, blood pressure control, cardiovascular prevention), it is particularly well known in glucose-lowering treatments [1].

Older patients with T2DM are at high risk of glucose-lowering over-treatment, (i.e. their 'level of glycaemia that is inappropriate to a patient's health status that places a high risk of unwanted adverse effects of glucose-lowering treatment, such as hypoglycaemia and/or its harmful consequences') [2]. Depending on the criteria used to define it, the setting or the country, the prevalence of over-treatment ranges from 22% (community-dwelling patients aged 75 years or more) to 57% (hospitalised patients aged 70 years or more with multimorbidity). Moreover, it has also been shown that glucose-lowering overtreatment increases the risk of a number of deleterious conditions, such as hospitalisation, admission to emergency departments or mortality [3, 4].

Besides overtreatment, which relates to iatrogenic risk, there are certain treatments from which no benefit can be expected. Guidelines suggest that treatment should be deintensified to avoid either a treatment that poses a risk or one that has no benefit. Deintensification of treatment should be defined as 'reducing the total dose or the number of drugs, including total discontinuation of the treatment' [5]. 'Deprescription', 'discontinuation' or 'reduction of treatment' are terms that broadly refer to the same concept of deintensification.

While this process is suggested by many guidelines, the recommendations relating to it are of very low quality [6]. This reflects the very limited evidence base for these recommendations, particularly with regard to the benefits and risks associated with reducing the dosage of glucose-lowering agents. The few available studies have shown that deintensification can be carried out safely. However, the benefits expected to be associated with the deintensification of glucose-lowering treatment (e.g. reduction in the number and intensity of hypoglycaemia) remain unknown. A gap exists in this area of clinical medicine and good-quality research is needed to inform future guidelines [7, 8].

The aim of this chapter is to highlight the key elements currently known about deintensification that are useful in clinical practice, with a view to incorporating deintensification into treatment where appropriate. This chapter focuses exclusively on the management of antihyperglycaemic therapy deintensification in older patients with T2DM.

Key Issues

- Integrating deintensification of glucose-lowering treatment into routine diabetes treatment management.
- Identifying patients who can benefit from a deintensification of glucose-lowering treatment (i.e. those at risk of iatrogenic events or those for whom no benefit is expected from the treatment).
- Deintensifying treatment using the appropriate strategy, supported by existing resources for healthcare professionals and patients.

Management

Of the various existing clinical guidelines on the deintensification of glucose-lowering treatment, those from Deprescribing.org and the European Geriatric Medicine Society/European Diabetes Working Party for Older People present the most usable algorithms for clinical practice, while also having a good methodological quality [1, 6, 9]. The elements developed in this chapter are therefore mainly adapted from these sources.

Deintensifying glucose-lowering treatment is part of the overall management of glycaemia in older people with T2DM. For each patient, at each assessment of their health status, it is essential to consider the place of the strategy of deintensification in the individualised care plan. The deintensification strategy must follow several successive stages, including the identification of patients who could benefit from deintensification, the deintensification actions themselves, and then the short-term evaluation of the effects of this deintensification (Figure 17.1).

Identifying Patients Who Might Benefit

Identification of patients who might benefit from deintensification of glucose-lowering treatment is the first step of the process. Deintensification should be proposed for patients to avoid either a treatment that poses a risk or a treatment that has no benefit (Figure 17.1). In more practical terms, the guidelines suggest deintensification for patients with one of the characteristics listed in Box 17.1.

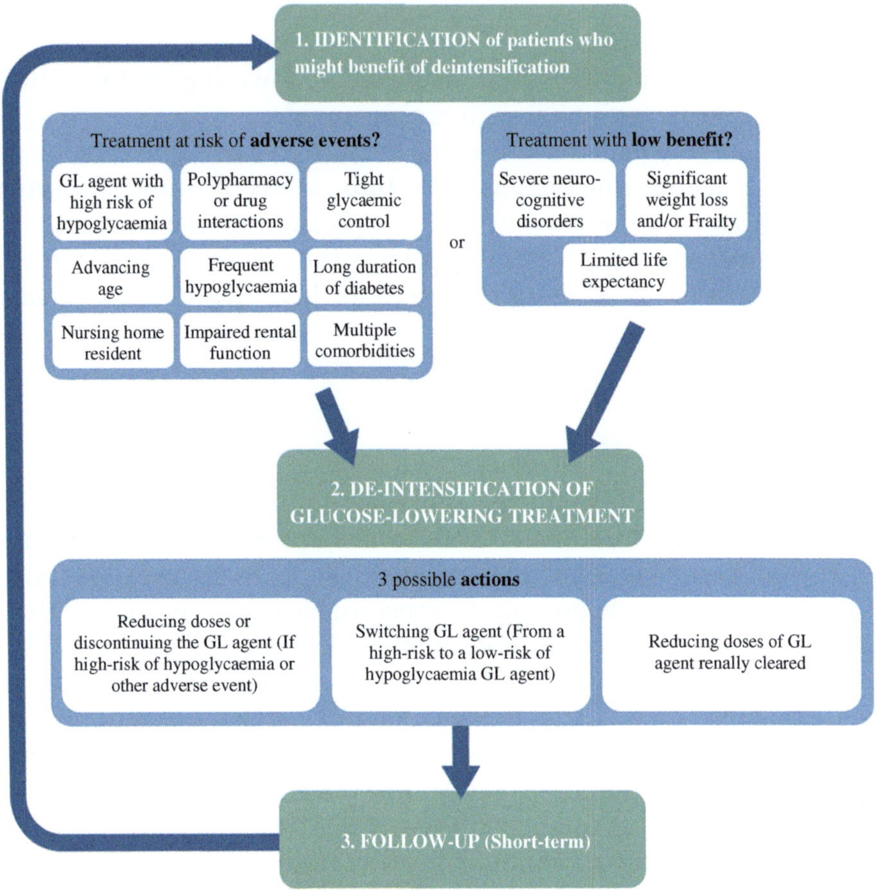

Figure 17.1: Steps to consider deintensification in older people with type 2 diabetes. GL, Glucose-lowering. Source: Adapted from Bourdel-Marchasson et al. [1] and Farrell et al. [9].

Nevertheless, it should be recognised that the list is not comprehensive. Other factors should be considered, such as the presence (sometimes temporary) of other drugs affecting glycaemic control; that is, those causing hyperglycaemia, for which the risk of hypoglycaemia exists after cessation in the presence of concomitant glucose-lowering treatment (e.g. corticosteroids, atypical antipsychotics, protease inhibitors, thiazides), causing hypoglycaemia (quinolones, quinin, beta-blockers, alcohol) or interacting with glucose-lowering drugs (e.g. trimethoprim sulfamethoxazole with sulfonylureas) [9].

The doctor's clinical experience, the aim of improving patient's quality of life or the patient's preference and values are all factors that

Box 17.1: Profiles of Patients for Whom Deintensification is Suggested

- Dementia, especially those with erratic eating pattern and abnormal behaviour
- Elderly, especially those ≥ 80 years old
- Impaired renal function, especially those with end stage renal disease
- Numerous comorbidities, especially those with ≥ 5 comorbidities
- Tight glycaemic control, especially those with HbA1c < 7%
- End of life phase, especially those with ≤ 1-year life expectancy
- Nursing home residents, especially those with multiple comorbidities
- Significant weight loss, especially unintentional indicating frailty
- Inappropriate medications, especially insulin or sulfonylureas
- Frequent hypoglycaemia, especially serious episodes needing assistance
- Long duration of diabetes, especially those > 20 years duration

Adapted from European Geriatric Medicine Society/European Diabetes Working Party for Older People [1].

may affect the decision to initiate deintensification. Moreover, the decision should obviously be based on a shared reflection between the patient and the doctor (or, more broadly, their healthcare team, where appropriate).

Deintensifying Glucose-lowering Treatment in Older Patients

Aiming to decrease the risks associated with glucose-lowering treatment and to simplify any treatment without benefits, the deintensification strategy can be achieved through three different, possibly complementary, actions [9]:

- Reducing doses or discontinuing the glucose-lowering agent if the glucose-lowering agent is at high risk of hypoglycaemia (e.g. sulfonylureas or insulin) or if the glucose-lowering agent is at high risk of other adverse effects.

- Switching the glucose-lowering agent from a high-risk to a low-risk agent (e.g. switching sulfonylureas to non-sulfonylureas, switching neutral protamine Hagedorn insulin to basal insulin such as detemir or glargine).
- Reducing doses of glucose-lowering agent renally cleared (e.g. metformin or sitagliptin).

After achieving deintensification, it is essential to offer the patient close follow-up (within one to two weeks after the change), to monitor the presence of symptoms (hyperglycaemia or hypoglycaemia) and to check blood glucose measurements (the frequency of which may be increased for capillary blood glucose measurements, or the temporary fitting of a continuous blood glucose sensor). It is also important to measure haemoglobin A1c (HbA1c), to check that average blood glucose levels are in line with recommendations. However, HbA1c testing will not be useful for several weeks.

Depending on the results of the monitoring, if hypoglycaemia is still demonstrated, it is necessary to continue the strategy of deintensification, for example by further reducing the doses. However, if hyperglycaemia is identified (symptoms or excessive level), the patient should return to the initial treatment, possibly replacing the molecules with a high risk of hypoglycaemia with other non-hypoglycaemic molecules.

Implementing Deintensification in Daily Clinical Practice

Finally, as numerous studies have shown, there are many barriers to deintensification. Among other factors, educating healthcare professionals and patients about deintensification is fundamental. Similarly, educating patients to recognise the symptoms of hypoglycaemia and hyperglycaemia is essential [10, 11].

Various resources are available to healthcare professionals to improve the implementation of glucose-lowering drugs deintensification. For example, in addition to the formal clinical practice guidelines, the deprescribing.org website provides a decision-support algorithm, a patient leaflet, infographic and whiteboard video [12].

Clinical Practice Questions

Q1. Mrs D is an 88-year-old patient, treated by her general practitioner for type 2 diabetes for over 25 years. As she has moderate-to-severe cognitive and functional impairments, she lives in a nursing home. She is currently treated by metformin and gliclazide (a sulfonylurea). The latest available measurement of her haemoglobin A1c, two weeks ago, was 148 mmol/mol (or 6.8%). For this patient, when the individualised care plan is drawn up, would you recommend reducing her glucose-lowering treatment?
Choose one option:

- **A.** Mrs D. may benefit from a deintensification of treatment, given her tight glycaemic control, advanced age, probable frailty, long duration of diabetes and use of sulphonylureas.
- **B.** Mrs D's treatment should not be deprescribed as she has many comorbidities.
- **C.** Mrs D's treatment should not be deprescribed as she is in the right glycaemic target level.

Q2. Mr E is a 78-year-old man treated by his general practitioner for a type 2 diabetes, among many other comorbidities. He complains of having had several falls (including one complicated by a wrist fracture) and episodes of confusion in the past few months, which were diagnosed as recurrent and severe episodes of hypoglycaemia. His daily (glucose-lowering) treatment includes gliclazide and metformin. How should this patient, who should theoretically benefit from deintensification, be treated?
Choose one option:

- **A.** Metformin and gliclazide should be replaced by insulin to simplify the glucose-lowering treatment.
- **B.** The strict avoidance of hypoglycaemic event should be the therapeutic priority for Mr E.
- **C.** Two different glucose-lowering agents are too much for Mr E's glycaemic control. The best solution might be to discontinue metformin.

References

Key references only are listed here. For a full list of references visit: https://www.wiley.com/go/sinclair/1e.

1. Bourdel-Marchasson, I., Maggi, S., Abdelhafiz, A. et al. (2023). Essential steps in primary care management of older people with type 2 diabetes: an executive summary on behalf of the European geriatric medicine society (EuGMS) and the European diabetes working party for older people (EDWPOP) collaboration. *Aging Clin. Exp. Res.* 35: 2279–2291.
2. Christiaens, A., Henrard, S., Boland, B., and Sinclair, A.J. (2023). Overtreatment of older people with type 2 diabetes-a high impact frequent occurrence in need of a new definition. *Diabetic Med.* 40 (2): e14994.
3. Christiaens, A., Baretella, O., Del Giovane, C. et al. (2023). Association between diabetes overtreatment in older multimorbid patients and clinical outcomes: an ancillary European multicentre study. *Age Ageing.* 52 (1): afac320.
4. Lega, I.C., Campitelli, M.A., Austin, P.C. et al. (2021). Potential diabetes overtreatment and risk of adverse events among older adults in Ontario: a population-based study. *Diabetologia* 64 (5): 1093–1102.
5. Niznik, J.D., Zhao, X., Slieanu, F. et al. (2022). Effect of Deintensifying diabetes medications on negative events in older veteran nursing home residents. *Diabetes Care* 45 (7): 1558–1567.
6. Christiaens, A., Henrard, S., Sinclair, A.J. et al. (2023). Deprescribing glucose-lowering therapy in older adults with diabetes: a systematic review of recommendations. *J. Am. Med. Dir. Assoc.* 24: 400–402.
8. Deng, Z., Thompson, W., Korenvain, C. et al. (2022). Benefits and harms of deprescribing antihyperglycemics for adults with type 2 diabetes: a systematic review. *Can. J. Diabetes* 46 (5): 473–479.
9. Farrell, B., Black, C., Thompson, W. et al. (2017). Deprescribing antihyperglycemic agents in older persons: evidence-based clinical practice guideline. *Can. Fam. Physician* 63 (11): 832–843.
10. Mellot, M., Jawal, L., Morel, T. et al. (2024). Barriers and enablers for Deprescribing glucose-lowering treatment in older adults: a systematic review. *J. Am. Med. Dir. Assoc.* 25: 439–447.
11. Pilla, S.J., Jalalzai, R., Tang, O. et al. (2023). A national survey of physicians' views on the importance and implementation of deintensifying diabetes medications. *J. Gen. Intern. Med.* 39: 992–1001.
12. Deprescribing.org (2023). Deprescribing guidelines and algorithms. https://deprescribing.org/resources/deprescribing-guidelines-algorithms. (accessed 10 August 2024).

18 Diabetes in End-of-Life Care

June James

Leicester Diabetes Centre, University Hospitals of Leicester NHS Trust, Leicester, UK

Key Points

- Diabetes is linked to the recognised main causes of death but is largely unreported on death certificates.
- Individuals likely or expected to die within a 12-month period are said to be entering their end of life.
- Glycaemic targets can be relaxed in end-of-life care.
- In type 2 diabetes therapies may require de-escalating as individuals approach the end of life.
- Insulin treatment should not be discontinued in the dying individual with type 1 diabetes.
- Health professionals should receive initial and the updated training and education relating to diabetes end-of-life care.

Introduction

Throughout a life span, the need to plan for major life events plays an integral part, prepregnancy care, pregnancy, birth, school life, further education, holidays, weddings, christenings, partnerships, relationship breakdowns, surgery and care in older age are all examples of when planning and preparation is key. In caring for people living with diabetes there are many guidelines and recommendations that underpin safe and

Care of Older People with Diabetes: A Manual for Healthcare Practice, First Edition.
Edited by Alan J. Sinclair and Ahmed H. Abdelhafiz.

Companion website: www.wiley.com/go/sinclair/1e

appropriate diabetes management; however, end of life care planning is often overlooked and there is a dearth of evidence-based guidance.

In this chapter we provide a practical approach to end-of-life care based on current resources while acknowledging that most sources used are formed from consensus recommendations.

Background

The overall global prevalence of adults with diabetes in 2021 was 537 million; this number is expected to increase to 643 million by 2031 [1] The prevalence of diabetes in older people is increasing and it is estimated that one third on people over the age of 65 years live with the condition [2]. In Europe, 10–30% of people accessing pensions have diabetes, and one quarter of care home residents in the UK have diabetes [3]

Having diabetes significantly reduces life expectancy compared with estimated death rates in the general population, and this is more apparent in remote geographical areas and low- or middle-income countries [1]. Death rates are underestimated; 35–40% of recorded deaths include diabetes on the death certificate; when audited, only 10–15% had it listed as the underlying cause of death [4,5]. Diabetes is one of the 10 top causes of death, and the death rates increase in line with prevalence [6]. In most deaths, diabetes is not given as the main cause of death. In the England and Wales in 2022, the main cause of death in was dementia and Alzheimer's disease. These conditions, together with cancer and chronic kidney disease, are intrinsically linked with diabetes [1]. People with diabetes are cared for in many healthcare settings including community care, hospitals, hospices and care homes. It is important the healthcare professionals providing that care are well trained, competent and have a working knowledge of how to manage diabetes.

What is End of Life and How is the Need for End-of-life Care Identified?

The General Medical Council UK [7] states that individuals are approaching the end of life when they are most likely expected to die within the next 12 months. This includes those whose death is imminent (expected within a few hours or days) and those with:

- advanced, progressive, incurable conditions

- general frailty and coexisting conditions which mean that they are expected to die within 12 months
- existing conditions if they are at risk of dying from a sudden acute crisis in their condition (e.g. dementia and chronic diseases such as diabetes where each crisis depletes the individuals' overall reserves)
- life-threatening acute conditions caused by sudden catastrophic events.

In 2016, the Gold Standards Framework in the UK identified three factors that can aid healthcare professionals in determining when the individual is entering the end-of-life phase of their life [8]:

1. The 'surprise question': would you be surprised if this person were to die in the next few months, weeks, days?

   The answer to this question should encompass a range of clinical, comorbidity, social, and other factors that give a whole picture of deterioration. If the healthcare professional would not be surprised, then it is important to consider what measures might be taken to improve the person's quality of life now and in preparation for possible further decline, and to check whether their advance care plan for end of life is still current.
2. General indicators of decline: deterioration, increasing need or choice for no further active care. These include:
   - Decreasing activity: functional performance status, declining limited self-care, in bed or in a chair 50% of day and increasing dependence in most activities of daily living.
   - Comorbidity, which is regarded as the biggest predictive indicator of mortality and morbidity.
   - General physical decline and increasing need for support.
   - Advanced disease with an unstable, deteriorating complex symptom burden.
   - Decreasing response to treatments.
   - Decreasing reversibility or exacerbations of underlying illnesses, which indicates reducing reserves.
   - The individual chooses to have no further active treatment.
   - Progressive weight loss (> 10%) in past six months.
   - Repeated unplanned or crisis admissions.
   - Sentinel event (e.g. serious fall, bereavement, transfer to nursing home).

- Serum albumin less than 25 g/l.
- Considered eligible for additional financial support and benefits.

3. Specific clinical indicators related to certain conditions.

   These indicators relate to specific conditions (e.g. cardiovascular disease). Although diabetes is not mentioned, it frequently occurs in association with those conditions that are specifically mentioned, including cancer, chronic obstructive airways disease, heart disease, renal disease, general and specific neurological disease, such as motor neurone disease, Parkinson's disease and multiple sclerosis, frailty, dementia, and stroke [1].

This framework defined four main stages of end of life (Box 18.1):

1. Stable from diagnosis (usually lasting years).
2. Unstable, advanced disease (usually lasting months).
3. Deteriorating, exacerbations (usually lasting weeks).
4. Last days of life pathway (usually lasting days).

Box 18.1: The four main stages of end of life care aligned to diabetes management

A. Blue: 'all' from diagnosis stable with year plus prognosis

- The use of cardioprotective therapies (e.g. angiotensin-converting enzyme inhibitors, angiotensin-receptor blockers, aspirin, statins) should be reviewed in the light of the diagnosis and the presence of other medical comorbidities, and dosage reductions (even withdrawal) of some of the therapies considered.
- Individuals may experience more gastrointestinal effects from aspirin with poor dietary intake or concurrent steroid use.
- Individuals on aspirin and steroids should be considered for gastrointestinal protection with a proton-pump inhibitor or suitable alternative.
- Oral hypoglycaemic agents (OHAs) and/or insulin should be reviewed and the targets for glucose control agreed. Weight loss may mean a reduced need for OHAs and/or insulin or offer potential for simplification of the glucose control regimen.

B. Green: 'benefits' unstable/advanced disease – months prognosis

- At this stage the aim is to keep drug interventions to a minimum that will control symptoms. All the above comments apply but complex regimens should be reviewed, especially where individuals are on combinations of oral hypoglycaemic agents with insulin. It is generally simpler for individuals to switch from combinations to insulin alone, once- or twice-daily insulin.
- Insulin alone is a simpler option than combinations of tablets and insulin.
- Insulin regimens should be simplified if possible. The likelihood of carers being involved in insulin therapy increases at this stage and may inform the choice of insulin regimen.
- If moving from twice-daily to once-daily insulin, the starting dose of long-acting insulin such as glargine or insulin degludec should be less than the total dose of twice-daily isophane analogue long-acting insulin or premixed insulin; 75% of total previous dose is recommended.
- Once-daily insulin is a simpler option if carers are involved and/or appetite is changing.

C. Yellow: 'continuing care' deteriorating weeks prognosis

- Individuals may present or be referred to the diabetes team at this time, in which case all the suggested changes above should be considered but keeping in mind that there may be little time to get used to a new insulin regimen. Intensive support can be needed for dose adjustments as wellbeing, activity and appetite can change day to day.
- Managing diabetes can be an added stress at an emotional time for individuals and carers. Relaxing targets for control may seem like 'giving up' for some while others may view managing diabetes in addition to their terminal illness as 'pointless'.

D. Red: 'terminal care' – days prognosis

- Ideally by this stage diabetes treatment has been minimised so that few changes are needed in the last days of life. If the stage is reached where the individual is bedbound, semi-comatose, no longer able to take tablets, no longer able to eat and only able to take sips of fluid, the use of a local protocol or advice from the specialist team may guide your decision making.
- At this stage, the *Flowchart for Diabetes at End of Life* describes how to manage diabetes in the dying individual. It can be reassuring for relatives and carers to know that this additional plan of care is being followed and that the diabetes is being managed differently rather than being 'ignored'.
- The flowchart has been devised to minimise symptoms of diabetes and keep invasive testing to the minimum needed to achieve that aim.

Source: Reproduced by kind permission of Trend Diabetes [20].

Australia adapted this model but included five stages with the inclusion of death and bereavement. Providing bereavement care to families is an integral part of care provision [9]:

1. Disease advancement.
2. Experiencing life-limiting illness.
3. Dependency and symptom increase.
4. Decline and last days.
5. Death and bereavement.

In Scotland, similar assessment tools were also produced, SPICT (Support and Palliative Care Indicators Tool) provides information for people from a variety of countries and in particular those from low-income setting (`www.spict.org.uk`). These tools are available in different languages [10].

Management of Diabetes in End-of-Life Care

End-of-life care planning should start early so the person can prioritise what they want to do in the time left and clearly document any decisions they may have regarding their care. Advanced care planning helps the individual, their families and healthcare professionals to make decisions when the individual no longer has the capacity to do so.

There remains a dearth of evidence-based guidance on end-of-life care in diabetes. Most guidance is based on consensus recommendations, with many offering generic recommendations relating to diabetes management in the last year. In 2010, Australian guidance was produced [11] and this used as a basis for Australia's national guidance in 2020 [12]. Other organisations include more generic guidance on end-of-life care in their recommendation documents [1,13,14]. In 2010, Diabetes UK commissioned a multidisciplinary working party with the aim of producing a consistent and high-quality approach to end-of-life care in diabetes [16]. In 2018, Diabetes UK requested that Trend Diabetes take on providing regular practical reviews, which are updated biannually.

Medicines Management and De-escalation of Therapies

In diabetes, the aim of treatment is to minimise symptoms of hypo- and hyperglycaemia, and the avoidance of acute diabetes emergencies such as hyperosmolar hyperglycaemic state, diabetic ketoacidosis and hypoglycaemia. Glycaemic targets are lower than in the general diabetes population, with glucose targets of 6–15 mmol/l (108–270 mg/dl) recommended to reduce the risk of hypo- or hyperglycaemia.

Many people with diabetes have striven to reach tighter glycaemic targets for many years and may feel that healthcare professionals are 'giving up' on them when targets are reduced. When considering reducing medications and targets it is important that there is a full discussion with the individual, carers and/or family so there is a mutually agreed treatment plan.

In type 2 diabetes, oral and non-insulin diabetes therapies can usually be reduced and discontinued depending on specific factors such as anorexia, weight loss, poor appetite [16]. The use of sulfonylureas in this stage of life is not recommended due to the risk of hypoglycaemia as appetite is reduced or when there is significant weight loss.

Insulin therapy doses may need to be significantly reduced or stopped. Table 18.1 provides a summary of specific glucose-lowering therapies, together with possible adverse effects and risks.

Table 18.1: Medicines Management: Non-insulin therapies

Drug	Risk of hypoglycaemia when used as monotherapy	General considerations
Metformin: standard metformin or metformin SR	No risk	Review dose according to changing renal function
		Withdraw if creatinine > 150 mmol/l or eGFR < 30 ml/l/1.73m^2
		Review if gastrointestinal disease is present or symptoms of nausea, heartburn, diarrhoea or flatulence are making individuals miserable with discomfort
Sulfonylureas: gliclazide, glipizide, glimepiride, repaglinide	Moderate risk	Review if dietary intake is reduced and/or there is significant weight loss
		Review dose if renal or liver function deteriorates and consider a switch to tolbutamide
		Review tolbutamide dose if liver function deteriorates as hypoglycaemia may occur
Pioglitazone	No risk	The risk–benefit ratio for pioglitazone in individuals with terminal disease requires review and should be only prescribed if benefits can clearly be identified
		Should not be used in individuals with or at risk of bladder tumour or heart failure

Table 18.1: Continued

Drug	Risk of hypoglycaemia when used as monotherapy	General considerations
Gliptins: alogliptin, linagliptin, saxagliptin, sitagliptin	Low risk	Review doses in accordance with individual licences if renal function deteriorates
		Some gliptins can be used for all stages of renal disease
		Combination with sulfonylurea increases the risk of hypoglycaemia
GLP-1 RA: dulaglutide exenatide, liraglutide, lixisenatide, semaglutide, tirzepatide	No risk	Review if eating patterns change or significant weight loss occurs
		Withdraw if abdominal pain or pancreatitis develops
		Refer to individual product SPC* for doses
SGLT2 inhibitors: dapagliflozin, empagliflozin, ertugliflozin and canagliflozin	Low risk	Refer to SPC for doses
		Refer to individual SPC for renal guidance
		Stop if evidence of clinical dehydration peripheral vascular disease/foot ulceration in acute illness and presurgery; test for ketones if there is acute illness

eGFR, estimated glomerular filtration rate
Source: Adapted by kind permission of Trend Diabetes [15].

In type 1 diabetes, insulin doses may need reducing or regimens simplified in line with glucose readings, but insulin should never be discontinued, because of the risk of diabetic ketoacidosis. In the last days of life, the giving of a once-daily longer-acting insulin such as insulin glargine or insulin degludec, which convey a lower risk of hypoglycaemia, may be beneficial. If the person is usually treated with an insulin pump and is able to manage it, they should be enabled to do so for as long as possible.

Glucose monitoring can be reduced in type 1 diabetes or in the case of type 2 diabetes not treated with insulin discontinued. The use of flash

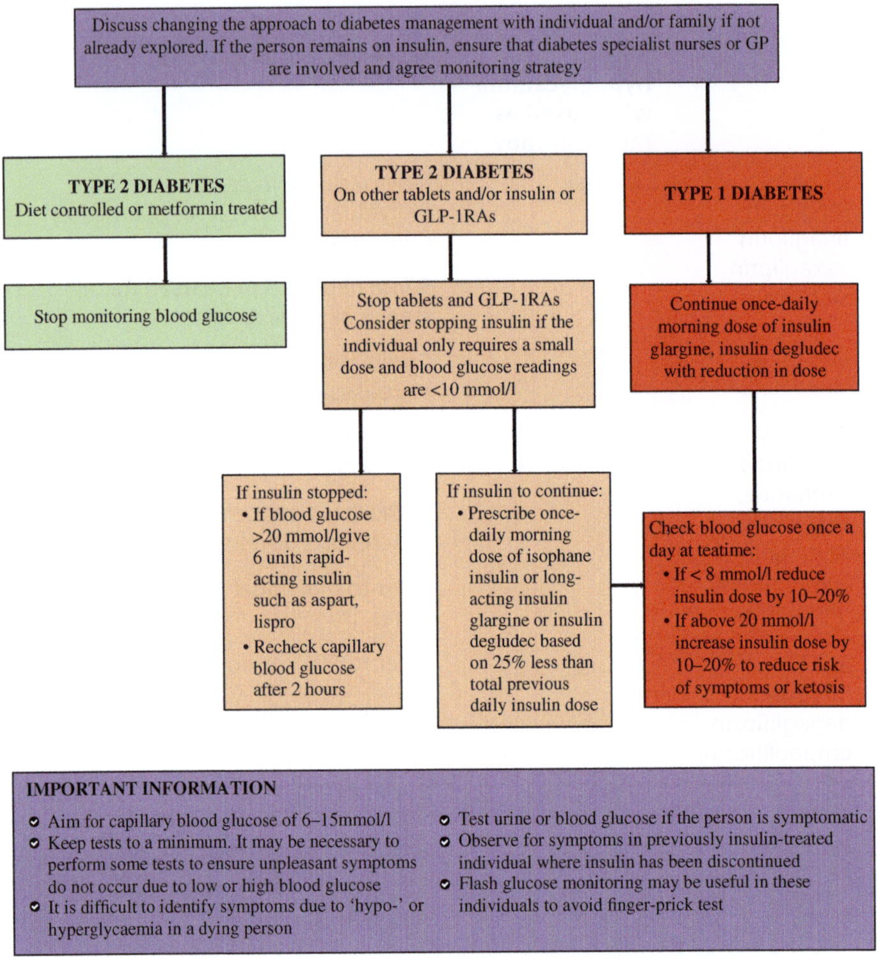

Figure 18.1: Algorithm for de-escalation of therapies at end of life. Source: reproduced by kind permission of Trend Diabetes [15].

glucose or continual glucose monitoring is less invasive and may be useful in these situations. An algorithm for de-escalation of therapies in the last days of life is given in Figure 18.1 [16].

Steroids and Cancer

Gluocorticosteroids are often used in the last year of life and particularly in people with cancer to stimulate appetite and improve quality of life (Figure 18.2) [16]. Prednisolone, given in the morning, is the

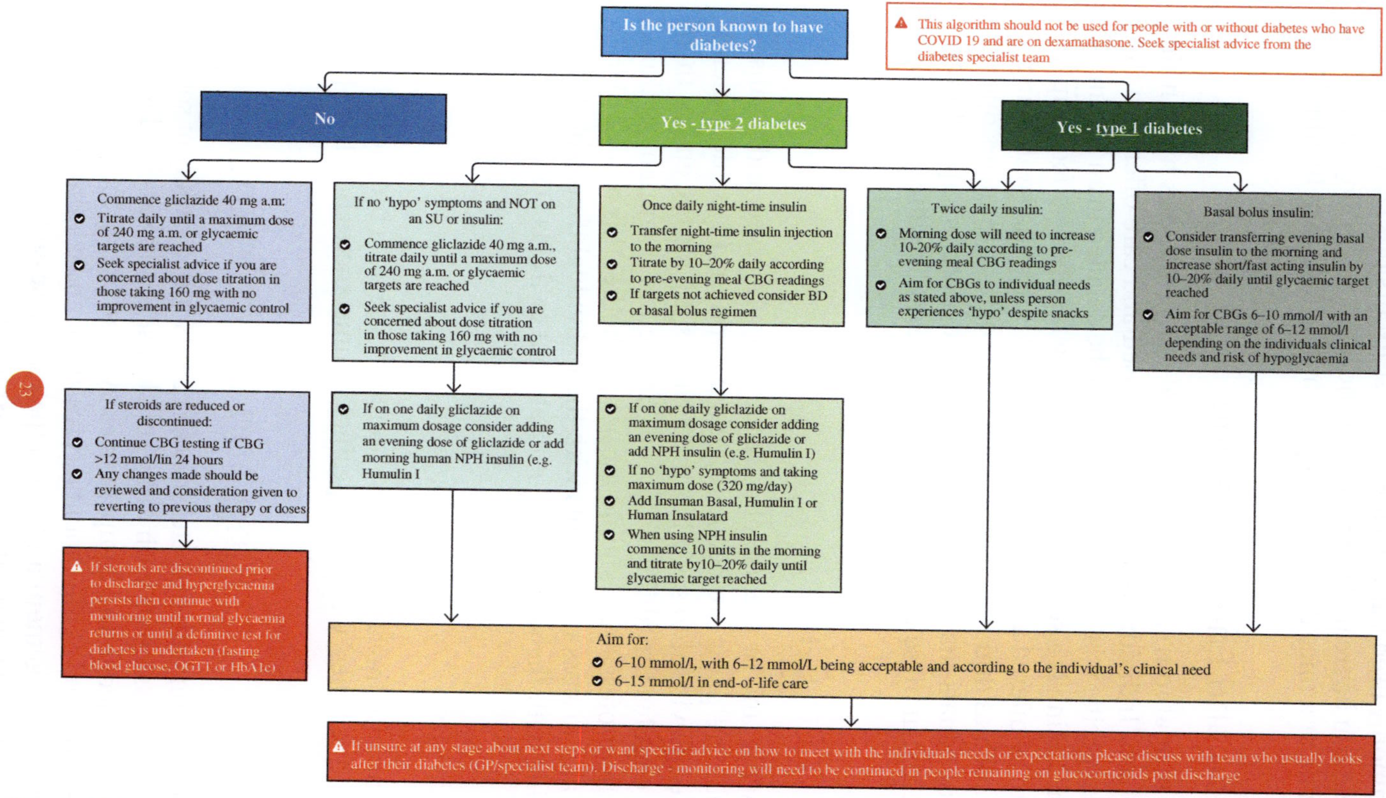

Figure 18.2: Algorithm for managing glucose with once-daily steroid therapy. CGMS, continuous glucose monitoring; CKD, chronic kidney disease; GIP, glucose-dependent insulinotropic polypeptide; GLP-1 RA, glucagon-like peptide-1 receptor analyst; isCGM, intermittently scanned continuous glucose monitoring; rtCGMS, real-time continuous glucose monitoring.

Source: reproduced by kind permission of Trend Diabetes [15].

most commonly used but will cause glucose excursions later in the day [16]. These can be treated with either a short acting sulfonylurea such as gliclazide or a once daily neutral protamine Hagedorn insulin [17].

Nutrition and Enteral Feeding

The risk of malnourishment and clinical dehydration is high in the dying person. Individuals should be assessed and care offered in line with their specific wishes. These wishes can be detailed in an 'advanced care plan'. Eating is a social activity for many families, so food supplements can be offered and treatment for factors affecting swallowing or appetite such as oral candidiasis, dry mouth or mouth ulcers offered. Some individuals may be receiving enteral feeding to support nutritional needs; in these instances, a dietetic referral is indicated [15].

Advanced Care Planning

Living 'wills' and or the use of a signed and witnessed and legalised advanced care plans are becoming more popular. These documents allow the individual to say what their wishes are for the end of their life and enables the ability to accept or decline treatment options. Healthcare professionals should ascertain whether this type of plan is in place and discuss its contents with the individual if possible before proceeding with the withdrawal of treatment or fluids [18–19].

Treatment Withdrawal

Treatment withdrawal can be considered in line with the individuals', carers' and families' wishes in specific circumstances (Box 18.2) [15].

Workforce Training and Competencies

The dying person with diabetes may be cared for in a variety of settings by health professionals with different skill sets and varying levels of diabetes knowledge and competencies. All staff caring for people with diabetes at the end of life should receive initial and continuing training in diabetes management and be competency assessed. An assessment tool is freely available to support assessment [20].

Box 18.2: Treatment Withdrawal

Treatment withdrawal can be considered:

- when the person with diabetes is entering the terminal phase of life
- where frequent treatment-related hypoglycaemia is causing distress and significant management difficulties
- where continued treatment with insulin poses an unacceptable risk of hypoglycaemia or where the benefits of stricter glucose management cannot be justified
- where continued use of blood-pressure or lipid-lowering therapy cannot be justified on health benefit considerations
- where continued food or fluids is not the choice of the individual who is dying
- where prescribing anti-infective therapy is unlikely to benefit the individual.

Source: Trend Diabetes [15].

Summary

Information provided in this chapter provides an overview of the care required for people with diabetes expected to die within a 12-month period. It is important that the dying individual is kept as the focus of care throughout that time and that their wishes are known and respected. Dame Tessa Jowell, a British Member of Parliament, had the last word when she stated in the House of Lords just prior to her death from cancer in May 2018 [21] 'In the end, what gives a life meaning is not only how it is lived, but how it draws to a close'.

Clinical Practice Questions

Q1. Which of these is the correct glucose target in diabetes end of life care?

A. 5–12 mmol/l
B. 4–12 mmol/l
C. 6–12 mmol/l
D. 6–15 mmol/l

Q2. Insulin therapy can be discontinued in end-of-life care in a person with type 1 diabetes. True or false?

References

Key references only are listed here. For a full list of references visit: https://www.wiley.com/go/sinclair/1e.

3. Sinclair, K., Dhatariya, O., Burr, D. et al. (2020). Guidelines for the management of diabetes in care homes during the Covid-19 pandemic. *Diabet. Med.* 37: 1090–1093.
6. World Health Organization. The top 10 causes of death. https://www.who.int/news-room/fact-sheets/detail/the-top-10-causes-of-death (accessed 5 September 2023).
7. Office for National Statistics. Census 2021: Death registration summary statistics, England and Wales 2022. www.ons.gov.uk/peoplepopulationandcommunity/birthsdeathsandmarriages/deaths/articles/deathregistrationsummarystatisticsenglandandwales/2022 (accessed 5 September 2023).
8. General Medical Council (2022). Treatment and care towards end of life: good practice in decision making. London: GMC. https://www.gmc-uk.org/ethical-guidance/ethical-guidance-for-doctors/treatment-and-care-towards-the-end-of-life (accessed 5 September 2023).
9. Thomas, K., Armstron-Wilson, J., and GSF Team (2016). The Gold Standards Framework Proactive Identification Guidance. London: GSF Centre. www.goldstandardsframework.org.uk/cd-content/uploads/files/General%20Files/Prognostic%20Indicator%20Guidance%20October%202011.pdf (accessed 14 September 2023).
12. SPICT-LIS Supportive and Palliative Care Indicators Tool. www.spict.org.uk/spict-lis (accessed 12 January 2022).
15. Trend Diabetes (2021). End of Life Guidance for Diabetes Care. Brixworth: Orange Juice Communications. https://trenddiabetes.online/portfolio/end-of-life-guidance-for-diabetes-care (accessed 14 September 2023).
16. Joint British Diabetes Society for Inpatient Care and UK Chemotherapy Board (2021). The Management of Glycaemic Control in Patients with Cancer: Guidance for the Diabetes and Oncology Multidisciplinary Teams. London: Diabetes UK. https://www.diabetes.org.uk/for-professionals/improving-care/good-practice/inpatient-and-hospital-care/joint-british-diabetes-society-for-inpatient-care (accessed 14 September 2023).

17. Joint British Diabetes Society for Inpatient Care (2023). Management of Hyperglycaemia and Steroid (Glucocorticoid) Therapy: A Guideline from the Joint British Societies for Inpatient Care. London: Diabetes UK. https://www.diabetes.org.uk/for-professionals/improving-care/good-practice/inpatient-and-hospital-care/joint-british-diabetes-society-for-inpatient-care (accessed 14 September 2023).
20. Trend Diabetes (2022). *An integrated Career and Competency Framework for Adult Diabetes Nursing*. 6e. Brixworth: Orange Juice Communications. https://trenddiabetes.online/portfolio/an-integrated-career-and-competency-framework-for-adult-diabetes-nursing-6th-edition (accessed 14 September 2023).

Answers to Clinical Practice Questions

Characteristics and Care Needs

A, B, D, E: She has multiple morbidities due to old age and long duration of diabetes, which affect her physical dysfunction leading to falls as one of the geriatric syndromes. Although her BMI is normal, her appetite is variable and her weight loss is likely reflecting early frailty and therefore, so she is at risk of further deterioration and disability. **C:** Although she has no history of dementia, her recent forgetfulness, vascular disease and long duration of diabetes are risk factors for cognitive impairment and her cognitive function should be assessed.

Chapter 1

H: Mrs Smith needs nutritional education and counselling, as her diet is high in simple carbohydrates and she is losing weight. Optimising her diet will decrease her glycaemic load and minimise further weight loss. She would also benefit from physical activity to improve her insulin sensitivity and decrease insulin resistance. Although her haemoglobin A1c and fasting blood sugars are elevated, Mrs Smith may be experiencing episodes of unrecognised hypoglycaemia, as she is on insulin therapy at bedtime (high-risk medication for hypoglycaemia). It would be important to increase monitoring of her blood sugars over a two-week period while implementing lifestyle changes before making changes to her medications.

Care of Older People with Diabetes: A Manual for Healthcare Practice, First Edition.
Edited by Alan J. Sinclair and Ahmed H. Abdelhafiz.

Companion website: www.wiley.com/go/sinclair/1e

Chapter 2

Q1. **D**
Q2. **B, C**
Q3. **E**

Chapter 3

D: This woman's body mass index is 37 kg/m^2 and is likely to have underlying sarcopenia considering her history of falls, weak handgrip and difficulty rising from a chair. She also has an unfavourable metabolic profile. In other words, she has sarcopenic obesity and high cardiovascular risk. Therefore, adequate nutrition with combined aerobic and resistance training are the ideal interventions for weight loss and improving her muscle mass and metabolic profile. **A:** A low-calorie diet alone may lead to loss of muscle mass, exacerbating her sarcopenia. **B:** Aerobic exercise without diet and resistance training is not ideal. **C:** Reduction of saturated fat may improve her lipid profile but will not increase her muscle mass or improve her overall risk. **E:** Increased dietary protein is not enough in the absence of exercise to improve muscle function and lower her cardiovascular risk.

Chapter 4

B, D and E: She is a sarcopenic obese with high risk of cardiovascular disease, and will benefit form SGLT-2 inhibitor therapy combined with weight reduction and resistance exercise training. Although her HbA1c is good, the benefits of SGLT-2 inhibitors are independent of glycaemic control. A. Metformin therapy alone is not enough considering her high cardiovascular risk. C. Although DPP-4 are well tolerated, they offer no additional cardiovascular benefits.

Chapter 5

C: In light of his age, comorbidities, severity of frailty and potential life expectancy, this patient's haemoglobin A1c and glucose levels are close to target; however, preventing hypoglycaemia is a major goal. Metformin cannot be used due to renal impairment (estimated glomerular filtration rate < 30 ml/minute). Gliclazide would be associated with a greater risk of hypoglycaemia. Reducing the dose of his current insulin would not necessarily eliminate the risk of hypoglycaemia and could lead to rise in glucose levels. An ultra-long-acting analogue is known to be associated to a lower risk of hypoglycaemia in older people. If his appetite improves a rapid acting analogue could be considered at breakfast and/or dinner (based on his glucose levels).

Chapter 6

A: An international consensus[1] recommends, for a 'high-risk' group (older adults with type 1 or 2 diabetes), a less-stringent time in range (3.9–10.0 mmol/l) target of more than 50% (vs > 70% general recommendation) and a time below range (<3.9 mmol/l) target of less than 1%.

Reference

1 Battelino, T., Danne, T., Bergenstal, R.M. et al. (2019). Clinical targets for continuous glucose monitoring data interpretation: recommendations from the international consensus on time in range. *Diabetes Care* 42 (8): 1593–1603.

Chapter 7

D: This woman will need a full assessment to determine her ability and dexterity in terms of insulin injection, hypoglycaemia treatment, assessment of cognitive ability, nutritional status, frailty and her own worries and concerns in relation to her diabetes treatment. Treatment options to be discussed may include switching to basal insulin only with oral anti-diabetic agents but this may depend on her preferences and personalised discussion of glycaemic targets in terms of any existing comorbidity or diabetes complications. It may also be appropriate to discuss using technology (e.g. use of continuous glucose monitoring to warn her of hypoglycaemia, and/or connected pens which could guide her in terms of how much insulin she has taken and when). She may or may not want to involve a carer, friend or family member in these discussions.

Chapter 8

A, B, C, E: This patient is having episodes of hypoactive delirium caused by hypoglycaemia. Her reduced eating and weight loss, which may be due to progression of dementia, has put her at risk of hypoglycaemia with her current doses of hypoglycaemic therapy. Therefore, encouraging frequent, even small feeding may help reduce this risk. The doses of her hypoglycaemic medications will need to be reduced following advice from health care professionals. Food supplementation will help her reduced calorie intake. Hospital admission is not indicated, as this condition can be managed in the community.

Chapter 9a

E: All the options are appropriate. **A:** Aspirin should be offered if peripheral arterial disease (PAD) is confirmed. Direct oral anticoagulants should be offered for prevention of atrial fibrillation-related vascular events. Since antiplatelets plus anticoagulants can increase bleeding risk, he should receive education about preventing falls, for example. **B:** Statins have shown some benefits improving walking claudication distance, which could improve our patient quality of life. **C:** There has been some concern in the past about the use of beta-blockers in the treatment of hypertension among patients with intermittent claudication, but there appears to be no adverse effect of beta-1 selective blockers on claudication symptoms. As a result, these drugs are not contraindicated in patients with PAD. **D:** Yes, he should be referred for vascular surgical advice after prior comprehensive geriatric assessment.

Chapter 9b

A: The clinical presentation of coronary artery disease in older patients with type 2 diabetes mellitus is often atypical, requiring a high degree of clinical suspicion and the need for additional tests.

Chapter 9c

C: Hypo- and hyperglycaemia can mimic acute stroke and need to be excluded before reperfusion therapies such as thrombolysis or thrombectomy can be considered. In the immediate phase following admission with stroke, close monitoring of blood glucose should be instituted, aiming for a target glucose level of between 5 and 12 mg/dl. Variable-rate insulin infusion for tight glycaemic control should be avoided because of the risk of early hypoglycaemia, which adversely affects outcomes.

Chapter 10a

Q1. **B:** We are satisfied that this man's diabetes and other risk factors for diabetic retinopathy are well controlled, and there are no signs of severe non-proliferative or proliferative diabetic retinopathy, so no acute action is required. However, this patient still requires regular retinal screening due to the risk of developing retinopathy, even in the absence of symptoms. He should be signposted and referred to his local retinal screening service. **A:** Urgent referral is not required in view of minimal changes on fundoscopy. **C:** Diabetic retinopathy is often asymptomatic. **D:** The presence of microaneurysms, although present in other retinal diseases, does not exclude diabetic retinopathy. **E:** Although he has controlled risk factors, his age and diabetes duration put him at increased risk of diabetic retinopathy.

Q2. **A:** Owing to the diagnostic uncertainty, ophthalmology referral is necessary. However, given the history and possibility of bilateral neovascularisation and of vitreous haemorrhage/retinal detachment in the left eye, this referral must be urgent. It would be appropriate to contact the eye clinic triage nurse or on-call ophthalmology registrar for advice if unsure about local pathways. **B:** Reduced visual acuity is probably due to proliferative diabetic retinopathy and needs ophthalmology assessment. **C:** Routine screening will be required afterward referral. **D:** Infection would be lower down the list of differentials given this vignette. Sight-threatening conditions should be excluded first. **E:** Routine bloods will be part of this patient's general care but not their acute management.

Chapter 10b

A, B, C, D: Metformin and ramipril should be withheld as he is likely to suffer from lactic acidosis and acute kidney injury. His potassium is dangerously high and should be urgently corrected. Gliclazide, together with insulin, increases the risk of hypoglycaemia, so should be stopped. A review of his medications and education are important as he may have used a non-steroidal anti-inflammatory drug, precipitating his acute kidney injury. **E:** Although his haemoglobin A1c is high, his hypoglycaemic therapy should be reviewed with consideration of using anti-diabetic medications with a lower hypoglycaemic risk and adjusting his insulin dose accordingly.

Chapter 10c

A: True – signs and symptoms of peripheral neuropathy can indeed be subtle or difficult to detect, especially in elderly care-home residents. Care staff may not have specialised training in identifying these symptoms, which can include numbness, tingling and pain in the extremities.

C: True – acupuncture can be used as an adjunct to drug therapy in treating peripheral neuropathy. Some studies suggest that acupuncture may help relieve pain and improve nerve function, although it is typically considered a complementary therapy rather than a primary treatment.

E: True – peripheral vascular disease (PVD) is a recognised risk factor for the development of peripheral neuropathy. Reduced blood flow to the nerves due to PVD can contribute to nerve damage, exacerbating the risk of neuropathy in individuals with diabetes.

B: False – peripheral neuropathy, once detected, can be challenging to manage and often has a significant impact on quality of life. It can lead to complications such as foot ulcers, infections and an increased risk of falls, all of which can severely affect the resident's future quality of life.

D: False – while a 256-Hz tuning fork is used to assess vibratory sensation and can help to detect sensory loss, it is not typically used to identify residents specifically at risk of developing peripheral neuropathy. It is more commonly employed in the diagnosis of established neuropathy.

Chapter 11a

E: Blood pressure of 112/78 mmHg is too low for this very old lady with dementia and frailty, which is likely contributing to her injurious fall despite no postural drop. **A.** Stopping ramipril alone will not be enough. **B.** She will be left at risk of further falls. **C.** Stopping ramipril and bendroflumethiazide will not be enough. **D.** Continuing a monotherapy of small dose of amlodipine 5 mg once daily is likely to keep her blood pressure lower than the required higher target of 150 mmHg and remained at risk of falling.

Chapter 11b

D: This man is very high risk of atherosclerotic cardiovascular events due to his history of established cardiovascular disease and the presence of cardiovascular risk factors. He has a metabolic syndrome and should be started on high-intensity statins with the aim to reduce low-density lipoprotein (LDL) to a target less than 1.4 mmol/l. A. His haemoglobin A1c level seems reasonable, and his lipid profile is unlikely to be corrected by adding an extra hypoglycaemic agent. **B:** Lifestyle modifications are advisable but he still needs pharmacological intervention. **C:** Increasing atorvastatin to a moderate intensity level of 20 mg will not be enough to reach LDL target. **E:** Although his triglyceride level is high, optimisation of LDL with high-intensity statin is required first, and triglyceride will also be reduced by increasing the statin dose.

Chapter 12a

D: The clinical picture is an of overlapping diabetic ketoacidosis (DKA)–hyperosmolar hyperglycaemic state, which requires correction of acidosis with fluids and insulin infusion given simultaneously following the DKA pathway. **A:** Patients should be admitted to intensive care unit if their Glasgow Coma Scale score is less than 12, sodium > 160 mmol/l and serum osmolality > 350 mOsm/kg. **B:** Combined insulin and fluid therapy is required due to acidosis. **C:** Starting insulin dose should be 0.1 units/kg/hour following DKA protocol.

Chapter 12b

C, D, E: are the correct answers. He has reasonably good renal function for his age and presence of diabetes, he is unlikely to have dementia, has no history given and he is self-managing his diabetes. Fatigue and weight loss are two key criteria for frailty and must be considered. A haemoglobin A1c level of 48 mmol/mol is often too low for older people with diabetes and may predispose them to hypoglycaemia, particularly in the presence of frailty. Undiagnosed malignancy (and associated weight loss/cachexia) can cause hypoglycaemia.

Chapter 13a

Q1. **A, B, C:** Oral semaglutide maximum dose, insulin and chronic kidney disease have contributed to hypoglycaemia.

Q2. **A, B, C:** Key factors as outlined in the Q1 answer, oral semaglutide maximum dose and no monitoring has led to significant weight loss due to loss of appetite which has hastened frailty, weakness with hypoglycaemia has led to falls.

Q3. **A–F:** Ensure regular monitoring and agree safe glucose targets in view of her age, frailty and chronic kidney disease. She will need dietetic review with possible food supplementation to build her back up and re-enablement team involvement for strength and resistance activities. Communication with all involved in her care to support and agree a plan going forward. Arrange recalls. Education regarding sick day rules if taking a sodium glucose transporter-2 inhibitor.

Q4. **A–C:** Stop semaglutide; review insulin, since fasting glucose levels are between 3 and 5 mmol/l, with a view to agreeing safe glucose maintenance targets (6–12 mmol/l) to reduce hypoglycaemia and hyperglycaemia with continuing monitoring in view of her chronic kidney disease. Consider an initial dose reduction of 20% with monitoring and regular review.

Chapter 13b

A–F: all the statements are true. Multiple factors are involved in increasing the risk of hypoglycaemia in a care-home resident with diabetes. There appears to be a reciprocal relationship between frailty and repeated hypoglycaemia also increasing the risk of frailty developing. The other risk factors shown are well documented.

Chapter 14

Q1. **C:** Both the Malnutrition Universal Screening Tool or Mini Nutritional Assessment are appropriate. Mary will also require blood tests (full blood count, urea, electrolytes folate, vitamin B_{12}, calcium, phosphate and magnesium levels).

Q2. B: Mary will probably require assistance with meals, given her cognitive impairment and residual weakness. Recognising her preferred meals and providing these regularly, as well as providing fortified food/drinks, would improve the quantity and quality of her meals.

Q3. B: Given her frailty, a haemoglobin A1c (HbA1c) level up to 75 mmol/mol is acceptable and capillary blood glucose targets range between 7 and 12 mmol/l. An HbA1c of 47 mmol/mol indicates that her glycaemic control is too tight.

Q4. A: Metformin has the potential to cause nausea, anorexia and changes in taste. Consequently, discontinuing its use may have a beneficial effect on food consumption. Considering her frequent episodes of hypoglycaemia, it is crucial to decrease her insulin dose.

Q5. A: Monitor capillary blood glucose every 6 hours: at 0, 6, 12 and 18 hours from the start of the feed.

Q6. B: The target blood glucose range is 6–12 mmol/l.

Q7. A: A safer option for this prolonged feed is isophane insulin (e.g. humulin I or insulatard) at the beginning and 10 hours after the start of the feed. Consider a small starting dose of 8–10 units twice a day and increase the doses by 2–4 units (or 10–20%) every day if blood glucose is persistently > 12 mmol/l. Given the increased risk of lactic acidosis, metformin should be held in acutely unwell patients.

Chapter 15

Q1. E: He is likely to have underlying metabolic syndrome and high cardiovascular risk presenting with erectile dysfunction as the first manifestation. He will therefore need a multidimensional intervention to reduce his overall cardiovascular risk. **A:** Increasing medications is only part of the treatment. **B:** A phosphodiesterase 5 inhibitor will be required only after correction of all other reversible factors. **C:** Testosterone level checking is not required at this stage. **D:** Reduction of alcohol is only part of the treatment.

Q2. C: She is likely to have underlying undiagnosed depression causing her physical symptoms of lack of energy and psychological symptom of lack of sex drive. These may improve by starting antidepressant medications. **A:** Her haemoglobin A1c is borderline but is unlikely to be the cause of her symptoms. **B:** Counselling the partner is not required. **D:** Although her blood pressure is mildly uncontrolled, it is unlikely to be the cause of her symptoms. **E:** Social support may help in her physical daily activities but will not treat her underlying condition.

Chapter 16a

Q1. **A–C:** He is likely to be frail in the spectrum of anorexic malnourished phenotype considering his low haemoglobin, albumin and cholesterol, which suggest malnutrition, and low creatinine, which suggests low muscle mass. **D, E:** Old age itself is not a cause of falls unless associated with frailty. Similarly, low haemoglobin A1c will lead to falls only if associated with hypoglycaemic episodes.

Q2. **A, B:** His falls are probably due to frailty, although recurrent hypoglycaemia is also possible considering his low haemoglobin A1c. He will benefit from a reduction or complete withdrawal of hypoglycaemic therapy and dietician review for a build-up supplements. He will need physiotherapy intervention with resistance exercise training to restore muscle strength and improve balance. **C:** Stopping all hypoglycaemic therapy at once is inappropriate but gradual deintensification is required.

Chapter 16b

A, B, D, E: He is likely to be developing depression. Screening for depression should be included in annual review of diabetes and when patients develop symptoms suggesting depression. Clustering of depression, hypertension and osteoarthritis may increase the risk of disability. Multidisciplinary follow-up that includes mental health service is required. Depression may lead to poor compliance with self-care tasks. **C.** Insulin dose should only be adjusted depending on his glycaemic control and risk of hypoglycaemia.

Chapter 16c

A, B, E: This woman is likely developing frailty, reduced and erratic oral intake, and difficulty in managing and controlling her blood glucose levels. continuous glucose monitoring equipped with an alarm system will help to better control her blood glucose levels, giving insulin before meals reduces the risk of hypoglycaemia, and carer education and involvement provides a safety net for early intervention when blood glucose levels are in extremis. **C** is incorrect since changes to the pre-mixed insulin regime increases the risk of hypoglycaemia given her irregular eating pattern. **D** is incorrect since reducing the bolus doses may lead to symptomatic and undesirable post-prandial peaks.

Chapter 16d

E: each of these options is an important treatment goal.

Chapter 16e

A, B, C, D: Establish that his symptoms are consistent with a recurrence of depression and he will benefit from lifestyle change by reducing alcohol excess, together with social interventions and pharmacological therapy by increasing mirtazapine dose. It is appropriate for him to be more educated about his mental health and wellbeing issues and offered access to further available local support services. **E**. He does not need urgent mental health referral as he is at low risk, with no suicidal thoughts at this stage.

Chapter 16f

Q1. Gangrenous second and third toes. Cellulitis of the whole dorsum of the foot. The foot is very swollen, which may indicate deep-seated infection and/or the presence of an abscess. There is pressure necrosis under the big toe and under the metatarsal head of the second toe.

Q2. **C:** Neuroischaemic foot. She has pressure necrosis in typical neuropathic sites and has peripheral neuropathy. Two of her toes are ischaemic. She is known to have ischaemic heart disease and is also very likely to have peripheral vascular disease.

Q3. Bed rest, pressure relief and pain control. Probe the pressure ulcers to check for a sinus/track. If there is an abscess, probing the ulcer might help it to drain by unblocking the sinus/track. Take microbiological specimens/swabs. Commence high-dose broad-spectrum intravenous antibiotics (e.g. ampicillin/clavulanate [co-amoxiclav]

1.2 g immediately, followed by 600 mg twice a day; renal dose because her estimated glomerular filtration rate is < 30 ml/minute/1.73 m^2). Request an urgent vascular assessment for vascular investigations, debridement and drainage of an abscess if present. While waiting for an urgent vascular assessment request urgent magnetic resonance imaging (MRI) of the foot. MRI is preferable to plain radiographs in this case, as it will detect both abscess formation and/or presence of osteomyelitis. She has an acute kidney injury, so ramipril and metformin should be omitted until renal function improves. Her insulin will need to be increased to improve glycaemic control.

Q4. This woman has already had an amputation of her left fifth toe (only four toes are seen in the photograph and there is evidence of previous surgery at the site of the fifth toe). This puts her feet in the high-risk category. Previous foot ulceration is the strongest predictor of future foot ulceration. She has diabetic peripheral sensory neuropathy (PSN) and possible peripheral vascular disease (PVD) in view of her ischaemic heart disease. PSN and PVD in combination would also put her feet in the high-risk category. Given her risk status, she should have been given foot-care advice and been referred to the foot protection service for regular foot checks.

Chapter 16g

A, B, D: Lipodystrophy could be the cause of erratic insulin absorption leading to erratic blood glucose levels and episodes of hypoglycaemia. This presents as soft fatty lumps under the skin at the site of injection and can be avoided by rotating injection sites. Regular eating pattern will help avoid hypoglycaemia. Although urinary incontinence could be related to high blood glucose, urinary tract infection needs to be excluded. **C**. No need to reduce insulin dose as hypoglycaemia could be due to erratic insulin absorption rather than high insulin dose. **E.** Metformin can be increased if his overall haemoglobin A1c is high in the context of a whole review of his hypoglycaemic therapy.

Chapter 16h

C: Take a thorough history of the fall, including previous falls and any risk factors for falls. Perform a clinical examination, checks routine bloods. Electrocardiogram can also be considered. Complete an online fracture risk assessment. The management plan should be drawn up based on this assessment. **A, B:** She will need assessment in community prior sending home and hospital admission is not required. **D, E:** Prophylactic treatment of vitamin D, calcium and alendronic acid will only be required after thorough assessment.

Chapter 16i

B: This woman was previously self-caring with good glycaemic control. She has probably developed cognitive impairment, causing self-care neglect and insulin administration errors and leading to dysglycaemia-related hospital visits and admission. **A:** Changing to long-acting insulin may reduce the risk of hypoglycaemia but will not address her underlying problem. **C:** Home help will be required for her care but will not address her recent diabetes problem. **D:** Insulin administration by the district nurse will ensure adequate dosage and timing but will not address the underlying problem. **E:** Adding another oral agent will increase polypharmacy and will not help compliance.

Chapter 16j

Q1. **A, B, C D:** All four options are relevant.

Q2. **A:** true. Older adults are a heterogenous population. Individuals may have drastically different priorities of care, capacity to use technology and attitudes towards its use and value for their diabetes management. Evaluating and incorporating these factors into the decision to initiate technology, and what type, can optimise long-term satisfaction and health outcomes.

Chapter 16k

A–E: All the options are appropriate. **A:** Medication review and compliance checking is needed. **B:** Cognitive decline or depression may lead to noncompliance or medication errors. **C:** Education and training for injection techniques, especially he has recently started insulin therapy is appropriate. **D:** Erratic eating and missing meals may lead to fluctuating glucose levels. **E:** Overall glycaemic control is required for further adjustment of his medications.

Chapter 16l

C and D: She is likely to have uncontrolled diabetes for some time, which increased her risk of oral infections, dental caries and tooth loss. Increasing her hypoglycaemic therapy to achieve better glycaemic control is indicated. Her white oral patches are probably due to fungal infection causing painful swallowing, which needs topical antifungal treatment. An educational dental care programme that is sensitive to her cultural background is required for her and her family. Antiseptic mouthwash, urgent dental review or speech and language referral are not required at this stage.

Chapter 16m

C: This woman will benefit from a comprehensive geriatric assessment and treatment of her pain holistically, considering her physical complaints (pain, reduced function, recurrent falls, frailty), psychological compromise (low mood) and social circumstances (living alone with no formal carers). In addition to drug therapy for pain, she will need screening and treatment for depression, physiotherapy for recurrent falls, physical exercise training and adequate nutrition for frailty and care need assessment for social care. Therefore, in this case, multidisciplinary approach, which addresses medical as well as psychosocial needs, is required to achieve optimal outcomes. **A:** Non-steroidal anti-inflammatory drugs may be useful in the short term but may further worsen her chronic kidney disease; similarly, capsaicin will be of partial benefit. **B:** Drugs for neuropathic pain will have some effect on her pain with little effect on prognostic outcomes. **D:** These procedures will address only part of the problem with no long-term impact.

Chapter 17

Q1. **A:** In accordance with recommendations, Mrs D may benefit from a deintensification of treatment, given her tight glycaemic control, advanced age, probable frailty (neurocognitive and functional impairments), long duration of diabetes and use of sulfonylureas. **B:** The presence of several comorbidities, is a very good reason for initiating deprescription. **C:** The recommended appropriate haemoglobin A1c target for older people with poor health status treated by drugs at high risk of hypoglycaemia is between 63.9 and 69.4 mmol/mol (or 8–8.5%).

Q2. **B:** Various options are possible; however, the strict avoidance of a hypoglycaemic event should be the therapeutic priority for this patient. Therefore, the cessation (discontinuation) of gliclazide (sulfonylureas) is suggested. Depending on the level of his haemoglobin A1c, a switch from sulfonylureas to a non-hypoglycaemic glucose-lowering agent (e.g. a dipeptidyl peptidase IV inhibitor) may be useful. A short-term reassessment is needed, after an increase of the number of capillary blood glucose measurement by day. **A:** Even if discontinuing gliclazide is a good option, replacing it with insulin is not necessarily required. Other non-hypoglycaemic agents could be tried first as second-line therapy. **C:** Hypoglycaemia should be avoided at all costs in this patient. Continuing gliclazide may therefore not be an appropriate option. On the other hand, metformin is a good therapeutic choice (as first-line therapy), unless contraindicated.

Chapter 18

Q1. **C:** 6–15 mmol/l. This is to protect from hypoglycaemia and symptomatic hyperglycaemia.

Q2. False: insulin should not be discontinued in type 1 diabetes because of the risk of diabetic ketoacidosis in these individuals.

Index

Note: Page numbers with figures in *italic* and tables in **bold**.

128-tuning fork test, 322

A

Abbey pain scale, 399–400
Acanthosis nigricans, 332, *330*
ACCORD-Blood Pressure study, 146
ACCORD-MIND trials, 182, 289, 291, 304
acidosis, 166, 171
  correction, 174
  lactic, 32, 60–61
  metabolic, 123–125, 165, 169
  severity of, 168
actinic cheilitis, 390
acupuncture, 136, 402
acute abdominal pain, 168
acute coronary syndrome (ACS), 90, 249
acute decompensation, 351–352
  identification, 72
  management, 382
  risk, 279
acute illness, 6, 150, 168, 181, 194, 216, 255, 392
  high frequency of, 206
  monitoring during, 280
  place policies for, 207
acute kidney injury, 126, 168, 192, 355–356, 381
  increased risk of, 356
  predisposing factors for, 36
  timely medication adjustment for, 380
acute metabolic decompensation, 352, 357
acute pain, 396
acute pseudomembranous candidiasis, 336
acute stroke, 102–104
  diagnosis, **103**
  management considerations in diabetes, **103**
adenosine triphosphate-sensitive potassium (K-ATP) channels, 36

Care of Older People with Diabetes: A Manual for Healthcare Practice, First Edition.
Edited by Alan J. Sinclair and Ahmed H. Abdelhafiz.

Companion website: www.wiley.com/go/sinclair/1e

adenosine triphosphate–citrate lyase inhibitors, 160
adiposity, 3–4, 6
adult-onset T1DM, 275–276
advanced care planning, 423, 428
advanced glycation end-products (AGE), 342
  formation, 342
  production of, 99, 392
ADVANCE trials, 182, 249, 293
aerobic activities, 66
aerobic exercise, 25–26, 257
  differences between resistance and, **26**
  improvement in insulin resistance, 26
ageing, 4, 57, 59, 62, 82, 98, 120, 266, 281, *305*, 330–331, 386
  age-related alterations in glucose metabolism, 3–5
  age-related oral changes, 386–387
  age-related skin changes, 330–331
  ageing-related atherosclerosis, 154
  ageing-related metabolic changes, 304
  ageing-related morbidities, 375
  anorexia of, 254
  clinical considerations, **8–9**
  clinical effects, **331**
  in diabetes, 319
  and diabetic foot ulcer disease, 319
  diabetic population, 135
  and lipid profile, 154
  normal, 12, 83, 230, 308
  peripheral neuropathy in, 132
  physiological changes with, 396
  populations, 130
  premature, 376
  and sexual function, 230
  synergistic effects, *156*
albumin–creatinine ratio (ACR), 121
alfacalcidol, 125
alpha-glucosidase inhibitors, 36–37
ambulatory care-sensitive conditions, 352
ambulatory hyperglycaemia pathway, 358
American Diabetes Association, 132, 142, 161, 296
  guidelines, 53
  Standards of Care, 53, 359
amputation, 82, 86, 318–319, 324
  minor or major, 318
  non-traumatic lower-extremity, 318
anaemia, 124
  iron deficiency, 122, 124
  renal, 125
  screening for, 124
anamnesis, 83–84
angiotensin converting enzyme (ACE) inhibitors, 91, 91, 122, 146–147
angiotensin receptor blockers (ARBs), 147
ankle–brachial index (ABI), 82, *85*, 90
ankle brachial pressure index (ABPI), 322
annual reviews, 327, 375
  cognition and mood, 380
  contents, 378–382, *379*
  demographics, 378
  diabetes phenotype in older people, 376–377
  diet and nutrition, 381

foot care, 381
functional implications, 377–378
history, 378
infection prevention, 382
medication review, 381–382
physical examination, 378–379
physical function and frailty, 381
sexual function, 380
template for, *383*
vascular complications, 380
anorexic malnourished (AM)
individuals, 22
phenotype, xlii, 254–255, 260–261
anti-diabetes oral and injectable agents, 60–62
anti-VEGF:
intravitreal, 115–116
therapies, 111
anticonvulsants, 135, 403, **401**
antidepressants, 217, 231
preferred, 312
tricyclic, 135, 313, 403
antioxidants, 235
antiplatelet therapy, 86
antipsychotic drugs, 217
anxiety, 50, 75, 192, 237, 269, 380, 400. *See also* depression
appetite, 45, 424, 426, 428
changes, 381
loss of, 216
reduction of, 254
aquatic exercise, 27, 257, 357
arterial wall stiffness, 142
artificial pancreas system. *See* automated insulin delivery (AID) systems
aspart, 44–45
aspirin, 86, 90, 105
asthaenia, 13–14
asymptomatic diabetes, 13
asymptomatic hypoglycaemia, 50, 280
asymptomatic PAD, 82, 84
atherosclerosis, 24, 57, 59, 64, 231, 319, 376
arterial, 154
coronary, 89–90
development, 82
diabetes-related, 153
increased risk of, 84, 155
atherosclerotic cardiovascular disease (ASCVD), 154
diabetes and risk of, 155
risk reduction, 156–157
atherothrombosis, 81
atrial fibrillation, 269
automated insulin delivery (AID) systems, 362–363, 367–368
challenges for, 368–369, **369**
clinical guidelines for, 368
evidence on automated insulin delivery for older adults, 368
automatic pancreas, 278–279
autonomic dysfunction, 59, 131–132, 144
autonomic neuropathy, 129, 142, 231, 342–343, 389

B

bacterial infections, 334
balanitis, 336–337
Barthel index, 381
basal bolus:
regimens, 41, 45–46, 222, 278–279
therapy, 45
basal insulin, 42, 45–46, 65, 224, 293–294, 414
analogues, 42–44

basal insulin (*cont'd*)
injection of, 62
use of, 42
behavioural activation, 313
Beijing Longitudinal Study of Ageing II, 244
benzodiazepines, 403
beta-blockers, 91, 146–147, 167, 231
beta cell, 61
function decline, 42
loss/hyperglycaemia, 62
mass and proliferation, 3–4
of pancreas, 36
residual, 276
biguanides, 60
biofeedback, 136
bisoprolol, 147
bisphosphonates, 125, 349, 403
blisters, 318–319, 333
blood glucose, 237
control, 335
high, 13, 16
homeostasis, 14
levels, 5, 12, 35, 223
management, 221–224
monitoring, 66, 185
readings, 221
time in range of, 279
blood pressure, 34, 59, 85, 104, 114, 144, 147
lowering, 92
reduction, 146
regulation, 132
blood pressure control, 104, 122–123, 149, 410
effect of, 92
escalation of, *146*
body mass index (BMI), 13, 22, 64, 237, 254
bolus calculator, 53
bolus intermittent feeding, 221
bone health, 125
assessment of bone health in community, 344–348
pathophysiology of fracture risk in diabetes, 341–342
bone mineral density (BMD), 341–342
bone mineralisation, 342
British Geriatrics Society, 202
bullae, 333
bullous diabeticorum. *See* bullous eruption of diabetes mellitus
bullous eruption of diabetes mellitus, 333, *331*
bunions, 318

C

calcitonin, 403
calcitriol, 125
calcium channel blockers (CCBs), 146
callus, 137, 318–320, 324, 327
canagliflozin, 258, 326
cancer, 16, 426–428
breast, 238
immune checkpoint inhibitor therapy in, 14
oral, 390–391
pancreatic, 14
skin, 331
steroids and, 426–428
Candida albicans, 390
Candida(l) intertrigo, 336, *337*
candidal skin infection, 336
Candida species, 335–336, 390
candidiasis, 390
genital, 336–337, *335*
oral, 336, *334*, 428
cannabinoids, 403

capillary blood glucose (CBG), 206, 221. *See also* blood glucose
measurements, 414
test, 210
capsaicin, 403
capsaicin patch, 135
cardiometabolic diseases, 269, 271
cardiovascular disease (CVD), 25, 59, 85, 294, 297. *See also* atherosclerotic cardiovascular disease (ASCVD); peripheral vascular disease (PVD)
in diabetes, 98
forms of, 83
incidence of, 157
prevalence, 154
secondary prevention, 90
Cardiovascular Health Study, 83, 90
cardiovascular risk factors, 160
management of, 92–93
pharmacological therapy of, 262
care:
acute phase of, **103**
benefit on outcomes, 74
care-home workforce, 202
organisation, xlvii
primary, 113–114
secondary, 115–117
care delivery, xlvi
care homes, xlviii
care organisation, xlvii
continuity of care, xlvii–xlviii
family support, xlvi–xlvii
care homes, xlviii, 27–28
communication and collaboration, 211
diabetes and older person, *202*
diabetes foot disease, 209
diabetes management in, 201
education, 210–211
frailty, 210
hypoglycaemia, 208–209
importance of monitoring glucose levels, 207
important considerations for diabetes care, 203–207
issues, 207–208
key areas of management in, **205**
key metrics for use in, **204**
measuring outcomes, 212–213
nutritional deficiency and weight loss, 209–210
pain in care-home residents, 400
providers, 212
setting, 357
staff, 203
teams, 208
use of audit, 211–212
workforce, 202
care needs:
diabetes, xliii
of older people with diabetes, 71–72
care plans, xliii, 355
ineffective or lacking, 206
patients, 375
systematic and multidisciplinary team approach to, xlviii
Care Quality Commission, 210
carers, xlvii, 66, 71, 193, 207, 282, 391, 423, 428
abilities, 356
caring for, 74–76
in caring for older people with diabetes, 74
groups, 73
increasing age and diabetes mellitus, *77*

carers (*cont'd*)
  knowledge requirement for carers of older people with diabetes, 72
  role of, 73–74
  syndrome, 75
  transmit data to, 280
caring for carers, 74
  carers' burden, 75
  supporting carers, 75–76
CARMELINA trial, 294
CAROLINA study, 294
carvedilol, 91, 147
catheters, 336
cell surface receptors, 342
cellulitis of left leg, 334, *332*
cerebral oedema, 175
cerebral small vessel disease (CSVD), 97, 99, 101–102
cerebrovascular disease, 97–98, 153, 243
  aetiology, 99–102
  epidemiology, 98
  management, 102–105
  pathophysiology, 99–102, *100*
  presentation, 99
  prognosis, 105–106
  risk factors, 98–99
  spectrum of cerebrovascular accident (CVA) presentation, *100*
  targets for risk reduction in diabetes, **105**
Charcot's neuroarthropathy, 318, 320
Charlson Comorbidity Index (CCI), 267–268
chewing, difficulty in, 217, 388
childhood-onset disease, 275–276
chlorpromazine, 217
cholesterol, 59
cholesterol-lowering medications, 154
chronic diseases, 74, 272
  management, 360–362
  occurrence of, 243
chronic hyperglycaemia, 111
chronic inflammation, 3, 57, 256, 342
  diabetes-related chronic inflammation, 377
  of vascular wall, 82
chronic kidney disease (CKD), 59, 120, 142, 243, 249, 269, 416. *See also* diabetic kidney disease (DKD)
  prognosis, *121*
  recognition and monitoring of, 380
chronic low-grade inflammation, 111–112, 243, 257
chronic pain, 60, 396–397
  complexities of managing, 401
  incidence of, 405
  mechanisms of, 397
  multidimensional approach for prevention of, *405*
cilostazol, 86
citalopram, 313
Clinical Frailty Index, 91
Clinical Frailty Scale, 210, 381
cognition, xlvii, 59, 191, 310, 380
  impact on, 182
  impaired, 181
  issues, 348
  periodic assessment, 52
cognitive behavioural therapy (CBT), 313, 401
cognitive decline, 59, 101, 145, 182, 210, 286, 295, 355

accelerated rate, 286–287
diabetes-specific interventions in, **292**
effects of, *288*
neuropsychological testing for early detection, 282
signs or symptoms, 380
cognitive deficits, 63–64, 289
cognitive dysfunction, xli, 65–66, 182, 277, 286, *286*, 296, 377
effect of current diabetes pharmacological agents on, 291, **292**
effect on self-care capacity, 288–290
implications, 287–288
knowledge gaps and future research, 296
population studies, 286
prevention and treatment, 291–295
risk factors for, 63
cognitive health agility, 288
assessment in older people with diabetes, 289–291
cognitive impairment, 52, 58, 63–64, 67, 101, 142, 209, 399
development, 39
progression of, 50
risks of, 270
substantive, 294
collaboration, 7, 95, 137, 211
Collaborative Atorvastatin Diabetes Study, 157
collaborative care, 311, 314
communication, 208, 211
effective communication channels, 206
problems, 398
community setting, 352, 356–357
comorbidity, 59, 65, 149, 242
burden, 229, 271
not specific to diabetes, 60
Comprehensive Geriatric Assessment (CGA), 84, 256, 344, 353
elements, 375–376
by general practitioners, 356
concordant multimorbidity, 269
confidence interval (CI), 34, 82, 155, 243, 247, 341, 355
continuity of care, xlvii–xlviii, 137
continuous feeding, 221
continuous glucose monitoring (CGM), 50–52, 62, 209, 279–280, 362, 366
challenges, 54, 367, **369**
clinical effects, 367
evidence for, 366–367
international consensus on time in range, **53**
in older people with diabetes, **51**
patient assessment, 52–54
continuous pump infusion, 278
contrast angiography, 85
corns, 318
coronary angiography, 91
coronary artery disease (CAD), 89. *See also* peripheral arterial disease (PAD)
epidemiology, 89–90
flowchart for referral to refer to specialist, *94*
frailty management, 93
indications for revascularisation, 91
management, 93–95
management of cardiovascular risk factors, 92–93
medical treatment, 90–91

coronary artery disease (CAD) (*cont'd*)
pathogenesis, 90
physical exercise and diet, 93
correction factor, 46
Country Standardised Substantive Cognitive Impairment (CS-SCI), 294
COVID-19 pandemic, 207, 369
C-peptide, 276
C-reactive protein, 6
creatinine, 120
cycling, 25
cyclooxygenase-2 inhibitor, 402

D

dapagliflozin, 258
Datix system, 196
debridement, 317, 324–325
de-escalation of therapies, 423–428
degludec, 42, 44, 46, 55, 425
deintensification of therapy, 262, 410
glucose-lowering treatment in older patients, 413–414
identification of patients, 411–413
implementation in daily clinical practice, 414–415
key issues, 411
management, 411–415
profiles of patients, 413
steps, *412*
delirium, 7, 13, 168
dementia, 34, 76, 99, 149, 179, 183, 204, 242, 286, 294
cerebral small vessel disease and, 101–102
implications, 287–288
incidence of, 182
population studies, 287
denosumab, 349
dental caries, 387–389, 392
dental diseases, 386
dentin, 386
deprescribing, 65–66
Deprescribing.org, 411, 415
deprescription. *See* deintensification of therapy
depression, 34, 59, 258, 269, 303
assessment, 308–310
barriers to patients at risk of depression accessing healthcare, 308
coexistence of, 355
collaborative care, 314
criteria for depression diagnosis, 307
depressed mood, 307
and diabetes, 304–305
diagnosis, 307–308
evaluation, 306–311
factors indicating patients at high risk of, 307
lifestyle, 311–312
management, 311–314, *312*
patients at high risk of suicide, 311
pharmacological therapy, 312–313
presentation, 304
psychotherapy, 313–314
relationship between ageing, diabetes mellitus and, *305*
screening tools, **309–310**
symptoms in younger compared with older people, **306**
depressive illness, xliii
detemir, 42, 44, 46
diabetes. *See* diabetes mellitus (DM)
diabetes care, 2, 178, 206, 230, 275, 302. *See also* end-of-life care

burden of, 273
general and regular education about, 76
important considerations for, 203–207
for older people, 201
strategies, 137
Diabetes Care Accreditation programme, 192
Diabetes Control and Complications Trial, 131, 287
diabetes mellitus (DM), xxxix, 1, 11, 110, 119, 130, 153, 229, 340, 375, 386, 386. *See also* type 1 diabetes mellitus (T1DM); type 2 diabetes mellitus (T2DM)
advice to prevention, 335
AVOID-HYPOS acronym in older people with, *184*
background, 12–14
bacterial infections, 334
care needs, xliii
champion, 210
characteristics, xli–xliii
clinical considerations, **8**
cognitive health agility assessment in older people with, 289–291
complications, 58–60
depression and, 304
diabetes-concordant comorbidities, 272
diabetes-related oral changes, 386–387
diabetes-related skin infections, 334–337
diabetes-specific admissions, 191
diabetes-specific interventions in cognitive decline, **292**
diabetes medications-related skin adverse effects, 338
diabetes mellitus-related skin conditions, 331
differences in presentation of new-onset, **17**
dyslipidaemia in, 154
effects of frailty, 244–255, *245*, *248*
epidemiology, 2
foot care in care homes, 136–137
foot disease, 209
fungal infections, 335–337
global prevalence of, 241
integration with remote patient monitoring, 369–370
interventions based on foot risk stratification in, **323**
key issues, 6–7, 14–17, 370–372, *371*
and lipid profile, 154–155
management, 7, 366–369
medications-related skin adverse effects, 338
multimorbidity effects on, 268–269, *271*
impact of old age and, xl, *xl*, 303
in older adults, *360*, 360–362,
older people with, 266
pathophysiology and risk factors for falls in, 342–343
pathophysiology in older adults, 3–6
pathophysiology of fracture risk in, 341–342
phenotype in older people, 376–377
population studies, 287
prevalence of, 71
prevention in older adults, 6–7

diabetes mellitus (DM) (*cont'd*)
primary skin conditions, 332–333
and risk of atherosclerotic cardiovascular disease, 155
self-management education for older people, 50, 67
and sexual dysfunction, 230–231
signs/symptoms and conditions, **15**, 334
specific for older people with, 218
symptoms of testosterone deficiency in older men with, 234
technologies, 362–363, **361**
therapies, 60
training, 210
Diabetes Prevention Program study, 7, 22
diabetic dermopathy, 333, *331*
diabetic eye disease, 59
epidemiology, 110
fundus photographs, *113*
management, 113–117
pathophysiology, 111–112
presentation, 110–111
diabetic foot problem, 212, 317–318
diabetic foot ulcer (DFU), 318
aetiology of, 318–319
ageing and, 319
assessment of diabetic foot, 320–322
diabetic ketoacidosis (DKA), 46, 165–166, 175, **176**, 276
classic laboratory findings, 169
recurrent, 175
risk of, 425
signs and symptoms, 62
diabetic kidney disease (DKD), 119–120
definitions and diagnoses, 120–121
diabetic kidney disease-related complications, 124–125
lifestyle, 121–122
management, 121–126
nephrology referral, 125–126
diabetic neuropathy, 120, 130, 138. *See also* peripheral neuropathy
diagnostic tests for assessing, **133–134**
individuals with, 132
management of, 135–136
pathophysiology of, 131
diabetic retinopathy (DR), 110–111
focused history, *115*
screening, 114
treatment for, *116*
United Kingdom national screening guidelines, **112**
Diagnostic and Statistical Manual of Mental Disorders V, 237, 307
Diamond study, 66, 362
DIAMOND trial, 51
diarrhoea, 32, 36, 150, 217
diastolic blood pressure (DBP), 142
diet, 2, 6, 22, 46, 93, 256–257, 381
healthy, 104, 157
liberalised, 28
low-protein, 121
low-salt, 125, 145
Mediterranean, 24, 67
and regular physical exercise, 93
dietary counselling, 219–220
digital symbol substitution test (DSST), 291
Digit Symbol Substitution Test score, 289
dipeptidyl peptidase-4 (DPP-4) inhibitors, 34, 37, 61, 258, 294

discontinuation. *See* deintensification of therapy
discordant multimorbidity, 269
dizziness, 61–62
Doppler ultrasonography, 237
dorsal root ganglia stimulation, 402
dressings, 320, 324
dry mouth, 389, 428
dual antiplatelet therapy, 90
duloxetine, 135
dyslipidaemia, 59, 110, 154, 254, 269
  ageing and lipid profile, 154
  atherosclerotic cardiovascular disease risk reduction, 156–157
  diabetes and lipid profile, 154–155
  diabetes and risk of atherosclerotic cardiovascular disease, 155
  goals in frailty, 162
  goals of therapy in old age, 160
  lipid-lowering agents, 157–160
  recommendations from guidelines, 160–161, **161**
  synergistic effects of ageing and diabetes on, *156*
dysphagia, 101, 103, **103**

E

Early Treatment of Diabetic Retinopathy Study (ETDRS), 111
e-cigarettes, 104
ecological momentary assessments, 370
Edinburgh Type 2 Diabetes Study, 182
education, 196–197, 210–211, 335
  in diabetes self-care, 358
  diabetes self-management education for older people, 67
  on foot care, 381
  key issues, 58–64
  management, 64–67
  about pain, 402
  strategies for, 372
elderly people. *See* older adults/people with diabetes
electroconvulsive therapy, 311
electrolytes, 223
  correction, 175
  serum, 171
electronic devices, 360
emergency setting, 357–359
end-of-life care, 418
  advanced care planning, 428
  algorithm for de-escalation of therapies, *426*
  identification, 418–422
  management of diabetes in, 423
  medicines management and de-escalation of therapies, 423–428
  stages, 420–422
  treatment withdrawal, 428–429
  workforce training and competencies, 428
endothelial dysfunction, 82, 231, 234
  pathways, 99
  vascular, 82
end-stage renal disease (ESRD), 120, 249, 260
enteral feeding, 221
  delivery options, 221
  nutrition and, 428
  type 1 diabetes on, 222
enteral nutrition, 218, 220–224

enteral tubes, 221
Enterococci, 324
Epidemiology of Diabetes Interventions and Complications study, 131
erectile dysfunction, 231, 378. *See also* cognitive dysfunction
  non-pharmacological interventions for, 235
  risk factors for, 232
  threefold increased risk of, 230
erythropoiesis stimulating agent (ESA), 124
escitalopram, 313
essential amino acids, 25, 27, 256
estimated glomerular filtration rate (eGFR), 60, 120, 126, 243, 442
European Diabetes Working Party for Older People, 411
European Geriatric Medicine Society, 411
European Society for Clinical Nutrition and Metabolism (ESPEN), 217
executive function, 63, 101, 287–288, 294
exercise, 25–27, 144, 378
  aerobic, 25, 257
  aquatic, 27, 257
  maintenance, 357
  modalities, 27
  physical, 66
  programmes, 5
  rehabilitation, 85
  resistance, 25
  synergy between nutrition and, 27
  training, 21, 27
ezetimibe, 123, 157, 161, 163

F

falls, 7, 50, 63, 148, 341
  assessment and management algorithm, *345*
  components of multifactorial assessment, 345–346
  epidemiology, 341
  management and prevention, 348–349
  pathophysiology and risk factors in diabetes, 342–343
  risk of, 63, 343–344
family support, xlvi–xlvii, 313
fast-acting analogues, 45
fatigue, resistance, ambulation, illness, and loss of weight (FRAIL) score, 65
feeds/feeding, **103**
  enteral feed delivery options, 221
  management of blood glucose, 221–222
  types of, 221
Female Sexual Function Index (FSFI), 237
fibrates, 123, 157, 159
finerenone, 123
finger-prick glucose testing, 42, 50
finished consultant episodes (FCEs), 191
Finnish Geriatric Intervention Study to Prevent Cognitive Impairment and Disability (FINGER) trial, 295, 355
flatulence, 32, 36
fluid retention, 35, 122, 124–125
food fortification, 220
foot care, 85–86, 381
  ageing and diabetic foot ulcer disease, 319

assessment, 193
diabetic foot assessment, 320–322
diabetic foot infection treatment, *326*
epidemiology, 318
foot problem, 317–318
interventions based on foot risk stratification in diabetes, **323**
management, 322–326
pathogenesis, 318–319
prevention, 326–327
severity assessment of diabetic foot infection, 325

Fracture Risk Assessment (FRAX) tool, 347, 381

fractures, 35, 50
clinical risk factors for, **346**
management and prevention, 349
risk assessment algorithm in older people, *347*
risk of, 63
risk pathophysiology in diabetes, 341–342

Frailty Index, 65, 256

frailty, xxxix, xlii, xliii, 11, 58, 90–91, 148, 241–242, 319, 381
in care homes diabetes management, 209–210
degrees of, 52
diabetes phenotype in older people, 376–377
effects on diabetes, 244–255, *248*
frailty–diabetes inter-relationship, 242–243
goals in, 162, 261–262
management, 93
metabolic effects, 249–255
metabolic phenotypes in older people with diabetes, **xlii**
multimorbidity and, 268
outcome effects, 249
prevention and management, 255–258
risk, 64–65
special considerations, 259–262
studies investigating frailty effects, **250–253**
studies investigating glycaemic effects, **246–247**

French community-based study, 12

G

gastrostomy tube, 221

General Medical Council UK, 418

genital candidiasis, 336–337, *335*

genital fungal infection, 237

Geriatric Depression Scale, 380

geriatric syndromes, xli, 1, 5, 52, 243, 276, 376–377

'get-up-and-go' test, 353

gingivitis, 386–388

glargine U-100 (Gla-100), 42–44

glargine U-300 (Gla-300), 42, 44, 46

glibenclamide, 37, 258

gliclazide, 37, 293, 428

glinides, 258

gliptins, 42

Global Registry of Acute Coronary Events (GRACE), 91

glucagon-like peptide-1 receptor agonists/analysts (GLP-1RA), 35, 37, 61, 92, 122, 217, 258, 294–295
in older people, 35
precautions with use of, 36

glucagon response, 4–5

glucocorticoids, 6, 149, 167

glucose:
age-related alterations in glucose metabolism, 3–5

glucose (*cont'd*)
control, 291–293
importance of monitoring glucose levels, 207
monitoring, 66
monitoring and insulin administration, **223**
variability, 51
Glucose Insulin in Stroke Trial, 102–103
Glucose Regulation in Acute Ischaemic Stroke Patients (GRASP) study, 101
gluocorticosteroids, 426
glutamate decarboxylase (GAD), 13
glutamic acid decarboxylase autoantibodies, 276
glycaemic control, 39, 122, 234, 259–260, 270, 326
effect on cardiovascular events, 92
mouth care, 392
glycaemic targets, 45, 183, 423
glyco-oxidation, 82
Gold Standards Framework in UK, 419

H

haemoglobin A1c (HbA1c), 12–13, 51, 59, 65, 101, 122, 206, 244, 270, 278, 378, 414
reduction, 259
targets, 53
haloperidol, 217
Hamilton Rating Scale for Anxiety, 380
healthcare providers, 73, 130, 138, 211, 359–360
healthcare system-related interventions, 356
care-home setting, 357
community setting, 356–357
emergency setting, 357–359
healthy diet, 67, 104, 157, 215, 388
hexosamine, 99
high-density lipoprotein (HDL), 154
high BMI, 13, 64
high hypoglycaemia risk agents, 36. *See also* low hypoglycaemia-risk agents
meglitinides, 37
sulfonylureas, 36–37
homeostasis model assessment estimated insulin resistance (HOMA-IR), 13
hormonal factors, 243
hospital/hospitalisation, 351
avoidance of, 353
considerations for care planning for older person with diabetes, 195
considerations for effective inpatient care, 192–193
considerations to reduce unscheduled admission, 193–197
diabetes management in, 190
education and training, 196–197
educational resources, 197
fundamentals of care, **190**, 190–192
healthcare system-related interventions, 356–359
hospital-acquired DKA, 166
inpatient care, 194
monitoring requirements, 196
patient-related interventions, 353–356, *354*

recommendations for reducing, 358–359
risk factors for, 352–353
hybrid closed loop (HCL) system, 54, 279, 368
hydroxymethylglutaryl coenzyme A reductase inhibitors, 157
hyperacute, **103**
hyperglycaemia, 3, 14, 59, 244, 342, 358
correction, 174
persistent, 231
prolonged, 342
hyperglycaemic crisis, 165
clinical presentation, 168–169
complications, 175
criteria for intensive care admission of older people, **173**
diagnosis, 169–171
diagnostic criteria, **171**
epidemiology, 166
management, 171–175, *172*
pathogenesis, 168, *169*
precipitating factors, 166–167
prevention, 176
hyperkalaemia, 123, 125
hyperlipidaemia, 59
hypernatraemia, 175
hyperosmolar hyperglycaemic state (HHS), 165–166, 192, 423
mortality in, 175
patients with, 171
hyperparathyroidism, secondary, 125, 342
hypertension, 6, 13, 59, 98, 110, 122, 141, 269
age-related blood pressure changes, 142
age-related vascular changes, *143*
considerations in older people, 147–150
definition, 142
diagnosis, 144
guidelines for blood pressure targets in diabetes, **143**
management, 145
medications, 146–147
prevalence of, 142
recommended targets, 145–146
types, 144–145, **145**
Hypertension in the Very Elderly Trial, 146
hypertension, resistant, 126, 144
hypnosis, 402
hypo-awareness, impairment of, 50
hypoalbuminaemia, 256
hypoglycaemia, xlviii, 7, 50, 57, 62–63, 179, 244, 289, 352
in care homes diabetes management, 208–209
characteristics of, *184*
clinical consequences, 181–182
difficulties in recognising, 180
epidemiology, 180
impact on cognition, 182
impact on frailty, 182–183
management, 183–185
in older adults with T2DM, 60
pathophysiology, 180–181
recognition, 179
reducing, 280–281
risk factors for, 181
unawareness, 281
hypoglycaemic agents, 32
anorexic malnourished phenotype, 260–261
choice of, 260
sarcopenic obese phenotype, 260

hypoglycaemic medications, 32, 258, 342
  adverse effects of, 330
  withdrawing, 183
hypokalaemia, 175
hyponatraemia, 173, 175
hypophosphataemia, 175
hypovolaemia correction, 172–173
hypoxia inducible factor (HIF), 124

I

incontinence, 336
incretin pathway, 61
Independent Diabetes Federation working group, 194–195
infection control, 324
inflammation, 3, 6, 83
innovative technologies, 362
inpatient setting, 192–193
insulin, 16, 258, 293–294, 338
  delivery technologies, 66
  doses, 425
  pumps, 53, 62, 278–279
  resistance, 13, 25, 57
  secretagogues, 37
  sensitivity, 4
insulinopoenia (HOMA2-B), 13
insulin, regular, 44–45, 107, 174
insulin therapy, 41, 174, 278–279
  basal insulin analogues, 42–44
  rapid-acting analogues, 44–45
  rapid acting and long-acting insulin for use, **43**
  treatment regimens, 45–46
interleukin-6, 6, 257
intermittent pain, 397
International Diabetes Federation (IDF), 2
International Index of Erectile Function, 232
International Verapamil SR-Trandolapril Study, 146
International Working Group on the Diabetic Foot, 132
interpersonal psychotherapy, 313
intracellular dehydration, severe, 14
intraocular steroids, 115–117
intravenous insulin infusion, 174, 223
intravitreal anti-VEGF, 115–116
invasive tests, 85
Ipswich touch test (IpTT), 320, 322
ischaemia:
  critical, 325
  relief, 325
ischaemic heart disease, 234–235, 243
ischaemic toe, *319*
isolated systolic hypertension, 144, 150
isophane. *See* neutral protamine Hagedorn (NPH)

J

Japanese cross-sectional study, 243
jogging, 25

K

ketone body testing, 174
ketosis, 165–166, 168
kidney disease, 59–60, 120. *See also* chronic kidney disease (CKD); diabetic kidney disease (DKD)
Kidney Disease Improving Global Outcome (KDIGO), 121
Kussmaul breathing, 168

L

lactic acidosis, 32, 60–61, 171
L-arginine, 235

laser photocoagulation, 111, 115–116
latent autoimmune diabetes in adults (LADA), 3, 13
leucine, 25, 27, 256
leukoplakia, 391
lichen planus, 387, 391
lidocaine, 403
lifestyle interventions, 7, 22–23
  care homes, 27–28
  goals, 24
  impact of lifestyle changes, 22–23, *23*
linagliptin, 34, 61
lipid control, 123–124
lipid-lowering:
  agents, 154, 157–160, **158–159**
  therapy, 85, 156–157, *163*
lipid monitoring, 93
lipid profile:
  ageing and, 154
  diabetes and, 154–155
lipoatrophy, 338
lipodystrophy, 338
lipohypertrophy, 237, 338
lipolysis, 168
liquid metformin, 221–222
lispro, 44–45
longitudinal studies, 131, 272
Look AHEAD (Action for Health in Diabetes) randomised controlled study, 22, 237–238, 249, 270, 311–312, 355
low-density lipoprotein (LDL), 123, 154
lower-extremity amputations, 318
low glucose suspend (LGS) system, 367–368
low hypoglycaemia-risk agents, 32
  alpha-glucosidase inhibitors, 36
  DPP-4, 34
  GLP-1, 35
  metformin, 32–34
  SGLT-2, 34–35
  TZD, 35
lubricants, 238
luseogliflozin, 258

M

macrovascular disease, 153, 269
magnesium, 5, 220
magnetic resonance imaging (MRI), 293
major adverse cardiovascular events (MACE), 141
malnutrition, 216, 256. *See also* nutrition
  causes and suggested interventions, **220**
  causes in elderly people, 216–217
Malnutrition Universal Screening Tool (MUST), 219, 381
mannitol infusion, 175
mastication, 386
  age-related oral changes, 387
  muscles of, 385
McGill Pain Questionnaire, 399
mechanical ventilation, 175
medication, 6
  classes of, 217
  review, 381–382
medicines management, 423–428, **424–425**
meditation, 402
Mediterranean diet, 24, 67
meglitinides, 37, 61
men, sexual dysfunction in, 231
  advantages and cautions of testosterone therapy, **235**

men, sexual dysfunction in (*cont'd*)
aetiology and pathogenesis, 231, *233*
diagnosis, 232–233
symptoms of testosterone deficiency in older men with DM, 234
treatment, 233–235
mental function, xliii–xlv, 355
mental health conditions, 269
Mental State Examination, 310
metabolic acidosis, 125
metabolic screen blood tests for osteoporosis, 348
metformin, 22, 32–34, 37, 42, 60, 217, 257–258. *See also* diabetes mellitus (DM)
methicillin-resistant *S. aureus* (MRSA), 324
Mexican Health and Nutrition Survey, 243
micronised NSAIDs, 403
micronutrients deficiencies, 216
microvascular:
damage, 111
disease, 269
MID-Frail study, 93
mindfulness, 402
mineral bone disorder, 124–125
minimal cognitive impairment (MCI), 286
Mini-Mental Status Examination (MMSE), 290, 293
Mini Nutritional Assessment, 219
mirtazapine, 313, 314, 441
mismanagement of diabetes, 191, 289
mitochondrial dysfunction, 57
mnemonic aids, 399
MOBILE study, 366
moisturisers, 238
monofilament test, 132, 209, 321, *319*
Montreal Cognitive Assessment (MoCA), 290–291, 380
mood:
cognition and, 380
depressed, 307
disorders, 303
monitoring, 313
morbidity, 1, 6, 58, 75, 242
burden, 376, 377
cardiovascular, 81
discordant, 266
due to hypoglycaemia, 182
reduction, 104
motor impairments, 131
motor neuropathy, 318
mouth care, 391
age-related oral changes, 386–387
diabetes-related oral changes, 386–387
education, 391
factors leading to oral complications, *393*
glycaemic control, 392
oral conditions in older people with diabetes, 388–391
preventative measures, 392–393
multidomain approach, 295–296
multifactorial falls assessment, components of, 345–346
multimorbidity, 266–267
adverse outcome predicted by, 269
clinical implications, 270–272
clinical manifestation, 242
clusters, 269–270
diabetes phenotype in older people, 376–377

effects on diabetes, 268–269
impact on diabetes management, *271*
multimorbidity–frailty interaction, 268
prevalence, 270
scales, **267**
multiorgan dysfunction concept, 242
muscle mass, 24–25
muscle relaxants, 403
myofascial release techniques, 402
myokines, 257

N

nasogastric tube, 220–222
National Advisory Panel on Care Home Diabetes, 206
National Diabetes Inpatient Audit, 197
National Health and Nutrition Examination Survey, 90
National Institute for Health and Care Excellence, 206
National Osteoporosis Guideline Group, 347
nausea, 32, 168, 217
nebivolol, 147
Necrobiosis lipoidica, 332, *333*
nephrology referral, 125–126
nerve decompression surgery, 402
Neuropad®, 209
neuropathic/neuropathy, 317
pain, 137
ulcer, *319*
neutral protamine Hagedorn (NPH), 42
nicotinic acid, 159–160
nicotinic stomatitis, 391
night time bruxism, 386
nitrates, 91
nocturnal hypoglycaemia, 44
nocturnal hypotension, 144–145
non-critical ischaemia, 325
non-healing foot ulcers, 318
non-iatrogenic hypoglycaemia, 179
non-invasive tests, 84
non-pharmacological therapy, 256–257, 401–402
non-steroidal anti-inflammatory drugs (NSAIDs), 356, 402, **403**
NuAge study, 27
nutrition, 24–25, 64, 215, 381, 426. *See also* malnutrition
assessments, 219
causes of malnutrition in elderly, 216–217
considerations for patients on nutritional support, 224
enteral nutrition, 221–222
feeding patterns, *222*
glucose monitoring and insulin administration, **223**
intervention, 219–220
nutritional deficiencies, 216
parenteral nutrition, 222–224
practical steps for nutritional care in elderly, 218–222
recommendations, 217–218
screening, 218–219
specific for older people with diabetes, 218
synergy between exercise and, 27
nutritional deficiency, 209–210
Nutritional Risk Screening (2002), 219
nutritional screening, 218–219
nystatin spray, 336

O

obesity, 4, 6, 64, 254, 269. *See also* sarcopenic obese/obesity (SO)
odds ratio (OR), 341
oedema of macula, 111
offloading, 324
older adults/people with diabetes, 12–13, 52, 83, 119, 137, 266, 362
  care planning for elderly people, 194–195
  causes of malnutrition in, 216–217
  practical steps for nutritional care in, 218–222
  AVOID-HYPOS, *184*
  characteristics of hypoglycaemia in, *184*
  cognitive health agility assessment in, 289–291
  competences for successful insulin therapy, 279
  depression presenting symptoms in younger compared with, **306**
  diabetes technology and remote patient monitoring in, 364–366
  diagnostic aids for T1DM in, 277
  difficulties in diagnosis of T1DM in, 277
  difficulties in recognising hypoglycaemia in, 180
  evidence on automated insulin delivery for, 368
  management of sexual dysfunction in, *236*
  pathophysiology of diabetes in, 3–6
  prevention of diabetes in, 6–7
  reducing hypoglycaemia in, 281
  risk factors for hypoglycaemia in, 181
  specific for, 218
oliguria, 168
omega-3 fatty acids, 25, 160
onychomycosis, 337, *335*
opioid analgesics, 402–403
opioids, **403**
optimisation, 65–66
oral cancer, 390–391
oral candida, 336
oral candidiasis, 336, *334*
oral cavity, 385–386
oral health, enquiries about, 392
oral hypoglycaemic therapy, 32
  advantages and disadvantages, **33**
  classes of, 32
  future perspectives, 39
  high hypoglycaemia risk agents, 36–37
  hypoglycaemic agents, 32
  low hypoglycaemia-risk agents, 32–36
  therapeutic approach, 37–38, *38*
oral nutritional supplements, 220
ORIGIN trial, 293, 295
orthostatic hypotension, 142, 144, 147–148
osmotic diuresis, 168
osteoblasts, 342
oxidative stress, 57, 82

P

pain, 396
  aetiology, 397
  algorithm of therapeutic options, *401*
  assessment, 397–400
  barriers to pain assessment, 398
  in care-home residents, 400

management, 401–405
multidimensional approach for prevention, *405*
pharmacological agents for pain control, **403–404**
prevention, 405
types, **398**
paracetamol, 402, **403**
parenteral nutrition, 220, 222–224
Patient Health Questionnaire (PHQ), 314
patient-related interventions, 353–356, *354*
pelvic floor physical therapy, 238
percutaneous coronary intervention, 90
percutaneous endoscopic gastrostomy (PEG) tube, 220
periodontal diseases, 386, 388–389
peripheral arterial disease (PAD), 81–82, 89. *See also* coronary artery disease (CAD)
consequences, 83
epidemiology, 81–82
investigations, 83–85
management, 85–86
pathogenesis, 82–83
prevalence, 82
risk factors, 81–82
peripheral autonomic neuropathy, 318
peripheral neuropathy, 59, 130, 317, 342
algorithm for approaching pain management, *136*
clinical manifestations and complications, 131–132
diabetes foot care in care homes, 136–137
diagnosis and assessment, 132–135
management of diabetic neuropathy, 135–136
prevalence and risk factors, 130–131
peripheral sensory neuropathy (PSN), 318
10-g monofilament test, 321, *319*
128-tuning fork test, 322
IpTT, 322
testing for, 320
peripheral vascular disease (PVD), 25, 105, 138, 317, 322
permission, limited information, specific suggestions and intensive therapy (PLISSIT), 238
persistent hyperglycaemia, 231
pharmacological therapy, 86, 257–258, 312–313, 402–404
pharmacotherapy (PhT), 135
phosphate, 24, 175, 220
phosphodiesterase 5 (PDE5) inhibitors, 234, 238
physical examination, 84, 310, 378–379
physical exercise, 66, 93
physical function, xliii, 26, 353–354, 381
pioglitazone, 35, 37
planning care, 193
pleasant activity scheduling, 313
polydipsia, 12–13
polyol, 99
polypharmacy, 60, 149, 166, 217, 343, 355–356, 381
polyuria, 12–13
population studies, 287

potassium, 24, 220
depletion, 175
potassium-lowering agents, 123
precision monitoring, 370
prediabetes, 155
predictive low glucose suspend (PLGS) system, 367–368
prednisolone, 426, 428
pregabalin, 135
pressure damage, 193
primary care, 113–114
primary skin conditions, 332
Acanthosis nigricans, 332, *330*
bullous eruption of diabetes mellitus, 333
diabetic dermopathy, 333
Necrobiosis lipoidica, 332, *333*
problem-solving treatment, 313
progressive resistance training, 25
proinflammatory cytokines, 6
proliferative diabetic retinopathy (PDR), 111
prolonged hyperglycaemia, 342
proprotein convertase subtilisin/kexin type 9 (PCSK9) inhibitors, 160–161
Prospective Study of Pravastatin in the Elderly at Risk (PROSPER), 157
protein–energy malnutrition, 216
protein kinase C pathways, 99
pseudohypertension, 144
psychotherapy, 313–314

R

raloxifene, 349
randomised controlled trials (RCTs), 293
rapid-acting analogues, 44–45
'reduction of treatment'. *See* deintensification of therapy
relative risk (RR), 155
remote activity monitoring (RAM), 360
remote patient monitoring (RPM) technologies, 358–360
integration of diabetes technologies with, 369–370
key issues, 370–372, *371*
in older adults, 360–362
renin–angiotensin–aldosterone system (RAAS), 122–123
repaglinide, 61
reperfusion therapies, 102
repetitive minor trauma, 318
resistance exercise, 25–26, **26**, 257
resistance training, 25, 66, 257
resistant hypertension, 126, 144
respiratory depression, 403
retinal neovascularisation, 111
retinal neurodegeneration, 112
retinal surgery, 117
retinopathy, 342
revascularisation, 86
indications for, 91
need for, 157
REWIND trial, 294
risk factor modification, 85
risk ratio (RR), 341
risperidone, 217
Rockwood cumulative deficit model, 256
Rockwood frailty scale. *See* Clinical Frailty Scale
roxadustat, 124

S

sarcopenia, xxxix, xliii, 217, 319
sarcopenic obese/obesity (SO), 64

individuals, 22
phenotype, xlii, 254, 260
screening, 255–256
depression, 306
for diabetes, 14
secondary care, 115–117
selective serotonin reuptake inhibitors (SSRI), 312–313
Self-Administered Gerocognitive Examination (SAGE), 290
self-care, 287–288
capacity, 286, 288–289
tasks, 237
self-management:
programmes, 402
in T1DM, 289
self-monitoring blood glucose monitoring (SBGM), 50
self-reported pain, 397–398
sensor-augmented pumps, 54
sensory manifestations, 131
serotonin–norepinephrine reuptake inhibitors, 403
sertraline, 313
sexual dysfunction, 229
diabetes and, 230–231
management, *236*
in men, 231–235
in women, 236–238
sexual function, 230, 380
sexual health, 229
ageing and sexual function, 230
diabetes and sexual dysfunction, 230–231
sexual dysfunction in men, 231–235
sexual dysfunction in women, 236–238
'share' feature, 52–53
Sheba Medical Center, 291, 295
short physical performance battery, 84
sildenafil, 234
silent infarcts, 101
sitagliptin, 34
six-metre walking speed, 84
skeletal muscle, 249
skin care, 330
age-related skin changes, 331
clinical effects of ageing on skin, **331**
diabetes mellitus-related skin conditions, 331–338
smart pens, 278
smartphone apps, 356–357
smoking, 24, 82
smoking cessation, 104
social care workforce, 207
sodium glucose transporter-2 (SGLT-2) inhibitors, 34–37, 42, 61, 92, 122, 258, 338
SOUL trial, 295
spinal cord stimulation, 402
spironolactone, 231
standard deviation (SD), 22, 243, 294, 314
Staphylococcus aureus, 324, *326*
statins, 123–124, 157, **159**
stem cell therapy, 235
steroids, 116–117, 426–428, *427*
stomatognathic system, 385
Strategic Document of Diabetes Care, A, 206
Streptococci, 324
stress, 6
stroke, 97, 99, 101
strontium, 349
subcutaneous insulin, 223, 363
substance abuse, 269

substantive cognitive
impairment, 294
sulfonylureas, 36–37, 61, 258, 424
Support and Palliative Care
Indicators Tool (SPICT), 422
supporting carers, 75–77
swallowing, difficulty in, 217
Swedish epidemiological study, 13
swimming, 25
symptomatic hypoglycaemia, 50
systolic blood pressure (SBP), 142, 145–146, 148, 150
systolic hypertension, 148
DBP for, 148
isolated, 144, 150
Systolic Hypertension in Europe trial, 145

T

Tachypnoea, 168
tadalafil, 234
tai chi, 27, 257, 312, 357
tapentadol, 135
taste impairment, 391
testosterone, 6
advantages and cautions of testosterone therapy, **235**
deficiency, 235
symptoms of testosterone deficiency in older men with DM, 234
Test Your Memory (cognitive assessment tool), 290
therapeutic approach of oral hypoglycaemic therapy, 37–38, *38*
thiamine, 220
thiazide diuretics, 231
thiazides, 146
thiazolidinediones (TZD), 35, 342
thiazolidinedione therapies, 61
thrombectomy, 102, **103**, 106, 435
thrombolysis, 102, **103**, 106, 434
Thrombolysis in Myocardial Infarction (TIMI), 91
thrush. *See* acute pseudomembranous candidiasis
tight glycaemic control, 270–271
"Timed Get Up and Go" assessment, 381
time in range (TIR), 278
trabecular bone score, 347
trace elements, 223
trail making test, 291
transcutaneous electrical nerve stimulation, 136, 402
transient ischaemic attack (TIA), 99, 101
treatment regimens of insulin therapy, 45–46
treatment withdrawal, 428–429
tricyclic antidepressants, 313, 403
tumour necrosis factor-α, 6
type 1 diabetes mellitus (T1DM), 3, 13, 41, 50, 58, 131, 165, 275, 287, 332, 341
characteristics and management, *278*
diagnostic aids for, 277
difficulties in diagnosis, 277
epidemiology and diagnosis, 276
goals of therapy, 282
insulin therapy, 278–279
management, 276–282
monitoring, 279–280
population of older people with, 275
reducing hypoglycaemia, 280–281
self-management in, 289

type 1 exchange programme, 289
type 2 diabetes mellitus (T2DM), 3, 13, 31–32, 41, 50, 58, 101, 131, 165, 182, 286, 333, 341, 409
age-related alterations in glucose metabolism, 3–5
diagnosis of, 13, 16
dyslipidaemia in, 154
factors, 6
genetics, 5
lifestyle and environmental factors, 5–6
in older adults, *4*
older people with, 32
type II fibres, 249, 254

U

ultrafast-acting insulin analogue, 279
United Kingdom (UK)
diabetes-related foot problems, 318
diabetes mellitus in, 110
UK-wide multidisciplinary initiative, 206
urinary calcium excretion, 342
urinary incontinence, 60, 237, 243, 339, 377, 442
urinary tract infection (UTI), 60, 225, 237, 442

V

vacuum erection devices, 235
vaginal lasers, 238
vaping, 104
vardenafil, 234
vascular:
complications, 380
conditions, 269
disease, 156, 231, 303, 377
endothelial dysfunction, 82
vascular endothelial growth factor (VEGF), 111
venlafaxine, 313
vibration, 27, 257, 357
vitamins, 223
vitamin B_{12} deficiency, 257, 354
vitamin D deficiency, 243
vitamin D supplementation, 257, 354
vitrectomy surgery, 115, 117
vomiting, 32, 61, 168, 217

W

walking, 25, 83–84, 377
assistance in, xliv
claudication distance, 434
weight-bearing exercise, 66, 349
weight loss, 13, 209–210, 254, 256–257, 270
weight loss therapy, 21
whey protein, 25, 256
white-coat hypertension, 144
Whitehall II Prospective Cohort Study, 243
whole-body electromyostimulation, 27, 257, 357
Wireless Innovation for Seniors with Diabetes Mellitus (WISDM) trial, 51, 362
Wnt signalling pathways, 342
women, sexual dysfunction in, 236
aetiology and pathogenesis, 236–237
diagnosis, 237
treatment, 237–238
Women's Health and Ageing Study, 341

Wong–Baker FACES tool, 399
workforce, 203
  care-home, 202
  social care, 207
  stumbling blocks of optimal
    diabetes management, 208
  training and competencies, 428
  turnover, 191

X

xerostomia, 217, 389
  diabetes-related, 391
  recommendations to reduce,
    389–390

Y

yoga, 27, 257, 357

Printed and bound by CPI Group (UK) Ltd, Croydon, CR0 4YY

22/01/2025

14630416-0001